T0202207

Apathy

Apathy

Clinical and Neuroscientific Perspectives from Neurology and Psychiatry

Edited by

André Aleman
Professor of Cognitive Neuropsychiatry,
University Medical Center Groningen and University of Groningen

Krista L. Lanctôt
Senior Scientist, Hurvitz Brain Sciences Program,
Sunnybrook Research Institute; Professor of Psychiatry and Pharmacology,
Vice Chair of Basic and Clinical Science, Department of Psychiatry,
University of Toronto

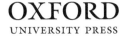

OXFORD
UNIVERSITY PRESS

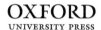

OXFORD
UNIVERSITY PRESS

Great Clarendon Street, Oxford, OX2 6DP,
United Kingdom

Oxford University Press is a department of the University of Oxford.
It furthers the University's objective of excellence in research, scholarship,
and education by publishing worldwide. Oxford is a registered trade mark of
Oxford University Press in the UK and in certain other countries

© Oxford University Press 2021

The moral rights of the authors have been asserted

First Edition published in 2021

Impression: 1

Published in the United States of America by Oxford University Press
198 Madison Avenue, New York, NY 10016, United States of America

British Library Cataloguing in Publication Data

Data available

Library of Congress Control Number: 2021932602

ISBN 978-0-19-884180-7

DOI: 10.1093/med/9780198841807.001.0001

Printed in Great Britain by
Ashford Colour Press Ltd, Gosport, Hampshire

Oxford University Press makes no representation, express or implied, that the
drug dosages in this book are correct. Readers must therefore always check
the product information and clinical procedures with the most up-to-date
published product information and data sheets provided by the manufacturers
and the most recent codes of conduct and safety regulations. The authors and
the publishers do not accept responsibility or legal liability for any errors in the
text or for the misuse or misapplication of material in this work. Except where
otherwise stated, drug dosages and recommendations are for the non-pregnant
adult who is not breast-feeding

Links to third party websites are provided by Oxford in good faith and
for information only. Oxford disclaims any responsibility for the materials
contained in any third party website referenced in this work.

Preface

Apathy, or a significant reduction of goal-directed activity, is a common and clinically relevant problem for many patients with a neurological or psychiatric condition. It is a prominent and severely debilitating aspect of many such disorders, including among others schizophrenia, depression, traumatic brain injury, stroke, and neurodegenerative diseases (e.g. Alzheimer's disease and Parkinson's disease). Patients with apathy show reduced initiative, indolence, and general passivity of thought and action. Apathy involves changes in affect, behaviour, and cognition. No wonder it impacts the lives of patients and their loved ones, especially affecting patients' independence and quality of life.

In recent years, there has been an increasing interest in studying apathy in its own right, given the prognostic value of apathy and its impact on daily functioning. Indeed, apathy can manifest itself independently from other neurological and psychiatric conditions and therefore deserves focused investigation. The advent of reliable measures and investigations of underlying mechanisms will also aid the development of novel treatment strategies.

The purpose of this book is to bring together current knowledge regarding apathy, ranging from conceptual insights to measurement, neurobiology, and treatment. For example, conceptual topics include the definition of apathy and the classification of dimensions pertaining to behaviour, cognition, and emotion. In addition, clinical observations suggest that a distinction can be made between different types of apathy. Measurement includes questionnaire and interview approaches, involving information obtained from self-report, informant (relative or close other), or clinician. Different brain circuits may be involved, such as frontoparietal, frontolimbic, and frontostriatal circuits. The neural structures subserving motivation and reward are highly relevant. Treatment has focused on diverse pharmacological approaches, and also psychosocial approaches such as behavioural activation therapy. More recently, neurostimulation has been introduced as a way of increasing brain activation of relevant circuits. Leading experts in the field have been asked to contribute a chapter on a diversity of topics, comprehensively covering different areas of apathy research. Despite the widespread presence of apathy across neurological and psychiatric disorders, much of the research has been done in artificial silos dictated by diseases. It is our hope that bringing together knowledge from across these disciplines will expand progress through cross-fertilization.

The book will be of interest to a wide range of professionals, including clinicians (psychiatrists, neurologists, psychologists, and psychiatric nurses) and researchers in the fields of neurology, psychiatry, and clinical psychology. We also trust that it will benefit students of psychiatry, neurology, clinical psychology, neuropsychology, and related disciplines.

We would like to take this opportunity to thank our colleagues for contributing to this book by accepting our invitation and for their scholarly, informative, and interesting chapters. We are very happy with the contribution of so many leading experts. We also want to thank Danielle Vieira (Sunnybrook Research Institute, Toronto) for her indispensable help in getting the chapters reviewed and sent to the publisher. Finally, we extend our gratitude to Oxford University Press and editor Lauren Tiley for their enthusiasm and help with this book.

Contents

Abbreviations

AA	Alzheimer's Association
AAD	auto-activation deficit
ACC	anterior cingulate cortex
ACT	acceptance and commitment therapy
AD	Alzheimer's disease
AES	Apathy Evaluation Scale
AES-C	Apathy Evaluation Scale Clinician reported
AES-I	Apathy Evaluation Scale Informant reported
AES-S	Apathy Evaluation Scale Self-reported
AI	Apathy Inventory
aMCI	amnestic mild cognitive impairment
APADEM-NH	Apathy in Dementia, Nursing Home
AS	Apathy Scale
BOLD	blood oxygen level-dependent
BPRS	Brief Psychiatric Rating Scale
CAINS	Clinical Assessment Interview for Negative Symptoms
CBSST	Cognitive Behavioral Social Skills Training
CBT	cognitive behavioural therapy
CI	confidence interval
CNS	central nervous system
CT	computed tomography
DAIR	Dementia Apathy Interview and Rating
DAS	Dimensional Apathy Scale
DFC	dynamic functional connectivity
DLPFC	dorsolateral prefrontal cortex
DSM-5	*Diagnostic and Statistical Manual of Mental Disorders*, fifth edition
DSM-IV	*Diagnostic and Statistical Manual of Mental Disorders*, fourth edition
DTI	diffusion tensor imaging
DWI	diffusion-weighted imaging
FA	fractional anisotropy
FDG	fluorodeoxyglucose
FrSBe	Frontal Systems Behaviour Scale
GABA	gamma-aminobutyric acid
GCS	Glasgow Coma Scale
GDB	goal-directed behaviour
HD	Huntington's disease
ICD-10	International Classification of Diseases, tenth revision
ISTAART	International Society to Advance Alzheimer Research and Treatment
LARS	Lille Apathy Rating Scale
LARS-i	Lille Apathy Rating Scale Informant

MBI	mild behavioural impairment
MBI-C	Mild Behavioural Impairment Checklist
MCI	mild cognitive impairment
MDD	major depressive disorder
MID	monetary incentive delay
MND	motor neuron disease
MOVE	Motivation and Enhancement
MR	magnetic resonance
MRI	magnetic resonance imaging
mTBI	mild traumatic brain injury
NAc	nucleus accumbens
naMCI	non-amnestic mild cognitive impairment
NCI	no cognitive impairment
NIMH	National Institute of Mental Health
NOSIE	Nurses' Observation Scale for Inpatient Evaluation
NPI	Neuropsychiatric Inventory
NPI-C	Neuropsychiatric Inventory Clinician
NPI-NH	Neuropsychiatric Inventory Nursing Home
NPI-Q	Neuropsychiatric Inventory Questionnaire
NPS	neuropsychiatric symptom(s)
OFC	orbitofrontal cortex
OR	odds ratio
PANSS	Positive and Negative Symptoms Scale
PAT	Positive Affect Treatment
PD	Parkinson's disease
PEPS	Positive Emotions Program for Schizophrenia
PET	positron emission tomography
PFC	prefrontal cortex
PRIME	personalized real-time intervention for motivational enhancement
PST	problem-solving therapy
PTA	post-traumatic amnesia
RDoC	Research Domain Criteria
RL	reinforcement learning
ROI	region of interest
RS-FC	resting-state functional connectivity
rTMS	repetitive transcranial magnetic stimulation
SANS	Scale for the Assessment of Negative Symptoms
SCIA	Structured Clinical Interview for Apathy
SMA	supplementary motor area
sMRI	structural magnetic resonance imaging
SNc	substantia nigra compacta
SNS	Self-evaluation of Negative Symptoms
SSRI	selective serotonin reuptake inhibitor
SST	social skills training
SVD	small vessel disease
TAU	treatment as usual

TBI	traumatic brain injury
tDCS	transcranial direct current stimulation
TEPS	Temporal Experiences of Pleasure Scale
UPDRS	Unified Parkinson's Disease Rating Scale
VS	ventral striatum
VTA	ventral tegmental area

Contributors

Ingrid Agartz
Division of Mental Health and Addiction,
University of Oslo and Diakonjemmet
Hospital, Oslo, Norway

André Aleman
Department of Neuroscience, University of
Groningen, Groningen, The Netherlands

Jozarni J. Dlabac-De Lange
University Medical Center Groningen,
University of Groningen, Groningen, The
Netherlands

Ann Faerden
Clinic of Mental Health and Addiction, Oslo
University Hospital, Oslo, Norway

Zahra Goodarzi
Departments of Medicine and Community
Health Sciences, University of Calgary,
Calgary, AB, Canada

Kyrsten M. Grimes
Department of Psychology, University of
Toronto Scarborough, Toronto, ON, Canada

Bradleigh Hayhow
School of Medicine, University of Notre
Dame Australia, Fremantle, WA, Australia

Jayna Holroyd-Leduc
Departments of Medicine and Community
Health Sciences, University of Calgary,
Calgary, AB, Canada

Masud Husain
Nuffield Department of Clinical
Neurosciences, University of Oxford, John
Radcliffe Hospital, Oxford, UK

Zahinoor Ismail
Departments of Psychiatry and Clinical
Neurosciences, Hotchkiss Brain Institute,
University of Calgary, Calgary, AB, Canada

Eliyas Jeffay
KITE, Toronto Rehabilitation Institute,
University Health Network, Toronto,
ON, Canada

Stefan Kaiser
Adult Psychiatry Division, Department
of Mental Health and Psychiatry, Geneva
University Hospitals, Geneva, Switzerland

Zuzana Kasanova
Katholieke Universiteit Leuven, Belgium

Krista L. Lanctôt
Sunnybrook Health Sciences Centre,
University of Toronto, Toronto, ON, Canada

Richard Levy
University Hospitals Pitié Salpêtrière,
Paris, France

Tania M. Lincoln
Department of Clinical Psychology and
Psychotherapy, University of Hamburg,
Hamburg, Germany

Celina Liu
Neuropsychopharmacology Research
Group, Hurvitz Brain Sciences Program,
Sunnybrook Research Institute, Toronto,
ON, Canada

Valeria Manera
University of Nice Sophia Antipolis,
Nice, France

Bria Mele
Department of Community Health Sciences,
University of Calgary, Calgary, AB, Canada

David Miller
Signant Health, Blue Bell, PA, USA

Lynn Mørch-Johnsen
NORMENT, Division of Mental Health
and Addiction, Oslo University Hospital
and Institute of Clinical Medicine,
University of Oslo, Oslo, Norway;
Department of Psychiatry and Department
of Clinical Research, Ostfold Hospital,
Graalum, Norway

Moyra Mortby
Neuroscience Research Australia, Randwick,
Sydney, NSW, Australia

Lisa Nobis
Oxford Centre for Human Brain
Activity, Wellcome Centre for Integrative
Neuroimaging, Department of Psychiatry,
University of Oxford, Oxford, UK

Prasad Padala
University of Arkansas for Medical Sciences,
Little Rock, AR, USA

Marcel Riehle
Department of Clinical Psychology and
Psychotherapy, University of Hamburg,
Hamburg, Germany

Philippe Robert
Institut Claude Pompidou, Nice, France

Gabriella Santangelo
Department of Psychology, University of
Campania 'Luigi Vanvitelli', Caserta, Italy

Florian Schlagenhauf
Charité – Universitätsmedizin Berlin, Berlin,
Germany

Sergio Starkstein
Division of Psychiatry, University of Western
Australia, Perth, WA, Australia

Danielle Vieira
Neuropsychopharmacology Research
Group, Hurvitz Brain Sciences Program,
Sunnybrook Research Institute, Toronto,
ON, Canada

Konstantine K. Zakzanis
Department of Psychology, University of
Toronto Scarborough, Toronto, ON, Canada

1
Definition of Apathy and Differential Diagnosis

Philippe Robert and Valeria Manera

Introduction

Apathy is prevalent across many neurodegenerative, neurological, and psychiatric disorders. It represents the most common behavioural and psychological symptom in people with Alzheimer's disease (AD), and is often observed in Parkinson's disease (PD), vascular dementia, stroke, traumatic brain injury, amyotrophic lateral sclerosis/motor neurone disease (MND), frontotemporal dementia, progressive supranuclear palsy, major depression, and schizophrenia (1). The definition and the diagnostic criteria for apathy have evolved over time, and the terminology employed to refer to apathy can vary in the context of different pathological conditions. In addition, the term apathy is employed to describe both a symptom and a syndrome (2).

Apathy Definition and Concept

The word apathy stems from the Greek *apatheia*, derived from *apathes*: 'a' (without) 'pathos' (feeling). In Stoic philosophy, the term described the state of a soul that has voluntarily become alien to the sensitive affections, which are also called 'passions' in the vocabulary of the Stoics. The term has undergone changes in meaning over the ages. The *Oxford English Dictionary* defines apathy as a lack of interest or enthusiasm, an approach emphasizing a 'cognitive' dimension (interest) and a 'feeling' or 'emotional' dimension (enthusiasm). The French Larousse dictionary defines apathy as indolence or indifference, slowness to act or react, passivity, inertia of a group, and of the economy.

Modern medicine conceptualizations of apathy reflect efforts to reconcile these various aspects of apathy. Despite differences, such as, for example, disagreements as to whether disturbances of motivation (3) or of initiative and self-generated voluntary and purposeful behaviour (4) are central features, most conceptualizations of apathy acknowledge that it is a multidimensional syndrome in which all these dimensions are prominent (Table 1.1).

Table 1.1 Concepts and definitions of apathy

Author	Concept/definition
Marin et al., 1990 (5)	Diminished motivation (not attributable to diminished level of consciousness, cognitive impairment, or emotional distress)
Cummings et al., 1994 (6)	Disorder of interest or motivation; it includes lack of emotion, lack of initiation, lack of enthusiasm
Stuss et al., 2000 (7)	Disorder of initiative, manifested as a lack of self-initiated action, which may be affective, behavioural, or cognitive; it includes 'social apathy'—a disorder of sense of self and of social awareness
Robert et al., 2002 (8)	Disorder of motivation including emotional blunting, lack of initiative, and lack of interest
Sockeel et al., 2006 (9)	Disorder of intellectual curiosity, action initiation, emotion, and self-awareness
Levy and Dubois, 2006 (4)	Disorder of voluntary and goal-directed behaviours; with three subtypes of disrupted 'signal' processing—emotional-affective, cognitive, and auto-activation
Starkstein and Leentjens, 2008 (10)	Disorder of motivation with diminished goal-directed behaviour and cognition
Ang et al., 2017 (11)	Disorder of motivation characterized by reduced behavioural initiation, emotional sensitivity, and social motivation, that is also apparent to varying degrees in healthy people
Husain and Roiser, 2018 (1)	Multicomponent entity; it is essential to understand the functional and brain mechanisms underlying the 'surface manifestations' of apathy
Robert et al., 2018 (12)	A quantitative reduction of goal-directed activity either in behavioural/cognitive, emotional, or social dimensions

Among the key figures that made it possible to move towards a better definition of apathy, we must first mention Robert Marin, who in 1990 defined apathy as a disorder of motivation (5). It is on this basis that Sergio Starkstein and colleagues provided a first assessment of the frequency of apathy in AD and other neuropsychiatric diseases (13). Finally, we should acknowledge that the interest in apathy increased in parallel with the renewed interest of neurologists and psychiatrists in dementia. Jeffrey Cummings' introduction of a specific area devoted to apathy into the Neuropsychiatric Inventory (6)—which has become the gold standard for assessing neuropsychiatric disorders—played a fundamental role in its recognition and the proliferation of scientific research.

Apathy Diagnostic Criteria

Starting from Marin's definition of apathy (3), Starkstein (14) and, in a second step, Starkstein and Leentjens (10) proposed a standardized set of diagnostic criteria for apathy. Based on these criteria, a patient is diagnosed with apathy if they present with a lack of motivation compared to the previous level of functioning or the standards of their age and culture (criterion A). Symptoms should be present for at least 4 weeks for most of the day, in at least one domain (goal-directed behaviour, cognition, and/or emotions; criterion B). These symptoms should cause significant impairment in important areas of functioning (criterion C). Finally, these symptoms should not be explained by a diminished level of consciousness or the direct effects of substances (criterion D). This represented the first attempt to structure the apathy criteria in four parts: A, the definition; B, the description of domains where the apathy symptoms can appear; C, the consequence of the symptoms in term of functioning; and D, the exclusion criteria. In this work, the authors strongly stressed the importance of reaching a consensus on such criteria to facilitate future research.

Another important reason for formulating formal consensus criteria regarding apathy in dementia and neuropsychiatry was the recognition of its growing importance to neuropsychiatric research and practice. Under the auspices of the Association Française de Psychiatrie Biologique and the European Psychiatric Association, a task force was set up in 2008 to revise Starkstein's original criteria and to develop criteria for apathy that could be widely employed, have clear operational steps, and could be easily applied in clinical practice and in research settings (15). There is wide acknowledgement that apathy is an important behavioural syndrome in AD and in various neuropsychiatric disorders. In light of recent research and the renewed interest in the correlates and impacts of apathy, and in its treatments, it is important to develop criteria for apathy that will be widely accepted, have clear operational steps, and will be easily applied in practice and research settings. Meeting these needs is the focus of the task force work reported here. The task force includes members of the Association Française de Psychiatrie Biologique, the European Psychiatric Association, the European Alzheimer's Disease Consortium, and experts from Europe, Australia, and North America. An advanced draft was discussed at the consensus meeting (during the European Psychiatric Association conference on 7 April 2008) and a final agreement reached concerning operational definitions and hierarchy of the criteria (published in 2009). Apathy is defined as a disorder of motivation that persists over time and should meet the following requirements. Firstly, the core feature of apathy, diminished motivation, must be present for at least 4 weeks; secondly, two of the three dimensions of apathy (loss of, or diminished, goal-directed behaviour, goal-directed cognitive activity, or emotions) must also be present; thirdly, there should be identifiable functional impairments attributable to the apathy. Finally, exclusion criteria are specified to exclude symptoms and states that mimic apathy (15). One of the principal characteristics of these criteria (presented in Box 1.1) was that change in motivation

Box 1.1 The 2009 apathy diagnostic criteria

For a diagnosis of apathy, the patient should fulfil the criteria A, B, C, and D.

A Loss of or diminished motivation in comparison to the patient's previous level of functioning and which is not consistent with his age or culture. These changes in motivation may be reported by the patient himself or by the observations of others.

B Presence of at least one symptom in at least two of the three following domains for a period of at least 4 weeks and present most of the time:

Domain B1. Loss of, or diminished, goal-directed behaviour as evidenced by at least one of the following:

- Loss of self-initiated behaviour (e.g. starting conversation, doing basic tasks of day-to-day living, seeking social activities, communicating choices).
- Loss of environment-stimulated behaviour (e.g. responding to conversation, participating in social activities).

Domain B2. Loss of, or diminished, goal-directed cognitive activity as evidenced by at least one of the following:

- Loss of spontaneous ideas and curiosity for routine and new events (i.e. challenging tasks, recent news, social opportunities, personal/family and social affairs).
- Loss of environment-stimulated ideas and curiosity for routine and new events (i.e. in the person's residence, neighbourhood, or community).

Domain B3. Loss of, or diminished, emotion as evidenced by at least one of the following:

- Loss of spontaneous emotion, observed or self-reported (e.g. subjective feeling of weak or absent emotions, or observation by others of a blunted affect).
- Loss of emotional responsiveness to positive or negative stimuli or events (e.g. observer reports of unchanging affect, or of little emotional reaction to exciting events, personal loss, serious illness, emotional-laden news).

C These symptoms (A–B) cause clinically significant impairment in personal, social, occupational, or other important areas of functioning.

D The symptoms (A–B) are not exclusively explained or due to physical disabilities (e.g. blindness and loss of hearing), to motor disabilities, to diminished level of consciousness, or to the direct physiological effects of a substance (e.g. drug of abuse, a medication).

Reproduced from Eur Psychiatry, 24(2), Robert P, Onyike CU, Leentjens AFG, et al., Proposed diagnostic criteria for apathy in Alzheimer's disease and other neuropsychiatric disorders, pp. 98–104, Copyright (2009), with permission from Elsevier Masson SAS.

could be observed (and measured) by examining a patient's responsiveness to internal or external stimuli. In this way, each of the three domains within criterion B (behaviour, cognition, and emotion) includes two types of symptoms. The first symptom pertains to self-initiated or 'internal' actions, cognitions, or emotions, and the second symptom to the patient's responsiveness to 'external' stimuli.

Several prevalence studies employed the Robert et al. criteria (15). In a cross-sectional, multicentre, observational study (16), the frequency of apathy was 55% in AD, 70% in mixed dementia, 43% in mild cognitive impairment, 53% in schizophrenia, and 94% in major depressive episodes. In another study focusing on PD (17), 17.2% of patients were diagnosed with apathy according to the criteria. Interestingly, the prevalence observed with the 2009 apathy diagnosis criteria is close to the overall pooled prevalence of apathy (49%) in AD observed across 25 studies reporting on 7671 persons (18).

The 2009 criteria were widely used in clinical and research practice (19) but research in the last decade has provided considerable advances in understanding the domain of apathy in brain disorders, including the biological and neural bases (20), which led a group of experts to propose a revision of the criteria. Several reasons emerged to update the diagnostic criteria of apathy. First, the definition of apathy as a disorder of 'motivation' has been extensively criticized, as 'motivation' (criterion A) is a psychological interpretation of behavioural internal states, which may be difficult to measure objectively (4). At the same time, the construct of goal-directed behaviour/activity—construed as a set of related processes by which an internal state is translated, through observable action, into the attainment of a goal—is increasingly used in the domain of neuroscience (2), and it has been proposed to be a useful way to operationalize apathy, particularly in clinical context. Second, the different apathy domains (criterion B) have been the subject of discussion, particularly the importance of adding 'social interaction' as a domain of apathy (11).

Using a Delphi panel methodology, a group of experts reached a consensus on the 2018 apathy diagnostic criteria (reported in Box 1.2) (12). The main modifications compared to the criteria published in 2009 included (i) replacing the term 'motivation' with goal-directed behaviour. This was a pragmatic choice, because 'goal-directed behaviours' are easier to observe and describe compared to motivation, which is an internal state that can only be inferred; and (ii) the modification of the dimensions in which symptoms can be observed (criterion B), to cognition/behaviour, emotion, and social interaction.

The new criteria were employed in a recent survey conducted in specialized memory settings (21), which showed that the frequency of apathy ranged from 25% in patients with mild neurocognitive disorders, to 57% in patients with affective disorders (depression, anxiety, and bipolar disorders), and to 77% in patients with major neurocognitive disorders. All subjects with apathy fulfilled the criteria for the behaviour/cognition dimension, 73.1% fulfilled the criteria for the emotion dimension, and 97.4% fulfilled the criteria for the social interaction dimension. Behaviour/cognition showed the highest sensitivity, and the co-presence of emotion and social interaction

Box 1.2 The 2018 apathy diagnostic criteria

For a diagnosis of apathy, the patient should fulfil the criteria A, B, C, and D.

Criterion A A quantitative reduction of goal-directed activity either in behavioural, cognitive, emotional, or social dimensions in comparison to the patient's previous level of functioning in these areas. These changes may be reported by the patient himself/herself or by observation of others.

Criterion B The presence of at least two of the three following dimensions for a period of at least 4 weeks and present most of the time:

B1. *Behaviour and cognition.* Loss of, or diminished, goal-directed behaviour or cognitive activity as evidenced by at least one of the following:

- *General level of activity*: the patient has a reduced level of activity either at home or work, makes less effort to initiate or accomplish tasks spontaneously, or needs to be prompted to perform them.
- *Persistence of activity*: he/she is less persistent in maintaining an activity or conversation, finding solutions to problems, or thinking of alternative ways to accomplish them if they become difficult.
- *Making choices*: he/she has less interest or takes longer to make choices when different alternatives exist (e.g. selecting TV programmes, preparing meals, choosing from a menu, etc.).
- *Interest in external issue*: he/she has less interest in or reacts less to news, either good or bad, or has less interest in doing new things.
- *Personal well-being*: he/she is less interested in his/her own health and well-being or personal image (general appearance, grooming, clothes, etc.).

B2. *Emotion.* Loss of, or diminished, emotion as evidenced by at least one of the following:

- *Spontaneous emotions*: the patient shows less spontaneous (self-generated) emotions regarding their own affairs, or appears less interested in events that should matter to him/her or to people that he/she knows well.
- *Emotional reactions to environment*: he/she expresses less emotional reaction in response to positive or negative events in his/her environment that affect him/her or people he/she knows well (e.g. when things go well or bad, responding to jokes, or events on a TV programme or a movie, or when disturbed or prompted to do things he/she would prefer not to do).
- *Impact on others*: he/she is less concerned about the impact of his/her actions or feelings on the people around him/her.
- *Empathy*: he/she shows less empathy to the emotions or feelings of others (e.g. becoming happy or sad when someone is happy or sad, or being moved when others need help).

- *Verbal or physical expressions*: he/she shows less verbal or physical reactions that reveal his/her emotional states.

B3. Social interaction. Loss of, or diminished engagement in social
interaction as evidenced by at least one of the following:
- *Spontaneous social initiative*: the patient takes less initiative in spontaneously proposing social or leisure activities to family or others.
- *Environmentally stimulated social interaction*: he/she participates
  less, or is less comfortable or more indifferent to social or leisure
  activities suggested by people around him/her.
- *Relationship with family members*: he/she shows less interest in
  family members (e.g. to know what is happening to them, to meet
  them, or make arrangements to contact them).
- *Verbal interaction*: he/she is less likely to initiate a conversation, or
  he/she withdraws soon from it.
- *Homebound*: he/she prefer to stays at home more frequently or
  longer than usual and shows less interest in getting out to meet
  people.

Criterion C These symptoms (A–B) cause clinically significant impairment in personal, social, occupational, or other important areas of functioning.

Criterion D The symptoms (A–B) are not exclusively explained or due to physical disabilities (e.g. blindness and loss of hearing), to motor disabilities, to a diminished level of consciousness, to the direct physiological effects of a
substance (e.g. drug of abuse, medication), or to major changes in the
patient's environment.

the highest specificity. The concordance between the 2009 and the 2018 criteria indicated an almost perfect agreement (more information concerning the criteria are
available at http://www.innovation-alzheimer.fr/assessment/).

Chapter 2 of this book is dedicated to the apathy assessment tools (scales, interviews) that can contribute to the diagnosis of apathy. Here we only want to recall the
main clinical principles to follow in order to fulfil the diagnostic criteria for apathy. As
with any evaluation in current practice, it is important to use the maximum number
of available elements regarding the behaviour and emotions of the patient. Several
sources of information may be available. Ideally, relying on all these sources should
allow the most accurate apathy diagnosis. The assessment of whether a patient meets
apathy diagnostic criteria should be done when the maximum of information has
been collected.

Here are some rules:

- *Always rely on the symptoms observed during the interview*: answers to questions, spontaneous expressions, attitude and involvement in the clinical relationship, the patient's subjective point of view, and scores on behavioural evaluation scales. These elements, in the absence of other information, should constitute the basis to complete the diagnostic criteria for apathy.
- *Always take into account the story of the subject* and their usual social relations, usual personality, and information given by the accompanying person (when present).
- *When a family or professional caregiver is present*, information on daily life or be-havioural disorders can be collected either spontaneously or using an interview such as the Neuropsychiatric Inventory (6) or Mild Behavioural Impairment Checklist (22), both of which represent good complements.
- *When a cognitive/behavioural assessment is performed*, it is also important to ob-serve or have information about the patient's involvement during the tests.
- *Observations of the patient in other situations* (use of serious games, individual or group stimulation sessions) or information obtained through new technolo-gies can also be useful. There is evidence that apart from the currently used as-sessment methods for apathy, information and communication technology approaches could provide clinicians with valuable additional information for apathy detection, and therefore a more accurate diagnosis of apathy. Actigraphy and methods used to monitor motor activity and rest–activity rhythms have al-ready been demonstrated to be accurate and related to apathy (23, 24). Other information and communication technology-based methodologies are already employed, but only in research settings at the moment. These include, for in-stance, voice analysis (25), video analysis (26), and the use of serious games and applications (an example of the Motivation Application (MotAp) is available at   http://www.innovation-alzheimer.fr/motivation-application-2/).   Motion-based technologies must be used and interpreted with caution in patients with movement disorders (e.g. PD, Huntington's disease, or progressive supranuclear palsy). These patients often have a reduction in total activity, related to their motor symptoms. In addition, they speak slowly, with a hypophonic voice, and have a low speech rate due to speech and respiratory disorders. They also have a hypomimic face which can give the incorrect impression that they do not react to emotion. Hence, the proposed measures need to be used with reservations.

It is important to have apathy diagnostic criteria for two main reasons: to promote re-search and to improve clinical practice.

In the research domain, having a better definition of apathy will contribute to a better understanding of the underlying biological mechanisms. In the context of clin-ical trials testing new pharmacological treatments, it is important to provide the sci-entific rational (biological basis) for targeting specific dimensions, and, if possible, to make the relation with the product intended for development explicit. These charac-teristics are difficult to reach if the pathological framework is not defined. In order to unify the definition, the 2018 diagnostic criteria for apathy have the advantage of addressing all brain diseases, including neurodegenerative, neurological, and psychiatric conditions. However, there is also a need to understand the peculiarities of apathy in each diagnostic category. This goal was achieved by a consensus group in 2021 (27), which defined diagnostic criteria for apathy focused only on neurocognitive disorders as defined by the fifth edition of the *Diagnostic and Statistical Manual of Mental Disorders* (DSM-5) (28) (see Chapter 3).

Clinical practice is also a crucial target of the diagnostic criteria, particularly in order to select the best non-pharmacological or ecopsychosocial approach (29). In fact, as indicated by Starkstein and Hayhow in a recent editorial (30), 'It is likely that a generic approach to activities may fail to produce positive changes in many patients. What is therefore required is a "tailor-made" approach, designing specific activities depending on individuals' interests and capacities'.

Differential Diagnosis

Apathy is frequently comorbid with other syndromes which may have symptoms of reduced interests/motivation/goal-directed behaviour, such as depression, anhedonia, and fatigue (1, 18, 31). Furthermore, terms such as avolition, abulia, and negative symptoms are sometimes used to describe apathy symptomatology (2). This raises the question of the extent to which apathy can be meaningfully distinguished from these other conditions. Overlaps also occur in terms of brain circuits: atrophy or functional disruption of the dorsal anterior cingulate cortex, ventromedial prefrontal cortex, orbitofrontal cortex, ventral striatum, and ventral tegmental area, as well as brain regions connected to these areas, can be found in apathy, anhedonia, fatigue, and depression, as well as in abulia and negative symptoms (1, 32, 33). Similarly, all these symptoms are mediated, among others, by dysfunctions of the dopaminergic system (see (1), and Chapters 11 and 12 in this book for more details). Table 1.2 provides examples of disorders/syndromes/symptoms that can partially overlap with apathy, focusing on their definitions and examples of disorders in which they have been more frequently investigated.

Anhedonia

In psychiatry, anhedonia is defined as an inability to experience pleasure (34). Recently, anhedonia has also been associated with a loss of interest or pleasure in doing previously rewarding activities (35). Similar to apathy, anhedonia might exist for different dimensions, with dissociable axes of loss of interest or pleasure in social activities, sensory experiences, and hobbies (36). Anhedonia is one of the core symptoms of major depressive disorder (MDD). According to the DSM-5 (28), patients meet criteria for MDD if they have five or more symptoms, one of which must

Table 1.2 Medical conditions overlapping with apathy

Condition	Definition	Examples of the most frequent diseases
Apathy	A quantitative reduction of goal-directed activity either in behavioural/cognitive, emotional, or social dimensions	Neurogenerative conditions (AD, PD, frontotemporal dementia, Huntington disease, vascular dementia, MND), psychiatric diseases (major depression, schizophrenia), neurological disorders (stroke, traumatic brain injury) (1)
Anhedonia	Consistently and markedly diminished interest or pleasure in almost all daily activities	Neurodegenerative conditions (PD (54)), psychiatric disorders (major depression, schizophrenia (55)), post-traumatic stress disorder (56), substance use disorders (57)
Negative symptoms	Thoughts, feelings, or behaviours normally present that are absent or diminished	Psychiatric diseases (e.g. schizophrenia, bipolar disorder) (2)
Aboulia	Reduced spontaneous verbal, motor, cognitive, and emotional behaviours	Neurodegenerative conditions (PD), psychiatric diseases (mania), neurological disorders (stroke, traumatic brain injury) (39)
Fatigue	Feeling of exhaustion caused by the exertion of effort, which is unrelated to actual exertion of energy by muscles	Neurodegenerative conditions (PD, MND, multiple sclerosis (58–60)), neurological disorders (stroke (61))
Depression	Mood disorder that causes a persistent feeling of sadness and loss of interest	Neurodegenerative conditions (AD, PD, frontotemporal dementia, vascular dementia, MND (62–64)), psychiatric diseases (schizophrenia (65)), neurological disorders (e.g. stroke (66))

be either depressed mood or anhedonia. However, anhedonia can occur outside of MDD. For example, it is included in the 'negative symptoms' of schizophrenia, and is also found in post-traumatic stress disorder, eating disorders, and substance use disorder (1). The overlap of apathy and anhedonia is evident in several conditions, such as PD and schizophrenia. This is also due to the fact that both apathy and anhedonia are assessed through clinical scales and questionnaires, and items used in the assessment of both syndromes are often overlapping (37). However, self-reports of apathy and anhedonia in the general population are not perfectly correlated, suggesting that there are also unique aspects of anhedonia not related to apathy, and vice versa (11).

Negative Symptoms

In the context of schizophrenia and other psychiatric disorders, negative symptoms include apathy, alogia (poverty of speech, increased latency of response), anhedonia, asociality (e.g. decreased ability to feel intimacy and closeness to other people), physical anergia, affective blunting, and attentional impairment (2). Apathy is thus included in the spectrum of negative symptoms. Clinical descriptions and empirical studies on the negative syndrome of schizophrenia suggest that apathy may be a key criterion of this syndrome (37). However, the negative syndrome of schizophrenia has more clinical complexity than apathy, both in terms of its phenomenology and putative mechanisms.

Abulia/Avolition

People with avolition or abulia encounter difficulty in initiating behaviours but can perform the same actions when verbally prompted to do so. Avolition can be a prominent negative symptom of schizophrenia. An extreme form of avolition is akinetic mutism, which is characterized by little or no self-generated movement or speech (38). In psychiatry, abulia is considered by some to be a severe form of apathy (10). Indeed, psychiatrists and neurologists responding to a survey considered aboulia to be a state characterized by difficulty in initiating and sustaining spontaneous movements, and reductions in emotional responsiveness, spontaneous speech, and social interaction (39), and acknowledged that the terms apathy and abulia were often used interchangeably in clinical practice. However, apathy as defined in the 2009 and the 2018 diagnostic criteria for apathy includes symptoms related to both self-generated behaviour and/or environment-stimulated behaviour. The definition of apathy thus encompasses a wider range of symptoms.

Fatigue

Fatigue is a common symptom, with up to half of the general population reporting fatigue. It is also reported by at least 20% of patients seeking medical care. Typically, fatigue is transient, self-limiting, and explained by prevailing circumstances. However, a minority of people experience persistent and debilitating fatigue. When the fatigue cannot be explained by a medical condition such as anaemia or hypothyroidism, it may represent chronic fatigue syndrome or myalgic encephalomyelitis (40). Despite the fact that there is still no clear consensus on its definition (41), myalgic encephalomyelitis/chronic fatigue syndrome is usually described as a disorder of more than 6 months' duration comprised of unexplained fatigue, post-exertional malaise, unrefreshing sleep, and either cognitive dysfunction or orthostatic intolerance. The diagnosis of myalgic encephalomyelitis/chronic fatigue syndrome requires the presence of a substantial reduction/impairment in the ability to engage in pre-illness activities (41). The definition of fatigue in terms of reduction in the ability to engage in pre-illness levels of activities constitutes the basis for the overlap with apathy, as well as with depression. Fatigue in terms of symptoms can be associated with apathy in clinical disorders such as PD, MDD, and multiple sclerosis (42, 43). The tenth revision of the International Classification of Diseases (44) criteria for MDD include fatigue or low energy as a cardinal symptom, in addition to anhedonia and depressed mood.

However, apathy and fatigue are distinguishable. For instance, emotional blunting is not a key feature of fatigue, while several fatigue features (e.g. unrefreshing sleep) are not core features in apathy diagnostic criteria.

Depression

Similar to apathy, depression can be described both at the level of a symptom (depressive mood, which can be found in several pathological conditions) and a syndrome (MDD, also simply defined as depression). The DSM-5 (28) outlines the following criteria to make a diagnosis of MDD. The individual must be experiencing five or more symptoms during the same 2-week period and at least one of the symptoms should be either (i) depressed mood or (ii) loss of interest or pleasure. In this definition, loss of interest is defined as a 'markedly diminished interest or pleasure in all, or almost all, activities most of the day, nearly every day'. Other symptoms include significant and unexplained weight loss/decrease in appetite, a slowing down of thought and a reduction of physical movement, fatigue or loss of energy, feelings of worthlessness, diminished ability to think or concentrate, recurrent thoughts of death, suicidal ideation, or suicide attempts. To receive a diagnosis of depression, these symptoms must cause the individual clinically significant distress or impairment in social, occupational, or other important areas of functioning. The symptoms must also not be a result of substance abuse or another medical condition.

Given that loss of interest is a central feature of a depression diagnosis, it is not surprising that apathy and depression often co-occur in several psychiatric, neurological, and neurodegenerative conditions. This is illustrated in a cross-sectional observational study of 734 subjects with probable mild AD, where depression was diagnosed using the diagnostic criteria for depression in AD (45), and apathy with the 2009 diagnostic criteria for apathy. Apathy and depression were associated in 32.4% of patients. The study confirms that two 'overlapping' symptoms are present in 62.9% of the patients presenting the depression criteria alone and in 81.3% of the patients presenting both apathy and depression diagnostic criteria. These symptoms are loss of goal-directed cognitive activity (apathy criteria indicating loss of or diminished interest that is most observed in leisure activities) and decreased positive affect symptoms (depression criteria indicating decreased interest or pleasure in things). Beyond the partial overlap in the definition, the clinical assessment scales employed to assess apathy and depression also show several common items (e.g. (46)).

Despite this overlap, there is also evidence that apathy and depression may be distinguishable (47). For instance, in the domain of affect, apathy is characterized by emotional blunting, while depression is an affective disorder characterized by negative mood and extreme emotional fluctuations (2). In apathy, contrary to depression, there is typically (i) an absence of subjective distress; (ii) an absence of negative thoughts about self, present, and future; and (iii) a general lack of responsiveness to positive and negative events (compared with the biased perception or response to the two types of events in depression) (2). Also, there is a robust association between the degree of apathy (but not depression) and the degree of cognitive impairment, particularly in executive function (48, 49). In PD, depression was found to be associated with less advanced pathology status and more intense motor features, while apathy was found to be associated with more advanced cognitive impairment (50). Similarly, apathy, but not depression, was found to be associated with executive dysfunction in cerebral small vessel disease (51). Furthermore, the brain areas involved in apathy and depression show only a partial overlap (52). For instance, in PD depression has been specifically associated with morphological and functional changes in prefrontal cortex, cingulate, and thalamus, as with 5-hydroxytryptamine transmission reduction in posterior cingulate and amygdala–hippocampus complex. Apathy has been related with grey matter volume reductions or functional deficits in many regions, such as anterior and posterior cingulate and dorsolateral or inferior frontal gyrus. Some of these deficits may be also related with a more pronounced reduction in striatal dopamine transmission (53). Distinguishing between apathy and depression is very important in order to put in place tailored pharmacological and non-pharmacological treatments.

Beyond the differences between syndromes, Table 1.2 emphasizes that the use of the terms also varies according to the disease, and probably according to the practice of the clinicians and researchers involved.

Apathy Theoretical Framework

Apathy is at the crossroads of several theoretical frameworks and it is important to briefly describe the main ones for a better understanding of the definitions. The first framework describes apathy in terms of motivation and reward systems in the mesolimbic cortex and neostriatum (see also Chapter 11). Dopamine projections have been suggested to mediate reward. Berridge and Robinson (67, 68) argue that reward is a constellation of multiple processes, many of which can be separately identified in behaviour. In animal studies, Berridge (69) suggested that dopamine-related neural systems mediate more specifically one component of reward. Their incentive salience hypothesis is built on the earlier incentive theory formulation of motivation (70). Incentive salience transforms the brain's neural representations of conditioned stimuli, converting an event or stimulus from a neutral representation into an attractive and wanted incentive that can 'grab attention' and is able to elicit voluntary action. Incentive salience can be dissociated into the complementary but separate components 'liking' and 'wanting', with dopamine systems mediating only the latter. In this theory, 'wanting' refers specifically to the underlying core process that instigates goal-directed behaviour, attraction to an incentive stimulus, and consumption of the goal object with behavioural manifestations evidenced by the interest of the animal in the goal object and the initiative to obtain it. This early animal evidence was gradually completed by a number of human studies emerging around 2000 that confirmed the dopamine-based liking/wanting distinction and were mostly applied to the addiction disorders such as cocaine, heroin, and food reward (for review, see (71)). Incentive salience, and 'wanting' concepts are at the level of the mesocorticolimbic biological processes. At the psychological level, there are cognitive forms of wanting. Cognitive wanting is goal oriented, and based on declarative memories and on cognitive expectations of act–outcome relations. The lack of initiative and interest frequently presented in several apathy descriptions are in some way clinical examples of incentive salience deficit.

The second important theoretical framework is that of goal-directed behaviour. The goal-directed behaviour model is related to goal-directed behaviour/activity defined as behaviour aimed towards a goal or towards completion of a task. Brown and Pluck (2) stated that 'the goal object can be immediate and physical such as relieving thirst, or long term and abstract, such as being successful in one's job or the pursuit of happiness. By "directed" it is meant that the action is mediated by knowledge of the contingency between the action and the outcome'. So central to the model is the functional integration of motivational, cognitive, and motor processes. In their article entitled 'Negative symptoms: the "pathology" of motivation and goal-directed behaviour', the authors link this model directly to schizophrenia but also to other pathologies. This is perfectly in line with the modern conceptualization of apathy and can be, as in the 2018 diagnostic criteria (12), applied to the three clinical dimensions that are cognitive/behaviour, emotion, and social interaction. We will not go into the details of this framework here because a chapter of this book is devoted to the topic (see Chapter 9). It should be noted that this fits perfectly with the presumed underlying pathophysiological mechanisms, indicating that apathy is the clinical consequence of various underlying dysfunctions of mental and biological processes required to elaborate, initiate, and control intentional/goal-directed behaviour.

Conclusion

The paradox of apathy is that it is a concept so difficult to capture and define at the theoretical level, and at the same time quite easy to understand and observe in clinical practice. For about 30 years the understanding of apathy has evolved considerably with a better knowledge of theoretical concepts and biological mechanisms but also interactions with other concepts used by clinicians and researchers. The recent definitions and diagnostic criteria are much more precise and easier to use in clinical practice, thus allowing a better evaluation. This is a great advance because the presence of apathy in many neuropsychiatric pathologies has considerable consequences on the functioning and quality of life of patients.

The next step consists of using these advances to inform pharmacological treatments, brain stimulation approaches, and ecopsychosocial interventions (72). The healthcare world is now experiencing changes in practice because information and communication technology and digital tools are transforming prevention, semiology, and treatments. This is very positive for individualizing the approach to treating apathy according to the individual interests and characteristics of each patient (72). In this context, future progress will come from the result of the collaboration between researchers and clinicians at the international level. Let's be motivated and do it now!

References

1. Husain M, Roiser JP. Neuroscience of apathy and anhedonia: a transdiagnostic approach. Nat Rev Neurosci. 2018;19(8):470–84.
2. Brown RG, Pluck G. Negative symptoms: the 'pathology' of motivation and goal-directed behaviour. Trends Neurosci. 2000;23(9):412–7.
3. Marin RS. Apathy: a neuropsychiatric syndrome. J Neuropsychiatry Clin Neurosci. 1991;3(3):243–54.
4. Levy R, Dubois B. Apathy and the functional anatomy of the prefrontal cortex-basal ganglia circuits. Cereb Cortex. 2006;16(7):916–28.
5. Marin RS. Differential diagnosis and classification of apathy. Am J Psychiatry. 1990;147(1):22–30.
6. Cummings JL, Mega M, Gray K, Rosenberg-Thompson S, Carusi DA, Gornbein J. The Neuropsychiatric Inventory: comprehensive assessment of psychopathology in dementia. Neurology. 1994;44(12):2308–14.
7. Stuss DT, Van Reekum R, Murphy KJ. Differentiation of states and causes of apathy. In: Borod J (Ed), The Neuropsychology of Emotion. New York: Oxford University Press; 2000, pp. 340–63.
8. Robert PH, Clairet S, Benoit M, Koutaich J, Bertogliati C, Tible O, et al. The apathy inventory: assessment of apathy and awareness in Alzheimer's disease, Parkinson's disease and mild cognitive impairment. Int J Geriatr Psychiatry. 2002;17(12):1099–105.
9. Sockeel P, Dujardin K, Devos D, Deneve C, Destee A, Defebvre L. The Lille apathy rating scale (LARS), a new instrument for detecting and quantifying apathy: validation in Parkinson's disease. J Neurol Neurosurg Psychiatry. 2006;77(5):579–84.
10. Starkstein SE, Leentjens AFG. The nosological position of apathy in clinical practice. J Neurol Neurosurg Psychiatry. 2008;79(10):1088–92.
11. Ang YS, Lockwood P, Apps MAJ, Muhammed K, Husain M. Distinct subtypes of apathy revealed by the Apathy Motivation Index. PLoS One. 2017;12(1):e0169938.
12. Robert P, Lanctôt KL, Agüera-Ortiz L, Aalten P, Bremond F, Defrancesco M, et al. Is it time to revise the diagnostic criteria for apathy in brain disorders? The 2018 international consensus group. Eur Psychiatry. 2018;54:71–6.
13. Starkstein SE, Mayberg HS, Preziosi TJ, Andrezejewski P, Leiguarda R, Robinson RG. Reliability, validity, and clinical correlates of apathy in Parkinson's disease. J Neuropsychiatry Clin Neurosci. 1992;4(2):134–9.
14. Starkstein SE. Apathy and withdrawal. Int Psychogeriatr. 2000;12(S1):135–7.
15. Robert P, Onyike CU, Leentjens AFG, Dujardin K, Aalten P, Starkstein S, et al. Proposed diagnostic criteria for apathy in Alzheimer's disease and other neuropsychiatric disorders. Eur Psychiatry. 2009;24(2):98–104.

16. Mulin E, Leone E, Dujardin K, Delliaux M, Leentjens A, Nobili F, et al. Diagnostic criteria for apathy in clinical practice. Int J Geriatr Psychiatry. 2011;26(2):158–65.
17. Drijgers RL, Dujardin K, Reijnders JSAM, Defebvre L, Leentjens AFG. Validation of diagnostic criteria for apathy in Parkinson's disease. Parkinsonism Relat Disord. 2010;16(10):656–60.
18. Zhao QF, Tan L, Wang HF, Jiang T, Tan MS, Tan L, et al. The prevalence of neuropsychiatric symptoms in Alzheimer's disease: systematic review and meta-analysis. J Affect Disord. 2016;190:264–71.
19. Radakovic R, Harley C, Abrahams S, Starr JM. A systematic review of the validity and reliability of apathy scales in neurodegenerative conditions. Int Psychogeriatr. 2015;27(6):903–23.
20. Le Heron C, Apps MAJ, Husain M. The anatomy of apathy: a neurocognitive framework for amotivated behaviour. Neuropsychologia. 2018;118(Pt B):54–67.
21. Manera V, Fabre R, Stella F, Loureiro JC, Agüera-Ortiz L, López-Álvarez J, et al. A survey on the prevalence of apathy in elderly people referred to specialized memory centers. Int J Geriatr Psychiatry. 2019;34(10):1369–77.
22. Ismail Z, Agüera-Ortiz L, Brodaty H, Cieslak A, Cummings J, Fischer CE, et al. The Mild Behavioral Impairment Checklist (MBI-C): a rating scale for neuropsychiatric symptoms in pre-dementia populations. J Alzheimers Dis. 2017;56(3):929–38.
23. David R, Mulin E, Friedman L, Le Duff F, Cygankiewicz E, Deschaux O, et al. Decreased daytime motor activity associated with apathy in Alzheimer disease: an actigraphic study. Am J Geriatr Psychiatry. 2012;20(9):806–14.
24. Zeitzer JM, David R, Friedman L, Mulin E, Garcia R, Wang J, et al. Phenotyping apathy in individuals with Alzheimer disease using functional principal component analysis. Am J Geriatr Psychiatry. 2013;21(4):391–7.
25. Konig A, Linz N, Zeghari R, Klinge X, Troger J, Alexandersson J, et al. Detecting apathy in older adults with cognitive disorders using automatic speech analysis. J Alzheimers Dis. 2019;69(4):1183–93.
26. Happy SL, Dantcheva A, Das A, Zeghari R, Robert P, Bremond F. Characterizing the State of Apathy with Facial Expression and Motion Analysis. In: 2019 14th IEEE International Conference on Automatic Face & Gesture Recognition (FG 2019). May 2019, Lille, France, pp. 1–8.
27. Miller DS, Robert P, Ereshefsky L, Adler L, Bateman D, Cummings J, et al. Diagnostic criteria for apathy in neurocognitive disorders. Alzheimers Dement. 2021 May 5. doi:10.1002/alz.12358. Epub ahead of print. PMID: 33949763.
28. American Psychiatric Association. Diagnostic and Statistical Manual of Mental Disorders (5th ed). Arlington, VA: American Psychiatric Association; 2013.
29. Zeisel J, Reisberg B, Whitehouse P, Woods R, Verheul A. Ecopsychosocial interventions in cognitive decline and dementia: a new terminology and a new paradigm. Am J Alzheimers Dis Other Demen. 2016;31(6):502–7.
30. Starkstein S, Hayhow B. Apathy in dementia: time to stand up. Am J Geriatr Psychiatry. 2019;27(4):406–7.
31. Seel RT, Kreutzer JS, Rosenthal M, Hammond FM, Corrigan JD, Black K. Depression after traumatic brain injury: a National Institute on Disability and Rehabilitation Research Model Systems multicenter investigation. Arch Phys Med Rehabil. 2003;84(2):177–84.
32. Pardini M, Bonzano L, Mancardi GL, Roccatagliata L. Frontal networks play a role in fatigue perception in multiple sclerosis. Behav Neurosci. 2010;124(3):329–36.
33. Gotlib IH, Hamilton JP. Neuroimaging and depression: current status and unresolved issues. Curr Dir Psychol Sci. 2008;17(2):159–63.

34. Rømer Thomsen K, Whybrow PC, Kringelbach ML. Reconceptualizing anhedonia: novel perspectives on balancing the pleasure networks in the human brain. Front Behav Neurosci. 2015;9:49.

35. Treadway MT, Zald DH. Reconsidering anhedonia in depression: lessons from translational neuroscience. Neurosci Biobehav Rev. 2011;35(3):537–55.

36. Rizvi SJ, Quilty LC, Sproule BA, Cyriac A, Michael Bagby R, Kennedy SH. Development and validation of the Dimensional Anhedonia Rating Scale (DARS) in a community sample and individuals with major depression. Psychiatry Res. 2015;229(1–2):109–19.

37. Leentjens AFG, Dujardin K, Marsh L, Martinez-Martin P, Richard IH, Starkstein SE, et al. Apathy and anhedonia rating scales in Parkinson's disease: critique and recommendations. Mov Disord. 2008;23(14):2004–14.

38. Nemeth G, Hegedus K, Molnar L. Akinetic mutism associated with bicingular lesions: clinicopathological and functional anatomical correlates. Eur Arch Psychiatry Neurol Sci. 1988;237(4):218–22.

39. Vijayaraghavan L, Krishnamoorthy ES, Brown RG, Trimble MR. Abulia: a Delphi survey of British neurologists and psychiatrists. Mov Disord. 2002;17(5):1052–7.

40. Afari N, Buchwald D. Chronic fatigue syndrome: a review. Am J Psychiatry. 2003;160(2):221–36.

41. Brurberg KG, Fonhus MS, Larun L, Flottorp S, Malterud K. Case definitions for chronic fatigue syndrome/myalgic encephalomyelitis (CFS/ME): a systematic review. BMJ Open. 2014;4(2):e003973.

42. Skorvanek M, Gdovinova Z, Rosenberger J, Saeedian RG, Nagyova I, Groothoff JW, et al. The associations between fatigue, apathy, and depression in Parkinson's disease. Acta Neurol Scand. 2015;131(2):80–7.

43. Cochrane GD, Rizvi S, Abrantes AM, Crabtree B, Cahill J, Friedman JH. The association between fatigue and apathy in patients with either Parkinson's disease or multiple sclerosis. Parkinsonism Relat Disord. 2015;21(9):1093–5.

44. World Health Organization. The ICD-10 Classification of Mental and Behavioral Disorders: Diagnostic Criteria for Research. Geneva: World Health Organization; 1993. Available at: https://apps.who.int/iris/handle/10665/37108

45. Olin JT, Schneider LS, Katz IR, Meyers BS, Alexopoulos GS, Breitner JC, et al. Provisional diagnostic criteria for depression of Alzheimer disease. Am J Geriatr Psychiatry. 2002;10(2):125–8.

46. Sheikh JI, Yesavage JA. Geriatric Depression Scale (GDS): recent evidence and development of a shorter version. Clin Gerontol J Aging Ment Health. 1986;5(1–2):165–73.

47. Radakovic R. Convergence and divergence of apathy and depression. Psypag Q. 2016;99:44–7.

48. Vloeberghs R, Opmeer EM, De Deyn PP, Engelborghs S, De Roeck EE. [Apathy, depression and cognitive functioning in patients with MCI and dementia]. Tijdschr Gerontol Geriatr. 2018;49(3):95–102.

49. Szymkowicz SM, Dotson VM, Jones JD, Okun MS, Bowers D. Symptom dimensions of depression and apathy and their relationship with cognition in Parkinson's disease. J Int Neuropsychol Soc. 2018;24(3):269–82.

50. Camargo CHF, Serpa RA, Jobbins VA, Berbetz FA, Sabatini JS. Differentiating between apathy and depression in patients with Parkinson disease dementia. Am J Alzheimers Dis Other Demen. 2017;33(1):30–4.

51. Lohner V, Brookes RL, Hollocks MJ, Morris RG, Markus HS. Apathy, but not depression, is associated with executive dysfunction in cerebral small vessel disease. PLoS One. 2017;12(5):e0176943.

52. Dan R, Růžička F, Bezdicek O, Růžička E, Roth J, Vymazal J, et al. Separate neural representations of depression, anxiety and apathy in Parkinson's disease. Sci Rep. 2017;7(1):12164.
53. Benoit M, Robert PH. Imaging correlates of apathy and depression in Parkinson's disease. J Neurol Sci. 2011;310(1–2):58–60.
54. Kaji Y, Hirata K. Apathy and anhedonia in Parkinson's disease. ISRN Neurol. 2011;2011:219427.
55. Fawcett J, Clark DC, Scheftner WA, Gibbons RD. Assessing anhedonia in psychiatric patients. Arch Gen Psychiatry. 1983;40(1):79–84.
56. Kashdan TB, Elhai JD, Frueh BC. Anhedonia and emotional numbing in combat veterans with PTSD. Behav Res Ther. 2006;44(3):457–67.
57. Leventhal AM, Kahler CW, Ray LA, Stone K, Young D, Chelminski I, et al. Anhedonia and amotivation in psychiatric outpatients with fully remitted stimulant use disorder. Am J Addict. 2008;17(3):218–23.
58. Patejdl R, Penner IK, Noack TK, Zettl UK. Multiple sclerosis and fatigue: a review on the contribution of inflammation and immune-mediated neurodegeneration. Autoimmun Rev. 2016;15(3):210–20.
59. Vucic S, Krishnan AV, Kiernan MC. Fatigue and activity dependent changes in axonal excitability in amyotrophic lateral sclerosis. J Neurol Neurosurg Psychiatry. 2007;78(11):1202.
60. Brown RG, Dittner A, Findley L, Wessely SC. The Parkinson fatigue scale. Parkinsonism Relat Disord. 2005;11(1):49–55.
61. Ingles JL, Eskes GA, Phillips SJ. Fatigue after stroke. Arch Phys Med Rehabil. 1999;80(2):173–8.
62. Alexopoulos GS, Abrams RC, Young RC, Shamoian CA. Cornell scale for depression in dementia. Biol Psychiatry. 1988;23(3):271–84.
63. Ownby RL, Crocco E, Acevedo A, John V, Loewenstein D. Depression and risk for Alzheimer disease: systematic review, meta-analysis, and metaregression analysis. JAMA Psychiatry. 2006;63(5):530–8.
64. Aarsland D, Påhlhagen S, Ballard CG, Ehrt U, Svenningsson P. Depression in Parkinson disease—epidemiology, mechanisms and management. Nat Rev Neurol. 2012;8(1):35–47.
65. Addington D, Addington J, Maticka-Tyndale E. Assessing depression in schizophrenia: the Calgary Depression Scale. Br J Psychiatry Suppl. 1993;(22):39–44.
66. Hackett ML, Yapa C, Parag V, Anderson CS. Frequency of depression after stroke: a systematic review of observational studies. Stroke. 2005;36(6):1330–40.
67. Berridge KC, Robinson TE. Parsing reward. Trends Neurosci. 2003;26(9):507–13.
68. Berridge KC, Robinson TE. What is the role of dopamine in reward: hedonic impact, reward learning, or incentive salience? Brain Res Brain Res Rev. 1998;28(3):309–69.
69. Berridge KC. Food reward: brain substrates of wanting and liking. Neurosci Biobehav Rev. 1996;20(1):1–25.
70. Blackburn JR, Phillips AG, Jakubovic A, Fibiger HC. Dopamine and preparatory behavior: II. A neurochemical analysis. Behav Neurosci. 1989;103(1):15–23.
71. Berridge KC. Evolving concepts of emotion and motivation. Front Psychol. 2018;9:1647.
72. Manera V, Abrahams S, Agüera-Ortiz L, Bremond F, David R, Fairchild K, et al. Recommendations for the nonpharmacological treatment of apathy in brain disorders. Am J Geriatr Psychiatry. 2020;28(4):410–20.

2
Measurement of Apathy

Moyra Mortby, Bria Mele, Zahinoor Ismail, and David Miller

Introduction

Apathy, primarily defined by marked loss of motivation, is the most frequently observed neuropsychiatric symptom (NPS) across neurocognitive disorders (1). Despite a lack of unified definition, apathy, whether considered a syndrome or symptom, is increasingly being diagnosed (2).

Marin (3) was the first researcher to describe apathy as a syndrome nearly three decades ago. Apathy is conceptualized by its measurement scales (4). In clinical and research settings, apathy is assessed using a variety of methods, including diagnostic criteria-based clinical interviews, administration of measurement scales, and observational ratings of behaviours by a trained specialist. These assessments are generally structured, drawing on patient and caregiver input, while some also consider a physician's perspective (5). Importantly, apathy assessment tools are required that allow for robust measurement of severity and change, and which demonstrate reliability in distinguishing apathy from other comorbid syndromes commonly observed in neurocognitive disorders (e.g. depression) (5).

This chapter provides a detailed overview of apathy measurement in neurocognitive disorders, placing a particular focus on diagnostic criteria and commonly used assessment tools (see Fig. 2.1 for an overview of the development timeline of apathy assessment methods).

Diagnostic Criteria of Apathy

While often thought of solely as a component or symptom of other diagnoses such as depression, schizophrenia, or Parkinson's disease (PD), apathy should also be thought of as a distinct entity or syndrome. Marin (3) first described apathy as a syndrome characterized by deficits in goal-directed behaviour, goal-directed cognitive activity, and emotions, which are measured as a singular concept. Apathy was understood to be a disorder of motivation that was both persistent and caused apparent impaired function.

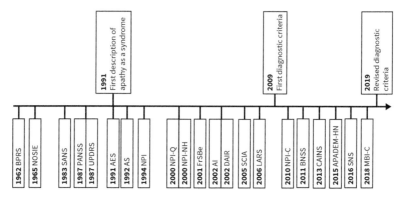

Fig. 2.1 Development timeline of apathy assessment methods. For abbreviations, see text.

The more recent appreciation that apathy can also be a distinct syndrome is important given its potential to impact the quality of life of both patients and their care-givers. While estimates of prevalence vary, it is clear that as patients progress from normal cognition to mild cognitive impairment (MCI) and to dementia (whether Alzheimer's disease (AD) or other types such as frontotemporal dementia), the prevalence of apathy increases (6). This is particularly relevant given that when present, apathy can accelerate the progression from normal cognition to MCI, and from MCI to AD (7).

Rooted in Marin's definition, Robert et al. (8) published the first diagnostic criteria for apathy in patients diagnosed with brain disorders. These are used in clinical and research settings (9), underpinning apathy assessment in many neurodegenerative and neuropsychiatric disorders (e.g. (10, 11–13)). According to these criteria, (A) patients had to demonstrate a loss or decrease of motivation compared to their norm; (B) the presence of symptoms in two of the following three symptoms—behaviour, cognition, and emotion—had to be present for most of the past 4 or more weeks; (C) the presence of A and B needed to result in clinically significant impairment; and (D) the symptoms could not be explained by other factors (e.g. substance abuse or ill-ness). While realizing that there is some overlap with depression, Robert et al. (8) described how apathy could be distinguished from depression, an important distinction when deciding how to treat it.

For the past decade, the Robert criteria have served as the gold standard. However, over time our understanding of both the clinical features and the underlying neuro-biology of apathy has improved, more sensitive assessments of apathy have been created, and some researchers have taken issue with the term motivation (as explained later). Additionally, as apathy gains traction as an identifiable treatment target for clinical trials, particularly within the context of dementia, it becomes increasingly important to reflect that understanding in diagnostic criteria that are acceptable to both researchers and regulators.

As a result, a group of experts led by Robert and Lanctôt organized a consensus conference in 2018 to revise the criteria (9). While they preserved the overall diagnostic criteria structure, the revisions are as follows:

Criterion A: (i) using the term 'goal-directed behaviour' in place of motivation. It was felt that 'goal-directed behaviour' could be measured more objectively compared to 'motivation', which is more often someone's psychological interpretation of another person's inner emotional state; (ii) removing the phrase 'which is not consistent with his age or culture' as it was deemed unnecessary given that apathy was considered to be present when there was a reduction compared to the patient's prior level of functioning; and (iii) listing the different apathy domains—behaviour, cognition, emotion, or social—in the definition.

Criterion B: (i) the 2009 criteria utilized three domains—behaviour, cognition, and emotion. In the revised criteria, two domains, behaviour and cognition, were combined into a single domain as it can be challenging to differentiate emotion from behavioural deficits as the cause for a decrease in observed behaviours. The emotion domain remained unchanged as blunted emotions were able to be separated from deficits in behaviour and cognition, and social interaction was added. The rationale for this addition is recent evidence from healthy people that it may represent a distinct element of apathy (14); (ii) the difference between environment-stimulated and self-initiated deficits was added; and (iii) examples of symptoms in each area of impairment were added.

Criterion C remained unchanged.

Criterion D was modified to include that significant changes to a person's environment are a potential reason for exclusion. This is in addition to the exclusion of conditions that can mimic apathy, and those that are transient and/or result from the effects of a medication (9).

These criteria revisions apply broadly to all neuropsychiatric disorders. There is a concurrent, related effort by the Apathy Interest Group of the International Society for CNS Clinical Trials and Methodology to determine whether there should be diagnostic criteria for apathy pertaining solely to neurocognitive disorders and, if so, whether they should include the social domain. Both of these efforts at criteria revision are the result of collaboration between representatives from academia, industry, and regulators. The ultimate goal is to develop criteria that are universally accepted, clear, reflective of the current and enhanced understanding of the underpinnings of apathy, and ultimately will serve as the basis for improved care and clinical trial investigation.

Apathy Measurement in Neurocognitive Disorders

Numerous psychometric measures to assess apathy are available, most having been derived from Marin's concept of apathy as a loss of motivation manifested in diminished emotions, interest/goal-setting cognitions and purposeful activity (15). These scales generally draw on structured or semi-structured interviews with patients and/ or caregivers (16); however, they differ in terms of content, reference timeframe, and target population (17).

When assessing apathy in neurocognitive disorders, the source of information is highly relevant. Self-report may not always be appropriate in neurocognitive disorders due to impaired capacity for self-observation (15, 18). Information should be elicited through direct patient behaviour/emotion examination and observation and/ or through an interview with a knowledgeable informant (15).

Apathy-Specific Measures

Several apathy-specific measures have been developed that facilitate apathy and apathy-domain assessment. Here we describe the most common apathy-specific measures.

Neuropsychiatric Inventory (NPI) and Variants

The NPI is available in four versions, including the original structured interview (NPI), an abbreviated informant report questionnaire (NPI-Q), a structured interview designed for use in nursing homes (NPI-NH), and a revised version of the NPI, based on clinician rating (NPI-C).

The original NPI (19) is a structured interview that assesses ten behavioural and two neurovegetative symptoms observed in AD and other dementias (19). The NPI focuses on new-onset behaviours and/or behavioural changes since diagnosis. Section G assessed apathy/indifference. This tool is well validated and commonly used in AD and PD populations (10).

The NPI is administered via scripted interview with a caregiver/informant, preferably one living with the patient. Ideally, the interview is conducted in the absence of the patient to facilitate open discussion of behaviours. Behavioural changes are assessed using a 4-week timeframe. The apathy screening question asks informants to determine whether the following applies: 'Has the patient lost interest in the world around him/her? Has he/she lost interest in doing things or does he/she lack motivation for starting new activities? Is he/she more difficult to engagement in conversation or in doing chores? Is the patient apathetic or indifferent?' Answers are coded using a 'yes'/'no' response. For negatively confirmed screening questions, the interviewer progresses to the next domain. In each domain, frequency, severity, and caregiver distress are only rated for problematic or aberrant behaviours. Scoring is based on frequency (rated on a scale of 1—'rarely (less than once per week)' to 4—'very often (once or more per day)') multiplied by severity (rated on a scale of 1—'mild' to 3—'severe'). Caregiver distress is assessed for each positive NPI domain, with scores ranging from 0—'no distress' to 5—'very severe or extreme'.

The NPI-Q (20) offers a shortened, self-administered version of the original NPI. The NPI-Q is given to a caregiver/informant who reports on patient behaviours. The NPI-Q assesses the same 12 domains as the NPI, using a screening question that covers core symptom manifestations (20). Apathy is assessed using a single screening question: 'Does the patient seem less interested in his/her usual activities or in the activities and plans of others?' and 'yes'/'no' responses recorded. The NPI-Q only assesses severity of positively confirmed symptoms, using the same three-point scale as in the NPI. The rationale for solely assessing severity is underpinned by research showing symptom severity more strongly correlates to caregiver distress than symptom frequency and that NPI-rated severity and frequency were highly correlated (19–21). Caregiver distress is rated identically to the original NPI. Only limited research validating the NPI-Q apathy domain in neurodegenerative disease is available. In a validation study of the NPI-Q, apathy was less frequently reported in AD using the NPI-Q when compared to the full NPI (20). Such limitations must be considered when selecting the appropriate apathy measure for research and clinical assessments.

The NPI-NH (22) was developed for use with professional caregivers in nursing homes. The scale is administered as an interview to nursing staff who report on behaviours of residents in their daily care. The NPI-NH can be used to ascertain behaviours using the traditional 4-week timeframe or for any other predefined period and is validated for use in clinical and research settings (22). While only limited research is available that validates the use of the NPI-NH to detect apathy in residents with neurodegenerative disease, it is one of the first scales designed for use within this setting/context (22). The NPI-NH assesses 12 domains as in the original NPI, and uses the same assessment format. The screening question of the NPI-NH apathy domain asks: 'Does the resident sit quietly without paying attention to things going on around him/her? Has he/she lost interest in doing things or lack motivation for participating in activities? Is it difficult to involve the resident in conversation or in group activities?' Frequency and severity are rated using the same rating scale as the original NPI. However, occupational disruptiveness (how much increased work, effort, time, or distress the behaviour causes them) as opposed to caregiver distress is assessed in the NPI-NH using a five-point scale ranging from (0—'not at all' to 5—'very severely or extremely').

The NPI-C (23) includes expanded domains and items and employs a clinician-rating methodology. The NPI-C uses a 4-week timeframe reference. For the apathy domain, additional items were added based on Robert et al.'s (8) diagnostic criteria for apathy. The apathy domain is assessed using a single 'yes'/'no' response to the following screening questions: 'Has (Subject) lost interest in the world around him/her? Has (Subject) lost interest in doing things or lack motivation for starting new activities? Is (Subject) more difficult to engage in conversation or in doing chores? Is (Subject) apathetic or indifferent?' On the NPI-C, the caregiver is asked to rate frequency, severity, and distress, the patient is asked about frequency, and the clinician incorporates these and their own observations to rate the severity of each behaviour. The sum of the clinician's frequency ratings constitutes the domain score. The rationale underpinning this change in rating each item individually was that the use of item scores was more suited to clinical trials where there is a need for finer detail to assess change (23). The use of a clinician rating approach also aims to reduce bias from the informant (23).

In conclusion, while the NPI and its versions are generally referred to as the gold standard assessment tool for NPS and are the most frequently used measures of apathy in research and clinical settings, they may not allow for complete consideration of apathy as a syndrome, encompassing all apathy domains (15).

Structured Clinical Interview for Apathy (SCIA)

This is the only structured clinical interview available to assess apathy. The SCIA (24) is rooted in Marin's (3) definition of apathy and Starkstein et al.'s (25) operationalized and validated criteria. It is validated for use within AD and PD populations (11, 24).

This clinician-based measure includes a series of questions that assess the domains of lack of motivation relative to previous levels of functioning, lack of effort to perform everyday activities, dependency on others to structure activities, lack of interest in learning new things or in new experiences, lack of concern about personal problems, unchanging or flat affect, and lack of emotional response to positive or negative personal events (24). All questions follow the *Diagnostic and Statistical Manual for Mental Disorders* (fourth edition) Structured Clinical Interview format (24).

The SCIA assesses each criterion using two key questions and follow-up questions are used to assess symptom severity. Criterion A (lack of motivation relative to the patient's previous level of functioning) is assessed by the following questions: 'Did you notice a lack of or diminished motivation to perform the activities of daily living?' and 'Does it happen most of the day, almost every day?' Follow-up questions elicit the rating of symptom frequency, approximate date of onset, progression patterns, and discrepancies between patient and caregiver information provided (24).

These follow-up questions are assessed for all positive responses to the following items: Criterion B1 (lack of effort or energy to perform everyday activities (e.g. grooming, work, social life)); Criterion B2 (dependency on prompts from others to carry out everyday activities); Criterion B3 (lack of interest in learning new things or in new experiences); Criterion B4 (lack of concern about one's personal problems); and Criterion B5 (unchanging or flat affect, lack of emotional response to positive or negative events) (24). Symptoms are scored as either 'absent', 'subclinical', or 'definitely present' based on the responses to the questions asked in Criterion B1 to B5 (24).

The extent of social and occupational dysfunction caused by the symptoms of apathy are assessed in Criterion C, while Criterion D is used to exclude organic causes of behavioural changes other than dementia (24).

A diagnosis of apathy is made when patients score 3 ('definitely present') for Criterion A, score 3 on at least three of the B criteria, and score 1 ('absent') for Criteria C and D.

Apathy Evaluation Scale (AES)

The first measure developed and validated to assess apathy severity, the AES (26), is considered an especially promising metric for apathy in AD (16), with sensitivity to differentiate patients with probable AD from cognitively normal elderly people based on apathy severity (26, 27). The AES is also used in other neuropsychiatric conditions, such as PD (28) and schizophrenia (29).

The AES consists of three versions. Each is scored based on the impression of a single rater. These include self-report (AES-S), informant-reported (AES-I), usually a family member or close friend, and clinician-reported (AES-C) versions. While the AES-I and AES-S are questionnaires, the AES-C is completed as a semi-structured interview (26). In the AES-C, the clinician takes into consideration both the self- and informant reports to generate a clinical judgement of each item. The three versions of the AES facilitate the consideration of potentially complementary sources of information, especially as apathy is often associated with impaired insight and dementia-related cognitive impairment (26). The three versions are identical, differing solely in terms of the pronoun used to refer to the subject/patient.

All three AES versions assess Marin's apathy domains of behavioural, cognitive, and emotional concomitants of goal-directed behaviour (26) and are consistent with the syndromic criteria. To date, it remains unclear whether any of the three AES versions provide a particular advantage above the others, especially as a predictor of MCI or AD (30).

This 18-item measure was developed for use within elderly populations specifically, as well as in those with AD, stroke, or major depression (26). Each item is scored on a four-point scale ranging from 1—'not at all' to 4—'a lot'. Scores range from 18 to 72 (26) and lower scores indicate greater apathy. The AES uses a 4-week reference timeframe. It was validated for use among elderly populations, people with stroke and/or major depression, and in PD populations. It has since been validated for use in dementia populations as well as with institutionalized patients (15).

Research has found limited usefulness of the AES in nursing home settings, with professional caregivers reporting (i) difficulties in judging items which were superimposed by severe cognitive deficits and which where therefore being rated in the same way for patients with dementia with and without comorbid apathy, and (ii) loss of specificity of apathetic behaviour items due to the externally driven daily structure in nursing homes (31). An abbreviated ten-item version of the AES (AES-10) has since been developed and validated, which is easier to complete, and is more relevant to the nursing home context (31). The AES-10 is administered as an interview to a caregiver who is familiar with the patient (31). Evaluation of the AES-10 yielded no substantial losses regarding internal consistency or construct validity compared to the full-length AES (31). The AES-10 provides a total score ranging between 10 and 40, with higher scores indicating more apathetic behaviour.

Apathy Scale (AS)

This is an abridged and modified version of Marin et al.'s (26) AES. It is intended to provide a brief and easier to administer version of the AES (32). The AS consists of 14 items scored by a caregiver/informant using a four-point scale ranging from 0—'not at all' to 3—'a lot'. Total scores range from 0 to 42 with higher scores indicating more severe apathy. The AS can be self-administered or administered through interview. While the AS was originally developed for use in PD populations, it is also validated for use in AD, Huntington's disease, and stroke, with good intra- and inter-rater reliability having been reported (32).

Apathy Inventory (AI)

The AI (33) was originally developed and validated in French and assesses global and subdomain apathy (emotional blunting, lack of initiative, and loss of interest) (4). The AI consists of three items (one per domain) and is validated as a self-report and informant interview (4). It is validated for use within PD, AD, and MCI populations (33).

In the self-report AI, the patient assesses their own behaviour using 'yes'/'no' responses and rates the severity of their behaviour on a continuum from 'mild' to 'severe' for each item/domain. A composite apathy score is calculated based on the three domain scores. The informant report follows the same approach as the NPI. Presence of a behaviour is recorded using 'yes'/'no' responses, while frequency is rated on a four-point scale (1—'occasionally' to 4—'very frequently') and severity is rated on a three-point scale (1—'mild' to 3—'marked'). Frequency and severity are multiplied to obtain the domain scores and to calculate the total score.

Dementia Apathy Interview and Rating (DAIR)

The DAIR (34) assesses dementia-related changes in motivation, emotional responsiveness, and engagement. It involves a structured interview with the primary caregiver that assesses the patient's initiation behaviour, interest, and engagement in the environment in the past 4 weeks (4). This clinician-administered scale consists of 16 items. Items are scored on a four-point scale ranging from 0—'no, almost never' to 3—'yes, almost always'. A mandatory follow-up question facilitates determination of whether the behaviours represent a change from pre-impairment behaviour (34). Only items that reflect a change in behaviour are included in the final score. The total score is a sum score of items reflecting change divided by the number of items completed (34). Higher scores indicate higher average apathy (34).

Lille Apathy Rating Scale (LARS)

Developed to address existing tool limitations and to include the assessment of the apathy domains, the LARS (35) is based on Marin et al.'s (26) conceptual principles of apathy and the authors' clinical experience (35). It provides a comprehensive assessment of apathy through a structured interview with either a patient (35) or with an informant (36). In the informant version (LARS-i), some items have been reworded for suitability as questions for informants; however, scoring is the same as the original patient version of the LARS. Both the patient and informant versions are validated for use in PD populations only (35, 37).

The LARS and the LARS-i consist of 33 items that underpin nine domains. Eight of the domains focus on the main clinical manifestations of apathy, namely reduction in everyday productivity, lack of interest, lack of initiative, extinction of novelty seeking and motivation, blunting of emotional responses, lack of concern, and poor social life (35). The ninth domain is extinction of self-awareness—a domain of apathy considered by Stuss et al. (38) to reflect a 'metacognitive ability, necessary to mediate information from a personal, social past and current history with projections to the future'—where apathy results in a reduction in ability to self-criticize and behavioural adjustment to social requirements (35). Items included in the self-awareness domain focus on a person's ability to question their decisions, change opinions or actions when needed, admit when they are wrong, and their feelings of guilt after being rude to others.

The first three items are coded using a five-point scale, while the rest are clinician-coded using a binary scale ('yes'/'no'). Non-classifiable answers or non-applicable answers can be scored as 'not available'. Each subscale contributes with equal weighting to the global score, which ranges from −36 to +36. Higher scores represent a greater degree of apathy.

The LARS is also available in a short form, consisting of 12 items that assess seven domains reflecting the clinical manifestations of apathy (39). The seven domains include everyday productivity, interests, taking the initiative, novelty seeking, motivation-voluntary actions, emotional responses, and social life. The short form is administered as a structured interview, focuses on the past 4 weeks, and is scored from −15 to +15 (39).

Apathy in Dementia, Nursing Home (APADEM-NH) Scale

The APADEM-NH scale assesses apathy in institutionalized patients with neurodegenerative dementia (40). This measure was developed to address ceiling effects which rendered commonly used apathy measures (e.g. AES, AI, and DAIR) insensitive when employed within a nursing home setting (15, 40). This measure considers the main characteristics of the most severe dementia stages as well as the distinctiveness of the institutional environment (15).

The APADEM-NH scale comprises 26 items, which assess three domains of apathy described by Levy and Dubois (41) and include deficit of thinking and self-generated behaviour, emotional blunting, and cognitive inertia (40). This is an interview-based scale, administered to a professional caregiver that works closely with the resident (40). The caregiver must have good knowledge of the resident's cognitive and functional status.

The APADEM-NH scale provides a general apathy score as well as three apathy domain scores. Items are scored on a three-point scale ranging from 0—'no apathy' to 3—'severe apathy'. Scoring takes into account the degree of stimulation needed to elicit a behaviour or emotion (15). Total scores range from 0 to 78, with higher scores indicating more severe apathy. Overall, this scale is reported to provide a satisfactory measure of apathy in those with advanced dementia living in institutionalized care (40).

General/Global Measures of Apathy

There are a number of scales that are specific to a variety of indications and/or settings. Many of these scales also assess apathy or symptoms related to apathy. They vary in the timeframes assessed, as well as the sources of information on which the ratings are based. Some scales were developed prior to Marin's (3) initial description of apathy as a syndrome and therefore do not reflect the most recent understanding of the symptom and/or syndrome. Among these scales are the following:

Frontal Systems Behaviour Scale (FrSBe)

The FrSBe (42), previously referred to as the Frontal Lobe Personality Scale (FLOPS) (43), is a 46-item scale designed for disorders of the frontal lobe. It comprises three subscales—apathy (14 items), executive dysfunction (17 items), and disinhibition (15 items)—that reflect three frontal behavioural syndromes most commonly seen with frontal lobe damage. The apathy items assess 'problems with initiation, psychomotor retardation, spontaneity, drive, persistence, loss of energy and interest, lack of concern about self/care, and/or blunted affective expression'.

The FrSBe can be administered in one of three forms: family version (rated by a family member or close caregiver), staff version (professional staff member caring for a patient), and self version (patient self-rating). The family version is most frequently used (44) and, in fact, is recommended when assessing patients with dementia as anosognosia, abulia, and amnesia are likely to impact self-ratings (45).

Items are rated on a five-point scale ranging from 1—'almost never' to 5—'almost always'. Each version provides a total score reflecting frontal lobe dysfunction, as well as subscale scores for apathy, disinhibition, and executive dysfunction—three distinctive frontal lobe syndromes (44). Scores are obtained for both premorbid and current behaviour. This allows for the measurement of change as a consequence of the neurological disease or insult. Research has shown the FrSBe to be sensitive to behavioural changes in AD, Huntington's disease, PD, vascular dementia, and MCI (45).

Scale for the Assessment of Negative Symptoms (SANS)

The SANS (46, 47), developed by Andreasen in 1983, devotes four questions to the assessment of 'avolition/apathy'. Under this heading, grooming and hygiene, impersistence at work or school, physical anergia, and a global rating are scored on a six-point scale ranging from 0—'none/not at all' to 5—'severe'. While emotion and social interactions are also rated, there does not appear to be any assessment of motivation or goal directed behaviours. For this reason, the SANS is not ideal for assessing apathy.

Brief Psychiatric Rating Scale (BPRS)

The BPRS (48, 49) is one of the most widely used instruments to assess the presence and severity of a number of psychiatric symptoms. The original 16-item scale was developed in 1962 (48) and was subsequently replaced by an 18-item version (49). In 1986, a 24-item version was introduced (BPRS-E) (50) which contains items not included in the 18-item version and addresses important criticisms of the older versions (e.g. change to semi-structured interview format from unstructured, inclusion of anchor points, and broader coverage of schizophrenia and mood disorders) (51). Exploratory factor analyses have identified a four-factor solution of the BPRS-E consisting of thought disturbance, animation, mood disturbance, and apathy (51). The apathy factor includes emotional withdrawal, blunted affect, motor retardation, and self-neglect—items associated with absence of emotion, drive, and affect (51). This apathy factor is proposed to reflect the emotional impoverishment aspect of Starkstein et al.'s (25) apathy model (52).

Positive and Negative Symptoms Scale (PANSS)

The PANSS (53) and BPRS are taken together since the PANSS was adapted from the BPRS (48) and the Psychopathology Rating Scale (54). This 30-item scale was developed to measure positive (e.g. hallucinations, delusions; seven items), negative (e.g. blunt affect, apathetic social withdrawal; seven items), and general psychiatric (e.g. depressed mood, anxiety; 16 items) symptoms in schizophrenia (53). The negative symptoms subscale (PANSS-NS) is used to measure apathy and apathy-related behaviours in schizophrenia (17). Items of the PANSS-NS that elicit apathy include the 'lack of spontaneity and flow of conversation' item which is scored based on cognitive-verbal processes observed during the interview and the 'passive/apathetic social withdrawal' item which is scored based on informant input. The 'disturbance of volition' item, which is scored based on thought content and behaviour expressed during the interview, also assesses apathy and is part of the General Psychopathology Scale.

The PANSS is scored on a seven-point scale ranging from 1—'absent' to 7—'extreme'. Completion of the PANSS relies on information obtained from patient reports, caregiver reports, and clinical observation (55) and is accompanied by a semi-structured interview (SCI-PANSS) which ensures all content domains are covered in the interview (56).

Brief Negative Symptoms Scale (BNSS)

The BNSS is a newer negative symptoms scale for schizophrenia (57, 58). It was designed for ease of use in clinical trials and is well validated (58). The BNSS covers the five core negative symptom domains of blunted affect, alogia, avolition, anhedonia, and asociality suggested by the 2005 National Institute of Mental Health Consensus Development Conference (57). It consists of 13 items which are organized into six subscales (anhedonia, distress, asociality, avolition, blunted affect, and alogia) (57). These can be clustered into two factors—Motivation-Pleasure (anhedonia, asociality, and avolition) and Emotional Expressivity (blunted affect and alogia) (59).

The BNSS is administered as a semi-structured interview and suggested prompts are available in the comprehensive manual and workbooks (57). Items are rated on a seven-point scale ranging from 0—'absent' to 6—'severe'. The total scores range from 0 to 78 and subscale scores are calculated by summing individual items within each subscale (57). The BNSS has been reported to correspond well with observer-rated apathy (60).

Clinical Assessment Interview for Negative Symptoms (CAINS)

The CAINS (61) is the second measure resulting from the 2005 National Institute of Mental Health Consensus Development Conference on negative symptoms. Items in this semi-structured interview assess the same five consensus negative symptom subdomains as assessed by the BNSS (57). In this clinician-rated instrument, ratings of asociality, avolition, and anhedonia are based on the interviewee's report of sub-jective experiences of motivation and emotion, as well as frequency of actual en-gagement in relevant activities (62). Blunted affect and alogia are assessed based on observable behaviours displayed throughout the interview (62). Ratings combine assessments of behavioural engagement in relevant activities with reported experi-ences of motivation and emotion to enable the comprehensive assessment of negative symptoms (61, 63).

The CAINS assesses internal experiences, including intensity of motivation and interest to engage in activities in social, vocational, and recreational areas, as well as actual behaviour manifested and differentiated between anticipatory and consummatory anhedonia (64). The CAINS comprises 13 items which form the same two subscales as the BNSS, namely motivation/pleasure (consisting of nine items) and expression (four items) (61, 62). Items are rated on a five-point scale from 0—'absent' to 4—'severe'. Overall, the CAINS shows good convergent and discriminant validity as well as good inter-rater reliability (62) and has to date not been significantly associ-ated with cognition (58, 61, 62).

Self-Evaluation of Negative Symptoms (SNS)

Apathy in schizophrenia can be screened for using a self-assessment measure of nega-tive symptoms—the SNS (65). The SNS was primarily designed for clinical evaluation and to help guide practitioners in treatment (e.g. cognitive or social therapy), but is also used during prodromal and early disease phases to identify negative symptoms (65). It assesses the five negative symptom dimensions using self-evaluation by the pa-tient, allowing them to express their deficits in motivation, pleasure, and loss of emo-tion independently of depressed mood (65). This short 20-item scale comprises of short and easily understandable sentences that allow for fast self-evaluation (less than 5 minutes) (66). Items are scored on a three-point scale ranging from 0—'strongly disagree' to 2—'strongly agree'. Total scores range from 0 (no negative symptoms) to

40 (severe negative symptoms). The five negative dimensions of the SNS reflect social withdrawal, diminished emotional range, alogia, avolition, and anhedonia (66). From these, a factor analysis has extracted two factors reflecting the dimensions of apathy (which include apathy, amotivation, asociality, and anhedonia) and emotion (65).

Unified Parkinson's Disease Rating Scale (UPDRS)

Apathy in PD is screened for in the UPDRS (67) using a single item (motivation/initiative item in section I—mentation, behaviour, and mood) (68, 69). This item is scored on a five-point scale ranging from 0—'normal' to 4—'withdrawn, complete loss of motivation'. This single-item apathy screen has been shown to be inadequately correlated with an AS cut-off of 14 points or greater for apathy, with the authors cautioning against using this item due to poor sensitivity (70).

Nurses' Observation Scale for Inpatient Evaluation (NOSIE)

The 30-item NOSIE (71) was developed by Honigfeld and Klett in 1965 to assess chronic schizophrenic patients in an inpatient setting. Apathy is assessed in the NOSIE under the negative factor of retardation items (item 5: 'Sits, unless directed into activity'; item 22: 'Sleeps, unless directed into activity'; item 27: 'Is slow-moving or sluggish') (72). Change since admission is assessed by joint raters. The lookback period is 3 days. This scale shows satisfactory inter-rater reliability, especially for positive symptoms compared to negative symptoms, such as apathy (72).

Assessing Apathy in Preclinical and Prodromal States

Mild behavioural impairment (MBI) is a validated neurobehavioral syndrome characterized by later life emergent and sustained NPS as an at-risk state for incident cognitive decline and dementia. MBI describes the neurobehavioural axis of pre-dementia risk states as a complement to the neurocognitive axis represented by subjective cognitive decline and MCI, both of which are well-known and established pre-dementia cognitive syndromes. Recent genetic evidence has demonstrated a common aetiology between MBI and AD, supporting the notion that neurodegeneration may contribute to the emergence of NPS, as it does with emergent neurocognitive symptoms (73). MBI can co-occur in those who have normal cognition, subjective cognitive decline, or MCI, and has been shown to significantly increase the progression rate to dementia in those with normal cognition or MCI, over a 3-year timeframe, compared to those without MBI (74).

MBI is a distinct entity from psychiatric illness that continues into late life. In a 5-year longitudinal study of older adults, MBI had a higher conversion rate to dementia than a psychiatric comparator group consisting of late-life psychiatric disorders (75), highlighting the prognostic utility of identifying MBI separately (76) and the fundamental importance of identifying age of onset of symptoms (77). MBI is detectable in community samples (78) and in clinical samples (79) where it is associated with greater caregiver burden. In both groups, MBI increases as cognition declines. More recently, in a large community cohort of 9931 cognitively normal older adults, MBI was associated with a faster decline in attention and working memory compared to those without MBI (80).

MBI consists of five domains: (i) impaired drive and motivation (apathy); (ii) affective/emotional dysregulation (mood and anxiety symptoms); (iii) impulse dyscontrol/agitation/abnormal reward salience (changes in response inhibition and self-regulation); (iv) social inappropriateness (impaired social cognition); and (v) abnormal thoughts/perceptions (psychotic symptoms). The presence of any domain qualifies as MBI.

Mild Behavioural Impairment Checklist (MBI-C)

The MBI-C is the case ascertainment tool developed to capture MBI criteria (available freely at https://mbitest.org/), including the mandated symptom duration of 6 months, and emergence of symptoms in later life. Validation studies of the MBI-C have determined cut-points in subjective cognitive decline (81) and in MCI (82, 83). Further, the MBI-C has demonstrated internal consistency, test–retest reliability (84), and discriminative validity from the NPI (84, 85). Factor analysis of the MBI-C has demonstrated a five-factor model, correlating with the five MBI domains, with appropriate mapping of domain member items (86), for both self- and informant-rated administrations. Self-rated MBI-C has correlated with cognitive decline when administered via an online portal (80). The MBI-C is also associated with subtle cognitive changes in those considered cognitively normal (87) and is associated with worsening cognition and temporal lobe atrophy in those with PD (88). Very recent data have correlated MBI-C score with beta-amyloid as measured by positron emission tomography in those with normal cognition, again supporting the utility of the MBI-C in case finding for early-stage neurodegenerative disease in advance of overt cognitive impairment (89). The sustained duration of symptoms in the criteria were included to decrease false positives from transient symptoms and reactive states, increasing the specificity of the criteria. Prevalence estimates have borne this out, as studies using the NPI to generate MBI prevalence have generated much higher estimates (78, 79) than those using the MBI-C (81, 83). This smaller, but more specific group is at high risk of incident cognitive decline and dementia, and may be biomarker-enriched for amyloid positivity (89).

Apathy in Mild Behavioural Impairment

Apathy is a prominent domain in MBI (domain 1). Importantly, apathy, as represented in the MBI-C is a syndromic rather than symptomatic measurement of apathy reflecting Marin (3), Starkstein (25), and ultimately Robert's International Consensus Criteria (8). In the MBI-C, there are six questions on apathy, two each mapping onto interest (cognitive apathy), initiative (behavioural apathy), and emotion (emotional apathy). The a priori development of the MBI-C was to capture apathy syndromically, as a pre-dementia manifestation, and to allow abstraction of each of the three apathy domains for subsequent research and clinical prognostication. The difference between the apathy syndrome captured by the MBI-C and the International Consensus criteria is that of duration. The apathy criteria require a minimum of 4 weeks' symptom duration, whereas for MBI, symptoms need to emerge for the first time in later life and be present, at least intermittently, for 6 months. Thus, the MBI-C can capture symptoms with confidence that these symptoms reflect an apathy syndrome. The rating for each of the apathy items is presence or absence, with a mild/moderate/severe rating for the present symptoms. However, the 6-month reference range of the MBI-C exceeds the minimum duration for the consensus criteria. Likely this is useful for ensuring case positivity, and thus the MBI-C may be a useful instrument to capture the apathy syndrome in older adults. However, further studies are required to determine the sensitivity and specificity of this tool for apathy case ascertainment as well as intervention studies to assess change in response to treatment.

Conclusion

In summary, there are many validated measures that can assist clinicians and researchers to assess apathy. Diagnostic criteria provide the framework for accurate apathy assessment. With recent scientific advances and proposed changes to the diagnostic criteria, it is necessary to review the psychometric properties of existing scales for quality of construction, reliability, validity, and sensitivity to change within the revised framework. New measures are needed which reflect the multidimensionality of the apathy and which assess these dimensions independently.

References

1. Lanctôt KL, Amatniek J, Ancoli-Israel S, Arnold SE, Ballard C, Cohen-Mansfield J, et al. Neuropsychiatric signs and symptoms of Alzheimer's disease: new treatment paradigms. Alzheimers Dement (N Y). 2017;3(3):440–9.
2. Starkstein SE, Leentjens AF. The nosological position of apathy in clinical practice. J Neurol Neurosurg Psychiatry. 2008;79(10):1088–92.
3. Marin RS. Apathy: a neuropsychiatric syndrome. J Neuropsychiatry Clin Neurosci. 1991;3(3):243–54.
4. Radakovic R, Harley C, Abrahams S, Starr JM. A systematic review of the validity and reliability of apathy scales in neurodegenerative conditions. Int Psychogeriatr. 2015;27(6):903–23.
5. Robert PH, Mulin E, Mallea P, David R. Apathy diagnosis, assessment, and treatment in Alzheimer's disease. CNS Neurosci Ther. 2010;16(5):263–71.

6. Hwang TJ, Masterman DL, Ortiz F, Fairbanks LA, Cummings JL. Mild cognitive impairment is associated with characteristic neuropsychiatric symptoms. Alzheimer Dis Assoc Disord. 2004;18(1):17–21.

7. Geda YE, Roberts RO, Mielke MM, Knopman DS, Christianson TJ, Pankratz VS, et al. Baseline neuropsychiatric symptoms and the risk of incident mild cognitive impairment: a population-based study. Am J Psychiatry. 2014;171(5):572–81.

8. Robert P, Onyike CU, Leentjens AF, Dujardin K, Aalten P, Starkstein S, et al. Proposed diagnostic criteria for apathy in Alzheimer's disease and other neuropsychiatric disorders. Eur Psychiatry. 2009;24(2):98–104.

9. Robert P, Lanctôt KL, Aguera-Ortiz L, Aalten P, Bremond F, Defrancesco M, et al. Is it time to revise the diagnostic criteria for apathy in brain disorders? The 2018 international consensus group. Eur Psychiatry. 2018;54:71–6.

10. Leentjens AF, Dujardin K, Marsh L, Martinez-Martin P, Richard IH, Starkstein SE, et al. Apathy and anhedonia rating scales in Parkinson's disease: critique and recommendations. Mov Disord. 2008;23(14):2004–14.

11. Drijgers RL, Dujardin K, Reijnders JS, Defebvre L, Leentjens AF. Validation of diagnostic criteria for apathy in Parkinson's disease. Parkinsonism Relat Disord. 2010;16(10):656–60.

12. Leontjevas R, Evers-Stephan A, Smalbrugge M, Pot AM, Thewissen V, Gerritsen DL, et al. A comparative validation of the abbreviated Apathy Evaluation Scale (AES-10) with the Neuropsychiatric Inventory apathy subscale against diagnostic criteria of apathy. J Am Med Dir Assoc. 2012;13(3):308.e1–6.

13. Mulin E, Leone E, Dujardin K, Delliaux M, Leentjens A, Nobili F, et al. Diagnostic criteria for apathy in clinical practice. Int J Geriatr Psychiatry. 2011;26(2):158–65.

14. Ang YS, Lockwood P, Apps MA, Muhammed K, Husain M. Distinct subtypes of apathy revealed by the Apathy Motivation Index. PLoS One. 2017;12(1):e0169938.

15. Lanctôt KL, Agüera-Ortiz L, Brodaty H, Francis PT, Geda YE, Ismail Z, et al. Apathy associated with neurocognitive disorders: recent progress and future directions. Alzheimers Dement. 2017:13(1):84–100.

16. Guercio BJ, Donovan NJ, Munro CE, Aghjayan SL, Wigman SE, Locascio JJ, et al. The Apathy Evaluation Scale: a comparison of subject, informant, and clinician report in cognitively normal elderly and mild cognitive impairment. J Alzheimers Dis. 2015;47(2):421–32.

17. Clarke DE, Ko JY, Kuhl EA, van Reekum R, Salvador R, Marin RS. Are the available apathy measures reliable and valid? A review of the psychometric evidence. J Psychosom Res. 2011;70(1):73–97.

18. Clarke DE, Reekum R, Simard M, Streiner DL, Freedman M, Conn D. Apathy in dementia: an examination of the psychometric properties of the apathy evaluation scale. J Neuropsychiatry Clin Neurosci. 2007;19(1):57–64.

19. Cummings JL, Mega M, Gray K, Rosenberg-Thompson S, Carusi DA, Gornbein J. The Neuropsychiatric Inventory: comprehensive assessment of psychopathology in dementia. Neurology. 1994;44(12):2308–14.

20. Kaufer DI, Cummings JL, Ketchel P, Smith V, MacMillan A, Shelley T, et al. Validation of the NPI-Q, a brief clinical form of the Neuropsychiatric Inventory. J Neuropsychiatry Clin Neurosci. 2000;12(2):233–9.

21. Kaufer DI, Cummings JL, Christine D, Bray T, Castellon S, Masterman D, et al. Assessing the impact of neuropsychiatric symptoms in Alzheimer's disease: the Neuropsychiatric Inventory Caregiver Distress Scale. J Am Geriatr Soc. 1998;46(2):210–5.

22. Wood S, Cummings JL, Hsu MA, Barclay T, Wheatley MV, Yarema KT, et al. The use of the neuropsychiatric inventory in nursing home residents. Characterization and measurement. Am J Geriatr Psychiatry. 2000;8(1):75–83.

23. de Medeiros K, Robert P, Gauthier S, Stella F, Politis A, Leoutsakos J, et al. The Neuropsychiatric Inventory-Clinician rating scale (NPI-C): reliability and validity of a revised assessment of neuropsychiatric symptoms in dementia. Int Psychogeriatr. 2010;22(6):984–94.

24. Starkstein SE, Ingram L, Garau ML, Mizrahi R. On the overlap between apathy and depression in dementia. J Neurol Neurosurg Psychiatry. 2005;76(8):1070–4.

25. Starkstein SE, Petracca G, Chemerinski E, Kremer J. Syndromic validity of apathy in Alzheimer's disease. Am J Psychiatry. 2001;158(6):872–7.

26. Marin RS, Biedrzycki RC, Firinciogullari S. Reliability and validity of the Apathy Evaluation Scale. Psychiatry Res. 1991;38(2):143–62.

27. Marin RS, Firinciogullari S, Biedrzycki RC. The sources of convergence between measures of apathy and depression. J Affect Disord. 1993;28(1):7–14.

28. Lueken U, Evens R, Balzer-Geldsetzer M, Baudrexel S, Dodel R, Graber-Sultan S, et al. Psychometric properties of the apathy evaluation scale in patients with Parkinson's disease. Int J Methods Psychiatr Res. 2017;26(4):e1564.

29. Servaas MN, Kos C, Gravel N, Renken RJ, Marsman JC, van Tol MJ, et al. Rigidity in motor behavior and brain functioning in patients with schizophrenia and high levels of apathy. Schizophr Bull. 2019;45(3):542–51.

30. Guercio BJ, Donovan NJ, Munro CE, Aghjayan SL, Wigman SE, Locascio JJ, et al. The Apathy Evaluation Scale: a comparison of subject, informant, and clinician report in cognitively normal elderly and mild cognitive impairment. J Alzheimers Dis. 2015;47(2):421–32.

31. Lueken U, Seidl U, Volker L, Schweiger E, Kruse A, Schroder J. Development of a short version of the Apathy Evaluation Scale specifically adapted for demented nursing home residents. Am J Geriatr Psychiatry. 2007;15(5):376–85.

32. Starkstein SE, Mayberg HS, Preziosi TJ, Andrezejewski P, Leiguarda R, Robinson RG. Reliability, validity, and clinical correlates of apathy in Parkinson's disease. J Neuropsychiatry Clin Neurosci. 1992;4(2):134–9.

33. Robert PH, Clairet S, Benoit M, Koutaich J, Bertogliati C, Tible O, et al. The apathy inventory: assessment of apathy and awareness in Alzheimer's disease, Parkinson's disease and mild cognitive impairment. Int J Geriatr Psychiatry. 2002;17(12):1099–105.

34. Strauss ME, Sperry SD. An informant-based assessment of apathy in Alzheimer disease. Neuropsychiatry Neuropsychol Behav Neurol. 2002;15(3):176–83.

35. Sockeel P, Dujardin K, Devos D, Deneve C, Destee A, Defebvre L. The Lille apathy rating scale (LARS), a new instrument for detecting and quantifying apathy: validation in Parkinson's disease. J Neurol Neurosurg Psychiatry. 2006;77(5):579–84.

36. Dujardin K, Sockeel P, Delliaux M, Destee A, Defebvre L. The Lille Apathy Rating Scale: validation of a caregiver-based version. Mov Disord. 2008;23(6):845–9.

37. Fernandez-Matarrubia M, Matias-Guiu JA, Moreno-Ramos T, Valles-Salgado M, Marcos-Dolado A, Garcia-Ramos R, et al. Validation of the Lille's Apathy Rating Scale in very mild to moderate dementia. Am J Geriatr Psychiatry. 2016;24(7):517–27.

38. Stuss DT, Van Reekum R, Murphy KJ. Differentiation of states and causes of apathy. In: Borod J (Ed), The Neuropsychology of Emotion. New York: Oxford University Press; 2000, pp. 340–63.

39. Dujardin K, Sockeel P, Carette AS, Delliaux M, Defebvre L. Assessing apathy in everyday clinical practice with the short-form Lille Apathy Rating Scale. Mov Disord. 2013;28(14):2014–9.

40. Aguera-Ortiz L, Gil-Ruiz N, Cruz-Orduna I, Ramos-Garcia I, Osorio RS, Valenti-Soler M, et al. A novel rating scale for the measurement of apathy in institutionalized persons with dementia: the APADEM-NH. Am J Geriatr Psychiatry. 2015;23(2):149–59.

41. Levy R, Dubois B. Apathy and the functional anatomy of the prefrontal cortex-basal ganglia circuits. Cereb Cortex. 2006;16(7):916–28.
42. Grace J, Malloy PF. Frontal Systems Behavior Scale (FrSBe): professional manual. Lutz, FL: Psychological Assessment Resources; 2001.
43. Grace J, Stout JC, Malloy PF. Assessing frontal lobe behavioral syndromes with the frontal lobe personality scale. Assessment. 1999;6(3):269–84.
44. Stout JC, Ready RE, Grace J, Malloy PF, Paulsen JS. Factor analysis of the frontal systems behavior scale (FrSBe). Assessment. 2003;10(1):79–85.
45. Malloy P, Tremont G, Grace J, Frakey L. The Frontal Systems Behavior Scale discriminates frontotemporal dementia from Alzheimer's disease. Alzheimers Dement. 2007;3(3):200–3.
46. Andreasen NC. The Scale for the Assessment of Negative Symptoms (SANS). Iowa City, IO: The University of Iowa; 1983.
47. Andreasen NC. The Scale for the Assessment of Negative Symptoms (SANS): conceptual and theoretical foundations. Br J Psychiatry. 1989;155(Suppl 7):49–52.
48. Overall JE, Gorham DR. The brief psychiatric rating scale. Psychol Rep. 1962;10:799–812.
49. Overall JE, Hollister LE, Pichot P. Major psychiatric disorders. A four-dimensional model. Arch Gen Psychiatry. 1967;16(2):146–51.
50. Lukoff D, Nuechterlien K, Ventura A. Manual for the expanded brief psychiatric rating scale. Schizophr Bull. 1986;13:261–76.
51. Thomas A, Donnell AJ, Young TR. Factor structure and differential validity of the expanded Brief Psychiatric Rating Scale. Assessment. 2004;11(2):177–87.
52. Zanello A, Berthoud L, Ventura J, Merlo MC. The Brief Psychiatric Rating Scale (version 4.0) factorial structure and its sensitivity in the treatment of outpatients with unipolar depression. Psychiatry Res. 2013;210(2):626–33.
53. Kay SR, Fiszbein A, Opler LA. The positive and negative syndrome scale (PANSS) for schizophrenia. Schizophr Bull. 1987;13(2):261–76.
54. Singh MM, Kay SR. A comparative study of haloperidol and chlorpromazine in terms of clinical effects and therapeutic reversal with benztropine in schizophrenia. Theoretical implications for potency differences among neuroleptics. Psychopharmacologia. 1975;43(2):103–13.
55. Opler MGA, Yavorsky C, Daniel DG. Positive and Negative Syndrome Scale (PANSS) training: challenges, solutions, and future directions. Innov Clin Neurosci. 2017;14(11–12):77–81.
56. Opler LA, Kay SR, Lindenmayer JP, Fiszbein A. The Structured Clinical Interview for the Positive and Negative Syndromes of Schizophrenia. New York: Multi-Health Systems; 1992.
57. Kirkpatrick B, Strauss GP, Nguyen L, Fischer BA, Daniel DG, Cienfuegos A, et al. The Brief Negative Symptom Scale: psychometric properties. Schizophr Bull. 2011;37(2):300–5.
58. Strauss GP, Gold JM. A psychometric comparison of the Clinical Assessment Interview for Negative Symptoms and the Brief Negative Symptom Scale. Schizophr Bull. 2016;42(6):1384–94.
59. Ang MS, Rekhi G, Lee J. Validation of the Brief Negative Symptom Scale and its association with functioning. Schizophr Res. 2019;208:97–104.
60. Bischof M, Obermann C, Hartmann MN, Hager OM, Kirschner M, Kluge A, et al. The brief negative symptom scale: validation of the German translation and convergent validity with self-rated anhedonia and observer-rated apathy. BMC Psychiatry. 2016;16(1):415.
61. Kring AM, Gur RE, Blanchard JJ, Horan WP, Reise SP. The Clinical Assessment Interview for Negative Symptoms (CAINS): final development and validation. Am J Psychiatry. 2013;170(2):165–72.
62. Horan WP, Kring AM, Gur RE, Reise SP, Blanchard JJ. Development and psychometric validation of the Clinical Assessment Interview for Negative Symptoms (CAINS). Schizophr Res. 2011;132(2–3):140–5.

63. Blanchard JJ, Kring AM, Horan WP, Gur R. Toward the next generation of negative symptom assessments: the collaboration to advance negative symptom assessment in schizophrenia. Schizophr Bull. 2011;37(2):291–9.

64. Rekhi G, Ang MS, Yuen CKY, Ng WY, Lee J. Assessing negative symptoms in schizophrenia: validity of the clinical assessment interview for negative symptoms in Singapore. Schizophr Res. 2019;206:177–82.

65. Dollfus S, Mach C, Morello R. Self-evaluation of Negative Symptoms: a novel tool to assess negative symptoms. Schizophr Bull. 2016;42(3):571–8.

66. Dollfus S, Delouche C, Hervochon C, Mach C, Bourgeois V, Rotharmel M, et al. Specificity and sensitivity of the Self-assessment of Negative Symptoms (SNS) in patients with schizophrenia. Schizophr Res. 2019;211:51–5.

67. Fahn S, Elton RL, UPDRS Program Members. Unified Parkinson's disease rating scale. In: Fahn S, Marsden C, Calne D, Liberman A (Eds), Recent Developments in Parkinson's Disease. Florham Park, NJ: Macmillan Health Care Information; 1987, pp. 153–63.

68. Starkstein SE, Merello M. The Unified Parkinson's Disease Rating Scale: validation study of the mentation, behavior, and mood section. Mov Disord. 2007;22(15):2156–61.

69. Pedersen KF, Larsen JP, Aarsland D. Validation of the Unified Parkinson's Disease Rating Scale (UPDRS) section I as a screening and diagnostic instrument for apathy in patients with Parkinson's disease. Parkinsonism Relat Disord. 2008;14(3):183–6.

70. Kirsch-Darrow L, Zahodne LB, Hass C, Mikos A, Okun MS, Fernandez HH, et al. How cautious should we be when assessing apathy with the Unified Parkinson's Disease Rating Scale? Mov Disord. 2009;24(5):684–8.

71. Honigfeld G, Klett CJ. The Nurses' Observation Scale for inpatient evaluation: a new scale for measuring improvement in chronic schizophrenia. J Clin Psychol. 1965;21:65–71.

72. Lyall D, Hawley C, Scott K. Nurses' Observation Scale for inpatient evaluation: reliability update. J Adv Nurs. 2004;46(4):390–4.

73. Andrews SJ, Ismail Z, Anstey KJ, Mortby M. Association of Alzheimer's genetic loci with mild behavioral impairment. Am J Med Genet B Neuropsychiatr Genet. 2018;177(8):727–35.

74. Cano J, Kan CN, Chen C, Hilal S, Venketasubramanian N, Xu X. Mild behavioral impairment: prevalence in clinical setting and cognitive correlates. Alzheimers Dement. 2018;14(7 Suppl): P639–40.

75. Taragano FE, Allegri RF, Heisecke SL, Martelli MI, Feldman ML, Sánchez V, et al. Risk of conversion to dementia in a mild behavioral impairment group compared to a psychiatric group and to a mild cognitive impairment group. J Alzheimers Dis. 2018;62(1):227–38.

76. Cieslak A, Smith EE, Lysack J, Ismail Z. Case series of mild behavioral impairment: toward an understanding of the early stages of neurodegenerative diseases affecting behavior and cognition. Int Psychogeriatr. 2018;30(2):273–80.

77. Ismail Z, Gatchel J, Bateman DR, Barcelos-Ferreira R, Chantillon M, Jaeger J, et al. Affective and emotional dysregulation as pre-dementia risk markers: exploring the mild behavioral impairment symptoms of depression, anxiety, irritability, and euphoria. Int Psychogeriatr. 2018;30(2):185–96.

78. Mortby ME, Ismail Z, Anstey KJ. Prevalence estimates of mild behavioral impairment in a population-based sample of pre-dementia states and cognitively healthy older adults. Int Psychogeriatr. 2018;30(2):221–32.

79. Sheikh F, Ismail Z, Mortby ME, Barber P, Cieslak A, Fischer K, et al. Prevalence of mild behavioral impairment in mild cognitive impairment and subjective cognitive decline, and its association with caregiver burden. Int Psychogeriatr. 2018;30(2):233–44.

80. Creese B, Brooker H, Ismail Z, Wesnes KA, Hampshire A, Khan Z, et al. Mild behavioral impairment as a marker of cognitive decline in cognitively normal older adults. Am J Geriatr Psychiatry. 2019;27(8):823–34.

81. Mallo SC, Ismail Z, Pereiro AX, Facal D, Lojo-Seoane C, Campos-Magdaleno M, et al. Assessing mild behavioral impairment with the mild behavioral impairment checklist in people with subjective cognitive decline. Int Psychogeriatr. 2019;31(2):231–9.

82. Mallo SC, Pereiro AX, Facal D, Lojo-Seoane C, Campos-Magdaleno M, Ismail Z, et al. Assessing mild behavioral impairment in people with subjective cognitive complaints (SCCS) with the Mild Behavioral Impairment Checklist (MBI-C): a pilot study. Alzheimers Dement. 2017;13(7):P364–5.

83. Mallo SC, Ismail Z, Pereiro AX, Facal D, Lojo-Seoane C, Campos-Magdaleno M, et al. Assessing mild behavioral impairment with the Mild Behavioral Impairment-Checklist in people with mild cognitive impairment. J Alzheimers Dis. 2018;66(1):83–95.

84. Mallo SC, Pereiro AX, Ismail Z, Lojo-Seoane C, Campos-Magdaleno M, Facal D, et al. Mild Behavioral Impairment Checklist (MBI-C): a preliminary validation study. Alzheimers Dement. 2018;14(7 Suppl):P1481

85. Kang Y, Juhee C, Noel H, Park J, Yeom J, Yang SJ, et al. Mild behavioral impairment (MBI) in MCi, SCD, and normal elderly: a pilot study for validation of the MBI Checklist (MBI-C). Alzheimers Dement. 2018;14(7 Suppl):P793.

86. Creese B, Brooker H, Ismail Z, Aarsland D, Corbett A, Khan Z, et al. Profile of mild behavioural impairment in a population-based sample of adults aged 50 and over: initial findings from the Protect Study. Alzheimers Dement. 2018;14(7 Suppl):P1335.

87. Brooker H, Creese B, Ismail Z, Khan Z, Megalogeni M, Corbett A, et al. The relationship between the Mild Behavioural Impairment Checklist (MBI-C) total score and core aspects of cognitive function in older adults. Alzheimers Dement. 2018;14(7 Suppl):P532.

88. Monchi O, Ismail Z, Kibreab M, Yoon E, Kathol I, Hammer T, et al. What can the mild Behavioral Impairment Checklist (MBI-C) tell us about cognition and behavior in Parkinson's disease? Alzheimers Dement. 2018;14(7 Suppl):P429.

89. Lussier F, Pascoal T, Chamoun M, Therriault J, Tissault C, Savard M, et al. Mild behavioral impairment is associated with β-amyloid but not tau in cognitively intact elderly individuals. Alzheimers Dement. 2020;16(1):192–9.

3

Apathy in Alzheimer's Disease

Danielle Vieira, Celina Liu, and Krista L. Lanctôt

Prevalence

Apathy is one of the most common neuropsychiatric symptoms (NPS) in Alzheimer's disease (AD). This has been demonstrated in both clinic and community AD samples. In an early study of 50 outpatients with AD, apathy was assessed using the Neuropsychiatric Inventory (NPI) and found to be the most common NPS with a prevalence of 72% (1). In clinic populations, the prevalence of apathy ranges from 51% to 78% (1–4). Similarly, in a longitudinal study of 177 memory clinic patients in Italy, apathy was also assessed using the NPI and found to be the most common NPS with a prevalence rate of 63.8% (2). Community-based studies have demonstrated prevalence rates ranging from 34% to 71% (5–11). For example, the Cardiovascular Health Study found apathy to be the most prevalent NPS in AD, affecting 36% of patients in 1 month based on the NPI (5). The Cache County Study reported an apathy 5-year period prevalence rate of 71% using the NPI scale (6). In summary, apathy is highly prevalent regardless of population.

Apathy is present throughout all stages of AD; however, data showing apathy increases with worsening dementia in both community and clinic samples have been reported (4, 9, 10). A community-based study in Brazil found that apathy was the only NPS that significantly differed with dementia severity as assessed by the Clinical Dementia Rating Scale (10). Similarly, a clinic-based study in Spain reported apathy to be more prevalent in moderate-to-severe AD with a rate of 78.4% compared to a prevalence rate of 64.6% in mild AD (4). Despite some variability in the apathy assessment used among studies, research has consistently reported high prevalence rates of apathy in AD.

Impact

Apathy has been associated with a higher risk of conversion from mild cognitive impairment (MCI) to AD and faster disease progression (Fig. 3.1). In a prospective study of 332 MCI patients, Pink et al. (12) reported that apathy in addition to agitation, night-time behaviours, and depression elevated the risk of incident dementia.

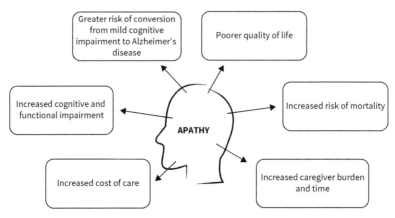

Fig. 3.1 Impact of apathy in Alzheimer's disease. Apathy is often associated with increased cognitive and functional decline, greater risk of conversion from mild cognitive impairment to Alzheimer's disease, poorer quality of life, increased risk of mortality, increased caregiver burden and time, and increased cost of care.

Another study found that patients with both apathy and amnestic MCI had an almost sevenfold risk of AD progression compared to those without apathy, after adjusting for age, sex, education, baseline global cognitive and functional status, and depression (13). The risk of developing AD also increased 30% with every point increase in apathy on the NPI. In a large longitudinal analysis including over 4900 MCI subjects, patients with apathy alone or with apathy and depression combined were at a significantly greater risk of developing AD compared to those without NPS (14). In another study with 397 MCI patients, the presence of apathy without symptoms of depressive affect increased the risk of progression from MCI to AD over 2 years in 41% of patients (15). In line with those findings, Vicini et al. (16) found that rates of conversion to AD were highest in apathetic MCI patients (60%) compared to MCI patients who were depressed-apathetic (19%), depressed (7.9%), or normal (24%).

Apathy has also been linked to greater cognitive and functional decline. Grossi et al. (17) demonstrated that AD patients with apathy had poorer performance than AD patients without apathy on frontal tasks. Another study found that persistent apathy in AD increased the probability of rapid functional decline, defined as a yearly drop of 4 points or more on the 14-point Instrumental Activities of Daily Living Lawton scale (18). In a large study including 395 MCI and 188 AD patients, greater hallucinations, anxiety, and apathy were also associated with greater global functional impairment at baseline. However, only hallucinations and apathy at baseline were associated with greater global functional impairment over time across all subjects (7). In accordance with those findings, Freels et al. (19) revealed that behavioural disorders and apathy were significantly associated with impairments in activities of daily living independent of age, sex, race, and cognitive impairment.

The presence of apathy was also independently associated with poorer quality of life (20). Apathy in dementia has been associated with an increased risk of mortality with studies reporting almost twice the risk of death in apathetic compared to non-apathetic AD patients (21, 22).

Together with poorer patient outcomes, apathy in AD also contributes to greater caregiver burden. Findings from a cross-sectional study in 310 patients with probable AD revealed that all 12 NPS in the NPI were significantly correlated with caregiver burden, but the three greatest neuropsychiatric predictors were depression, apathy, and anxiety (23). Terum et al. (24) also found that apathy, in addition to irritability, agitation, sleep disturbances, anxiety, and delusion, exerted the most impact on caregiver burden. Another prospective study of 1497 community-dwelling AD patients revealed that higher scores for apathy and psychosis were associated with greater caregiver supervision time (25). Similarly, a study in 613 AD patients, in which apathy was the most common NPS (47%) (26), reported that NPS were significantly associated with caregiver time after adjusting for age, education, cognitive function, and comorbidity. In that study, researchers found that every point increase in NPS was associated with a 10-minute increase in caregiver time.

This impact is reflected in cost. In a recent population-based sample of 218 patients with dementia, cost analyses revealed an adjusted informal care cost increase of 13% for every point increase in the apathy subdomain of the NPI (27). The percentage increase for apathy was greater than that for psychosis (5.6%), affective (6.4%), and agitation/aggression (7.6%) subdomains, suggesting that apathy management may improve patient and caregiver outcomes in addition to reducing the informal care costs of dementia.

Measurement

Apathy was first defined by Marin as diminished motivation (28). That definition was the basis for the diagnostic criteria for apathy in AD and other neuropsychiatric disorders published in 2009 (29). In those criteria, apathy was defined as a disorder of motivation in which diminished motivation was present for at least 4 weeks, had two of three dimensions of apathy (reduced goal-directed behaviour, goal-directed cognitive behaviour, and emotion), caused functional impairments, and was not caused by another symptom that could resemble apathy. Mulin and colleagues tested these diagnostic criteria in an observational study in multiple populations, including AD, and found that the NPI apathy subscore was significantly higher for those who met the diagnostic criteria (30). They reported that each domain—goal-directed behaviour, goal-directed cognition, and emotion—and the overall diagnostic criteria had high inter-rater reliability.

Based on advancements in the understanding of apathy, an expert panel revised the criteria for apathy in 2018 and expanded them to encompass brain disorders (31). These criteria defined apathy as a reduction in goal-directed activity present for a minimum of 4 weeks, affecting two of the three apathy dimensions (behaviour and cognition, emotion, and social interaction), causing functional impairments, and which was not caused by another symptom that could resemble apathy. The revised criteria replaced motivation with goal-directed activity and added social interaction as a dimension. An expert panel has also developed specific diagnostic criteria for apathy in neurocognitive disorders (32). These criteria defined apathy as a reduction in goal-directed activity present for a minimum of 4 weeks, affecting two of the three apathy dimensions (initiative, interest, and emotional responsiveness), causing functional impairments, and which was not caused by another symptom that could resemble apathy.

Several scales have been used to assess apathy in dementia and have been validated in AD populations (reviewed in (33)). These scales differ in administration; some scales are self-reported by the caregiver or patient and others are based on an interview between a clinician and caregiver and/or patient. The most commonly used scales for the assessment of apathy in clinical trials are the Apathy Evaluation Scale (AES) and NPI apathy subscale (33). The AES has three versions—clinician, informant, and self-rated—which have all been validated in many populations, including AD (34, 35). This scale has 18 questions and was developed based on Marin's definition of apathy; it, therefore, includes the subdomains behavioural, cognition, and emotional concomitants of goal-directed behaviour. A short version of the AES has also been developed, reducing the number of questions to ten to be more time efficient (36).

The NPI (37, 38) is a widely used, caregiver-rated measure of NPS in AD. It includes 10–12 subdomains, one of which is apathy. Total score (frequency multiplied by severity) and caregiver distress are recorded. Other versions of this scale have been developed including the NPI Clinician (NPI-C) and NPI Questionnaire (NPI-Q) (33, 39). The NPI-C assesses NPS with caregiver and patient interviews and a clinician rating. The NPI-Q is self-administered by the caregiver and assesses severity only. While the NPI is widely used in research, the apathy subscale has not been validated for use on its own.

The Dementia Apathy Interview and Rating (DAIR) scale is the only scale developed specifically for AD (40). The DAIR is a 16-item caregiver interview with questions of behaviour, interest, and engagement. Each item asks how often a certain behaviour occurred over the past month, rating it on a four-point scale. A follow-up question is then administered to identify if that behaviour was a change since developing memory loss. Only items that are reported as a change are included in the apathy score. This scale has demonstrated high positive test–retest reliability and excellent overall quality (33, 39).

Other scales that are also used in the measurement of apathy in AD include the Lille Apathy Rating Scale (LARS) (41), Dimensional Apathy Scale (DAS) (42), Apathy Inventory (AI) (43), Person Environment Apathy Rating (PEAR) (44), Structured Interview for Apathy (45), and the Apathy in Dementia, Nursing Home (APADEM-NH) scale (46). The LARS, AI, DAS, and Structured Interview for apathy assess apathy through patient and informant interview while the APADEM-NH scale uses only informant interview and the PEAR assesses apathy through patient observation.

Most of these scales were compared to the AES or NPI apathy subscale to assess convergent validity. They have demonstrated adequate to good quality (33, 39).

Information and communication technologies have been recommended for use in AD as they are objective and provide real-time data (47). Currently, there is limited evidence for information and communication technologies in measuring apathy in AD. Actigraphy has been used to assess apathy in AD in a few research studies and data have shown that apathy is associated with reduced motor activity during the day (48, 49). David and colleagues investigated 107 AD outpatients and found that those who had apathy based on the NPI apathy subscale had significantly lower daytime mean motor activity than those without apathy (48). Actigraphy may be a promising technique in measuring a dimension of apathy; however, it is limited as it does not assess other dimensions of apathy such as cognitive goal-directed behaviour and emotion (50). Evidence for other forms of technology remains limited. One study used eye tracking to measure visual scanning behaviours to assess apathy in AD and reported that apathetic patients showed reduced duration and fixation frequency on social images (51). Automatic speech analysis may also be of value in the assessment of apathy. Konig et al. (52) recorded speech from AD patients and found differences in temporal aspects of speech in apathetic and non-apathetic patients. These findings suggest an alternative method to assess apathy without the use of patient and caregiver interviews, although further validation is needed.

Appropriate diagnostic criteria and validated scales are necessary to properly identify apathy in AD. Further research should be conducted using the revised diagnostic criteria for apathy. More research needs to be conducted on information and communication technologies in assessing apathy to determine if there could be an appropriate objective measure of apathy in addition to the subjective scales currently being used. Improved methods of detecting and assessing apathy can assist in evaluating treatments.

Neurobiology

Structural and Metabolic Neuroimaging Correlates of Apathy in Alzheimer's Disease

The neurobiology of apathy in AD is frequently investigated in neuroimaging studies. Structural and metabolic correlates of apathy in AD have been consistently linked to abnormalities in prefrontal regions and the anterior cingulate (53). Damage to these structures is associated with impairments in decision-making, planning, and is related to emotional blunting and loss of motivation (54). Using magnetic resonance imaging data, Apostolova et al. (55) examined 35 AD patients and found a significant linear association between apathy severity and cortical grey matter atrophy in the bilateral anterior cingulate and left medial frontal cortex. Bruen et al. (56) also reported that apathy was significantly correlated with decreased density in the right putamen, bilateral inferior frontal gyrus, bilateral anterior cingulate, left caudate, and left putamen in 31 mild AD patients. Another study using structural magnetic resonance imaging assessed 111 AD patients and found that patients with apathy (57%) had greater cortical thinning in the left caudal anterior cingulate cortex, left lateral orbitofrontal cortex, and left superior ventrolateral frontal regions compared to non-apathetic AD patients (57), suggesting a relationship between apathy and dysfunction of the frontal–subcortical cingulate circuit in AD. Using single-photon emission computed tomography, Starkstein and colleagues also demonstrated a significant association between apathy and reduced activation of key neural regions responsible for emotion and memory (58). They found that apathy correlated with reduced perfusion in the prefrontal, anterior temporal, temporoparietal, and cingulate regions of 79 patients with probable AD (58). Jeong et al. (59) reported that AD patients with apathy, compared to those without, had reduced regional cerebral blood flow in the bilateral orbitofrontal cortex, left putamen, left nucleus accumbens, left thalamus, and bilateral insula. Additional positron emission tomography studies have reported that apathy was associated with reduced metabolic activity in the anterior cingulate gyrus (60) and orbitofrontal regions (60, 61).

Beta-amyloid and neurofibrillary tangles (NFTs), pathological hallmarks of AD which are associated with dysfunctional brain connectivity, have also been investigated in the development and progression of apathy. Vergallo et al. (62) found that beta-amyloid concentrations in cerebrospinal fluid were negatively correlated with apathy scores. However, another study (63) using positron emission tomography reported that beta-amyloid deposition was greater in the bilateral frontal cortex of 28 patients with AD compared to those without apathy. Marshall and colleagues found that chronic apathy and total NPS composite scores correlated with greater anterior cingulate NFT burden (64). Similarly, Tekin et al. (65) examined the association between NPS, including agitation, aberrant motor behaviours, and apathy, with NFT burden. They found that agitation and aberrant motor behaviour were correlated with greater NFT pathology in the orbitofrontal cortex in AD, whereas increasing apathy was related to greater NFT burden in the anterior cingulate.

Apathy severity in AD may also be associated with deficits in other cortical regions. Moon et al. (66) reported a significant negative correlation between apathy and the volume ratio of the bilateral anterior insular cortex and right posterior insular cortex in 40 AD subjects. In accordance with that study, Stanton et al. (67) found that apathy was associated with atrophy of the left insula in addition to the ventromedial orbitofrontal cortex in 17 AD patients. Other studies have demonstrated that reduced baseline inferior temporal cortical thickness was predictive of increasing apathy over time in 188 AD patients (68). Recently, a study measuring white matter integrity through fractional anisotropy (FA) found that those with apathy had significantly reduced FA values in the genu of the corpus callosum compared to those without apathy. Moreover, apathy severity was negatively correlated with FA values of the left anterior and posterior cingulum, right superior longitudinal fasciculus, splenium, body and genu of the corpus callosum, and bilateral uncinate fasciculus in the apathy group.

A multimodal magnetic resonance imaging study in 37 patients with moderate to severe AD revealed that apathy severity and emotional blunting were also associated with bilateral damage to the corpus callosum and internal capsule (69), suggesting that impaired brain connectivity contributes to apathy progression in AD and may be of particular relevance during later disease stages.

Neurotransmitter Systems in Apathy in Alzheimer's Disease

Preclinical and clinical studies have demonstrated that intact dopaminergic systems are essential for motivation, behavioural activation, exert of effort, and effort-related decision-making (70). Impaired dopaminergic neurotransmission caused by neuronal loss may be associated with apathetic symptoms in AD. David et al. (71) demonstrated a relationship between decreased bilateral putamen dopamine transporter density and greater apathy in 14 AD patients. Pharmacotherapy trials in AD have demonstrated improvements in apathy with dopamine-stimulating agents and dopaminergic agonists such as modafinil, amantadine, methylphenidate, and dextroamphetamine (72).

In addition to dopamine, a number of other neurotransmitters including acetylcholine, serotonin, and gamma-aminobutyric acid (GABA) have been implicated in the regulation of effort-related choice and motivation (73). Expression levels of the serotonin transporter gene in 43 AD subjects was found to be higher than in healthy controls and was significantly correlated with greater apathy (74). Lanctôt et al. (75) found that plasma GABA was positively correlated with depression and apathy scores on the NPI in 14 severe AD patients. Intervention studies reported that depression, anxiety, and apathy were significantly decreased in AD subjects treated with the acetylcholine-enhancing pharmacotherapies, donepezil and choline alphoscerate (76). Taken together, those findings suggest that multiple neurotransmitter systems may be involved in the development and progression of apathy.

Genetics of Apathy in Alzheimer's Disease

Evidence supporting the relationship between genetics and apathy in AD is mixed. While some studies have reported that the apolipoprotein E (ApoE) ε4 allele is associated with apathy in AD (12, 77, 78), others have found no relationship (79, 80). A recent meta-analysis found no evidence that ApoE ε4 carriership or zygosity was associated with the presence of depression, anxiety, apathy, agitation, irritability, or sleep disturbances in cognitively impaired subjects (81).

Similarly, association studies examining other hypothesized genetic correlates of apathy have reported a lack of association. David et al. (82) investigated the relationship between single nucleotide polymorphisms in catechol-O-methyltransferase, an enzyme involved in the degradation of dopamine, epinephrine, and norepinephrine, and also found no connection between these polymorphisms and apathy in AD. As a result, genetic determinations of apathy remain limited and unclear. Additional longitudinal studies with standardized apathy measurements are required to identify the relationship between genetics and apathy in AD.

Treatments

There are currently no approved therapies for the treatment of apathy in AD. However, some clinical trials have investigated potential pharmacological and non-pharmacological therapies for treatment of apathy in AD. A meta-analysis in 2018 identified 21 studies that investigated apathy as a primary or secondary outcome in double-blinded, placebo-controlled, randomized controlled trials (RCTs) (83).

Four pharmacological RCTs using methylphenidate or modafinil have investigated apathy as a primary outcome measure and recruited for participants with clinically significant apathy at baseline (83).

Modafinil has been investigated in a case study (84) and an RCT (85). The case study in an elderly gentleman with dementia showed improvements on the AES after treatment with modafinil (84). However, in the RCT of 23 apathetic AD participants, modafinil treatment did not significantly reduce apathy as assessed using the Frontal Systems Behavior Scale (85). Further RCTs could be conducted using a validated apathy scale, such as the AES or NPI apathy subscale, to determine the efficacy of modafinil.

Methylphenidate treatment has shown improvements in apathy in placebo-controlled studies (86–88). The Apathy in Dementia Methylphenidate Trial (ADMET) reported clinically significant improvements in apathy with methylphenidate compared to placebo on the NPI apathy subscale and the Alzheimer's Disease Cooperative Study–Clinical Global Impression of Change (ADCS-CGIC) but not on the AES (88). Currently ADMET 2, a multicentre RCT in a larger sample, is active and investigating the safety and efficacy of methylphenidate as a treatment for apathy in AD over 6 months (89). If positive, that study could confirm that methylphenidate is an effective and safe treatment for apathy.

Some cholinesterase inhibitor studies have reported apathy as a secondary or exploratory outcome measure (90–93). Those studies did not require apathy to be clinically significant at baseline. Donepezil treatment has been reported to significantly reduce apathy (92) or apathy emergence (90) compared to placebo in AD participants assessed with the NPI. Herrmann et al. (91) pooled data from three larger trials investigating the effect of galantamine on behaviour in mild to moderate AD. They reported that the NPI apathy subscale alone did not significantly differ between galantamine and placebo; however, the cluster of hallucinations, anxiety, apathy, and aberrant motor behaviours significantly improved with galantamine treatment. An open-label study of rivastigmine reported that patients that had baseline apathy saw statistically significant improvements in apathy at 26 weeks (94). Antidepressant treatment for apathy has not been shown to be effective (83, 95). While trials with cholinesterase inhibitors have shown some benefits, there is a need for more RCTs that recruit specifically for clinically significant apathy and measure apathy as a primary outcome.

Non-pharmacological interventions that treat apathy individually with therapeutic activities have shown some promise. Non-pharmacological treatments that have been investigated include occupational and sports therapy (96), music and art therapy with psychomotor activity (97), and functional performance enhancement (98). Music and art therapy along with psychomotor activity was found to be significantly beneficial for those with moderate apathy as measured by the DAIR, but reported no differences between groups on the NPI-Q (97). Studies that focus on occupational therapy have reported improvements in apathy during the intervention; however, these improvements were not sustained following termination of the intervention (96, 98). While non-pharmacological interventions look promising, additional research needs to be conducted. Future studies should also investigate the use of non-pharmacological treatments in combination with pharmacological treatments for apathy in AD.

Neuromodulation is another therapeutic that has recently gained interest in the treatment of apathy in AD (see Chapter 15 for more about neurostimulation). One study used transcranial direct current stimulation (tDCS), a non-invasive neuromodulatory technique that emits low, constant currents to treat apathy in AD (99). This study enrolled 40 moderate AD participants with apathy, as defined by the Apathy Scale, who received six sessions of tDCS over 2 weeks. NPI was measured as a secondary outcome. No significant difference in apathy change scores between active and sham stimulations was found. There is currently an RCT investigating the use of tDCS and cognitive remediation in mild to moderate AD over ten sessions (100). The results of that study could provide details as to whether tDCS could be an effective treatment for apathy in AD.

Apathy was also investigated as a secondary outcome in an open label study using repetitive transcranial magnetic stimulation, another non-invasive neuromodulatory technique that uses magnetism to alter synaptic activity in AD participants (101). Apathy scores on the AI significantly improved after receiving cognitive training and repetitive transcranial magnetic stimulation for 5 weeks, one session a day for 5 days. However, the NPI apathy subscale did not show improvements. More research should be conducted investigating the use of neuromodulatory treatments for apathy in AD.

Future Directions

The prevalence of AD will continue to rise over the upcoming decades. Apathy, which has a significant negative impact on patient and caregiver outcomes, is expected to become increasingly prominent in the geriatric population and is an important treatment target in AD trials. Research should focus on validating scales of apathy in order to properly identify the symptom and mitigate symptom progression. Additional mechanisms underlying the neurobiology of apathy in AD need to be investigated. Future genome-wide association studies should explore the relationship between dopaminergic and GABAergic genetic polymorphisms and apathy. Pharmacological, non-pharmacological, and neuromodulatory clinical trials should be targeting apathy as a primary outcome measure. Future studies should also consider using neuroimaging and biomarkers to better understand and predict apathy treatment response.

References

1. Mega MS, Cummings JL, Fiorello T, Gornbein J. The spectrum of behavioral changes in Alzheimer's disease. Neurology. 1996;46(1):130–5.
2. Palmer K, Lupo F, Perri R, Salamone G, Fadda L, Caltagirone C, et al. Predicting disease progression in Alzheimer's disease: the role of neuropsychiatric syndromes on functional and cognitive decline. J Alzheimers Dis. 2011;24(1):35–45.
3. Hwang TJ, Masterman DL, Ortiz F, Fairbanks LA, Cummings JL. Mild cognitive impairment is associated with characteristic neuropsychiatric symptoms. Alzheimer Dis Assoc Disord. 2004;18(1):17–21.
4. Fernández-Martínez M, Molano A, Castro J, Zarranz JJ. Prevalence of neuropsychiatric symptoms in mild cognitive impairment and Alzheimer's disease, and its relationship with cognitive impairment. Curr Alzheimer Res. 2010;7(6):517–26.
5. Lyketsos CG, Lopez O, Jones B, Fitzpatrick AL, Breitner J, DeKosky S. Prevalence of neuropsychiatric symptoms in dementia and mild cognitive impairment: results from the cardiovascular health study. JAMA. 2002;288(12):1475–83.
6. Steinberg M, Shao H, Zandi P, Lyketsos CG, Welsh-Bohmer KA, Norton MC, et al. Point and 5-year period prevalence of neuropsychiatric symptoms in dementia: the Cache County Study. Int J Geriatr Psychiatry. 2008;23(2):170–7.
7. Wadsworth LP, Lorius N, Donovan NJ, Locascio JJ, Rentz DM, Johnson KA, et al. Neuropsychiatric symptoms and global functional impairment along the Alzheimer's continuum. Dement Geriatr Cogn Disord. 2012;34(2):96–111.
8. Benoit M, Berrut G, Doussaint J, Bakchine S, Bonin-Guillaume S, Fremont P, et al. Apathy and depression in mild Alzheimer's disease: a cross-sectional study using diagnostic criteria. J Alzheimers Dis. 2012;31(2):325–34.
9. Tanaka H, Hashimoto M, Fukuhara R, Ishikawa T, Yatabe Y, Kaneda K, et al. Relationship between dementia severity and behavioural and psychological symptoms in early-onset Alzheimer's disease. Psychogeriatrics. 2015;15(4):242–7.
10. Tatsch MF, Bottino CM, Azevedo D, Hototian SR, Moscoso MA, Folquitto JC, et al. Neuropsychiatric symptoms in Alzheimer disease and cognitively impaired, nondemented elderly from a community-based sample in Brazil: prevalence and relationship with dementia severity. Am J Geriatr Psychiatry. 2006;14(5):438–45.
11. Geda YE, Smith GE, Knopman DS, Boeve BF, Tangalos EG, Ivnik RJ, et al. De novo genesis of neuropsychiatric symptoms in mild cognitive impairment (MCI). Int Psychogeriatr. 2004;16(1):51–60.

12. Pink A, Stokin GB, Bartley MM, Roberts RO, Sochor O, Machulda MM, et al. Neuropsychiatric symptoms, APOE epsilon4, and the risk of incident dementia: a population-based study. Neurology. 2015;84(9):935–43.
13. Palmer K, Di Iulio F, Varsi AE, Gianni W, Sancesario G, Caltagirone C, et al. Neuropsychiatric predictors of progression from amnestic-mild cognitive impairment to Alzheimer's disease: the role of depression and apathy. J Alzheimers Dis. 2010;20(1):175–83.
14. Ruthirakuhan M, Herrmann N, Vieira D, Gallagher D, Lanctôt KL. The roles of apathy and depression in predicting Alzheimer disease: a longitudinal analysis in older adults with mild cognitive impairment. Am J Geriatr Psychiatry. 2019;27(8):873–82.
15. Richard E, Schmand B, Eikelenboom P, Yang SC, Ligthart SA, Moll van Charante EP, et al. Symptoms of apathy are associated with progression from mild cognitive impairment to Alzheimer's disease in non-depressed subjects. Dement Geriatr Cogn Disord. 2012;33(2–3):204–9.
16. Vicini Chilovi B, Conti M, Zanetti M, Mazzu I, Rozzini L, Padovani A. Differential impact of apathy and depression in the development of dementia in mild cognitive impairment patients. Dement Geriatr Cogn Disord. 2009;27(4):390–8.
17. Grossi D, Santangelo G, Barbarulo AM, Vitale C, Castaldo G, Proto MG, et al. Apathy and related executive syndromes in dementia associated with Parkinson's disease and in Alzheimer's disease. Behav Neurol. 2013;27(4):515–22.
18. Lechowski L, Benoit M, Chassagne P, Vedel I, Tortrat D, Teillet L, et al. Persistent apathy in Alzheimer's disease as an independent factor of rapid functional decline: the REAL longitudinal cohort study. Int J Geriatr Psychiatry. 2009;24(4):341–6.
19. Freels S, Cohen D, Eisdorfer C, Paveza G, Gorelick P, Luchins DJ, et al. Functional status and clinical findings in patients with Alzheimer's disease. J Gerontol. 1992;47(6):M177–82.
20. Andrieu S, Coley N, Rolland Y, Cantet C, Arnaud C, Guyonnet S, et al. Assessing Alzheimer's disease patients' quality of life: discrepancies between patient and caregiver perspectives. Alzheimers Dement. 2016;12(4):427–37.
21. Nijsten JMH, Leontjevas R, Pat-El R, Smalbrugge M, Koopmans R, Gerritsen DL. Apathy: risk factor for mortality in nursing home patients. J Am Geriatr Soc. 2017;65(10):2182–9.
22. Vilalta-Franch J, Calvo-Perxas L, Garre-Olmo J, Turro-Garriga O, Lopez-Pousa S. Apathy syndrome in Alzheimer's disease epidemiology: prevalence, incidence, persistence, and risk and mortality factors. J Alzheimers Dis. 2013;33(2):535–43.
23. Lou Q, Liu S, Huo YR, Liu M, Liu S, Ji Y. Comprehensive analysis of patient and caregiver predictors for caregiver burden, anxiety and depression in Alzheimer's disease. J Clin Nurs. 2015;24(17-18):2668–78.
24. Terum TM, Andersen JR, Rongve A, Aarsland D, Svendsboe EJ, Testad I. The relationship of specific items on the Neuropsychiatric Inventory to caregiver burden in dementia: a systematic review. Int J Geriatr Psychiatry. 2017;32(7):703–17.
25. Haro JM, Kahle-Wrobleski K, Bruno G, Belger M, Dell'Agnello G, Dodel R, et al. Analysis of burden in caregivers of people with Alzheimer's disease using self-report and supervision hours. J Nutr Health Aging. 2014;18(7):677–84.
26. Chen P, Guarino PD, Dysken MW, Pallaki M, Asthana S, Llorente MD, et al. Neuropsychiatric symptoms and caregiver burden in individuals with Alzheimer's disease: the TEAM-AD VA Cooperative Study. J Geriatr Psychiatry Neurol. 2018;31(4):177–85.
27. Rattinger GB, Sanders CL, Vernon E, Schwartz S, Behrens S, Lyketsos CG, et al. Neuropsychiatric symptoms in patients with dementia and the longitudinal costs of informal care in the Cache County population. Alzheimers Dement (N Y). 2019;5:81–8.
28. Marin RS. Differential diagnosis and classification of apathy. Am J Psychiatry. 1990;147(1):22–30.

29. Robert P, Onyike CU, Leentjens AF, Dujardin K, Aalten P, Starkstein S, et al. Proposed diagnostic criteria for apathy in Alzheimer's disease and other neuropsychiatric disorders. Eur Psychiatry. 2009;24(2):98–104.

30. Mulin E, Leone E, Dujardin K, Delliaux M, Leentjens A, Nobili F, et al. Diagnostic criteria for apathy in clinical practice. Int J Geriatr Psychiatry. 2011;26(2):158–65.

31. Robert P, Lanctôt KL, Aguera-Ortiz L, Aalten P, Bremond F, Defrancesco M, et al. Is it time to revise the diagnostic criteria for apathy in brain disorders? The 2018 international consensus group. Eur Psychiatry. 2018;54:71–6.

32. Miller DS, Robert P, Ereshefsky L, Adler L, Bateman D, Cummings J, et al. Diagnostic criteria for apathy in neurocognitive disorders. Alzheimers Dement. 2021.

33. Mohammad D, Ellis C, Rau A, Rosenberg PB, Mintzer J, Ruthirakuhan M, et al. Psychometric properties of apathy scales in dementia: a systematic review. J Alzheimers Dis. 2018;66(3):1065–82.

34. Marin RS, Biedrzycki RC, Firinciogullari S. Reliability and validity of the Apathy Evaluation Scale. Psychiatry Res. 1991;38(2):143–62.

35. Clarke DE, Reekum R, Simard M, Streiner DL, Freedman M, Conn D. Apathy in dementia: an examination of the psychometric properties of the apathy evaluation scale. J Neuropsychiatry Clin Neurosci. 2007;19(1):57–64.

36. Lueken U, Seidl U, Volker L, Schweiger E, Kruse A, Schroder J. Development of a short version of the Apathy Evaluation Scale specifically adapted for demented nursing home residents. Am J Geriatr Psychiatry. 2007;15(5):376–85.

37. Cummings JL, Mega M, Gray K, Rosenberg-Thompson S, Carusi DA, Gornbein J. The Neuropsychiatric Inventory: comprehensive assessment of psychopathology in dementia. Neurology. 1994;44(12):2308–14.

38. Cummings JL. The Neuropsychiatric Inventory: assessing psychopathology in dementia patients. Neurology. 1997;48(5 Suppl 6):S10–6.

39. Radakovic R, Harley C, Abrahams S, Starr JM. A systematic review of the validity and reliability of apathy scales in neurodegenerative conditions. Int Psychogeriatr. 2015;27(6):903–23.

40. Strauss ME, Sperry SD. An informant-based assessment of apathy in Alzheimer disease. Neuropsychiatry Neuropsychol Behav Neurol. 2002;15(3):176–83.

41. Fernandez-Matarrubia M, Matias-Guiu JA, Moreno-Ramos T, Valles-Salgado M, Marcos-Dolado A, Garcia-Ramos R, et al. Validation of the Lille's Apathy Rating Scale in very mild to moderate dementia. Am J Geriatr Psychiatry. 2016;24(7):517–27.

42. Radakovic R, Starr JM, Abrahams S. A novel assessment and profiling of multidimensional apathy in Alzheimer's disease. J Alzheimers Dis. 2017;60(1):57–67.

43. Robert PH, Clairet S, Benoit M, Koutaich J, Bertogliati C, Tible O, et al. The apathy inventory: assessment of apathy and awareness in Alzheimer's disease, Parkinson's disease and mild cognitive impairment. Int J Geriatr Psychiatry. 2002;17(12):1099–105.

44. Jao YL, Algase DL, Specht JK, Williams K. Developing the Person-Environment Apathy Rating for persons with dementia. Aging Ment Health. 2016;20(8):861–70.

45. Starkstein SE, Ingram L, Garau ML, Mizrahi R. On the overlap between apathy and depression in dementia. J Neurol Neurosurg Psychiatry. 2005;76(8):1070–4.

46. Aguera-Ortiz L, Gil-Ruiz N, Cruz-Orduna I, Ramos-Garcia I, Osorio RS, Valenti-Soler M, et al. A novel rating scale for the measurement of apathy in institutionalized persons with dementia: the APADEM-NH. Am J Geriatr Psychiatry. 2015;23(2):149–59.

47. Robert PH, Konig A, Andrieu S, Bremond F, Chemin I, Chung PC, et al. Recommendations for ICT use in Alzheimer's disease assessment: Monaco CTAD Expert Meeting. J Nutr Health Aging. 2013;17(8):653–60.

48. David R, Mulin E, Friedman L, Le Duff F, Cygankiewicz E, Deschaux O, et al. Decreased daytime motor activity associated with apathy in Alzheimer disease: an actigraphic study. Am J Geriatr Psychiatry. 2012;20(9):806–14.

49. Kuhlmei A, Walther B, Becker T, Muller U, Nikolaus T. Actigraphic daytime activity is reduced in patients with cognitive impairment and apathy. Eur Psychiatry. 2013;28(2):94–7.

50. Lanctôt KL, Aguera-Ortiz L, Brodaty H, Francis PT, Geda YE, Ismail Z, et al. Apathy associated with neurocognitive disorders: recent progress and future directions. Alzheimers Dement. 2017;13(1):84–100.

51. Chau SA, Chung J, Herrmann N, Eizenman M, Lanctôt KL. Apathy and attentional biases in Alzheimer's disease. J Alzheimers Dis. 2016;51(3):837–46.

52. Konig A, Linz N, Zeghari R, Klinge X, Troger J, Alexandersson J, et al. Detecting apathy in older adults with cognitive disorders using automatic speech analysis. J Alzheimers Dis. 2019;69(4):1183–93.

53. Tascone LDS, Bottino CMC. Neurobiology of neuropsychiatric symptoms in Alzheimer's disease: a critical review with a focus on neuroimaging. Dement Neuropsychol. 2013;7(3):236–43.

54. Stella F, Radanovic M, Aprahamian I, Canineu PR, de Andrade LP, Forlenza OV. Neurobiological correlates of apathy in Alzheimer's disease and mild cognitive impairment: a critical review. J Alzheimers Dis. 2014;39(3):633–48.

55. Apostolova LG, Akopyan GG, Partiali N, Steiner CA, Dutton RA, Hayashi KM, et al. Structural correlates of apathy in Alzheimer's disease. Dement Geriatr Cogn Disord. 2007;24(2):91–7.

56. Bruen PD, McGeown WJ, Shanks MF, Venneri A. Neuroanatomical correlates of neuropsychiatric symptoms in Alzheimer's disease. Brain. 2008;131(Pt 9):2455–63.

57. Tunnard C, Whitehead D, Hurt C, Wahlund LO, Mecocci P, Tsolaki M, et al. Apathy and cortical atrophy in Alzheimer's disease. Int J Geriatr Psychiatry. 2011;26(7):741–8.

58. Starkstein SE, Mizrahi R, Capizzano AA, Acion L, Brockman S, Power BD. Neuroimaging correlates of apathy and depression in Alzheimer's disease. J Neuropsychiatry Clin Neurosci. 2009;21(3):259–65.

59. Jeong H, Kang I, Im JJ, Park JS, Na SH, Heo Y, et al. Brain perfusion correlates of apathy in Alzheimer's disease. Dement Neurocogn Disord. 2018;17(2):50–6.

60. Marshall GA, Monserratt L, Harwood D, Mandelkern M, Cummings JL, Sultzer DL. Positron emission tomography metabolic correlates of apathy in Alzheimer disease. Arch Neurol. 2007;64(7):1015–20.

61. Holthoff VA, Beuthien-Baumann B, Kalbe E, Ludecke S, Lenz O, Zundorf G, et al. Regional cerebral metabolism in early Alzheimer's disease with clinically significant apathy or depression. Biol Psychiatry. 2005;57(4):412–21.

62. Vergallo A, Giampietri L, Pagni C, Giorgi FS, Nicoletti V, Miccoli M, et al. Association between CSF beta-amyloid and apathy in early-stage Alzheimer Disease. J Geriatr Psychiatry Neurol. 2019;32(3):164–9.

63. Mori T, Shimada H, Shinotoh H, Hirano S, Eguchi Y, Yamada M, et al. Apathy correlates with prefrontal amyloid beta deposition in Alzheimer's disease. J Neurol Neurosurg Psychiatry. 2014;85(4):449–55.

64. Marshall GA, Fairbanks LA, Tekin S, Vinters HV, Cummings JL. Neuropathologic correlates of apathy in Alzheimer's disease. Dement Geriatr Cogn Disord. 2006;21(3):144–7.

65. Tekin S, Mega MS, Masterman DM, Chow T, Garakian J, Vinters HV, et al. Orbitofrontal and anterior cingulate cortex neurofibrillary tangle burden is associated with agitation in Alzheimer disease. Ann Neurol. 2001;49(3):355–61.

66. Moon Y, Moon WJ, Kim H, Han SH. Regional atrophy of the insular cortex is associated with neuropsychiatric symptoms in Alzheimer's disease patients. Eur Neurol. 2014;71(5-6):223–9.

67. Stanton BR, Leigh PN, Howard RJ, Barker GJ, Brown RG. Behavioural and emotional symptoms of apathy are associated with distinct patterns of brain atrophy in neurodegenerative disorders. J Neurol. 2013;260(10):2481–90.

68. Donovan NJ, Wadsworth LP, Lorius N, Locascio JJ, Rentz DM, Johnson KA, et al. Regional cortical thinning predicts worsening apathy and hallucinations across the Alzheimer disease spectrum. Am J Geriatr Psychiatry. 2014;22(11):1168–79.

69. Aguera-Ortiz L, Hernandez-Tamames JA, Martinez-Martin P, Cruz-Orduna I, Pajares G, Lopez-Alvarez J, et al. Structural correlates of apathy in Alzheimer's disease: a multimodal MRI study. Int J Geriatr Psychiatry. 2017;32(8):922–30.

70. Salamone JD, Yohn SE, Lopez-Cruz L, San Miguel N, Correa M. Activational and effort-related aspects of motivation: neural mechanisms and implications for psychopathology. Brain. 2016;139(Pt 5):1325–47.

71. David R, Koulibaly M, Benoit M, Garcia R, Caci H, Darcourt J, et al. Striatal dopamine transporter levels correlate with apathy in neurodegenerative diseases. A SPECT study with partial volume effect correction. Clin Neurol Neurosurg. 2008;110(1):19–24.

72. Mitchell RA, Herrmann N, Lanctôt KL. The role of dopamine in symptoms and treatment of apathy in Alzheimer's disease. CNS Neurosci Ther. 2011;17(5):411–27.

73. Le Heron C, Holroyd CB, Salamone J, Husain M. Brain mechanisms underlying apathy. J Neurol Neurosurg Psychiatry. 2019;90(3):302–12.

74. Yamazaki K, Yoshino Y, Mori T, Okita M, Yoshida T, Mori Y, et al. Association study and meta-analysis of polymorphisms, methylation profiles, and peripheral mRNA expression of the serotonin transporter gene in patients with Alzheimer's disease. Dement Geriatr Cogn Disord. 2016;41(5-6):334–47.

75. Lanctôt KL, Herrmann N, Rothenburg L, Eryavec G. Behavioral correlates of GABAergic disruption in Alzheimer's disease. Int Psychogeriatr. 2007;19(1):151–8.

76. Carotenuto A, Rea R, Traini E, Fasanaro AM, Ricci G, Manzo V, et al. The effect of the association between donepezil and choline alphoscerate on behavioral disturbances in Alzheimer's disease: interim results of the ASCOMALVA trial. J Alzheimers Dis. 2017;56(2):805–15.

77. Monastero R, Mariani E, Camarda C, Ingegni T, Averna MR, Senin U, et al. Association between apolipoprotein E epsilon4 allele and apathy in probable Alzheimer's disease. Acta Psychiatr Scand. 2006;113(1):59–63.

78. Park HK, Choi SH, Park SA, Kim HJ, Lee Y, Han SH, et al. Cognitive profiles and neuropsychiatric symptoms in Korean early-onset Alzheimer's disease patients: a CREDOS study. J Alzheimers Dis. 2015;44(2):661–73.

79. Levy ML, Cummings JL, Fairbanks LA, Sultzer DL, Small GW. Apolipoprotein E genotype and noncognitive symptoms in Alzheimer's disease. Biol Psychiatry. 1999;45(4):422–5.

80. van der Flier WM, Staekenborg S, Pijnenburg YA, Gillissen F, Romkes R, Kok A, et al. Apolipoprotein E genotype influences presence and severity of delusions and aggressive behavior in Alzheimer disease. Dement Geriatr Cogn Disord. 2007;23(1):42–6.

81. Banning LCP, Ramakers I, Deckers K, Verhey FRJ, Aalten P. Apolipoprotein E and affective symptoms in mild cognitive impairment and Alzheimer's disease dementia: a systematic review and meta-analysis. Neurosci Biobehav Rev. 2019;96:302–15.

82. David R, Friedman L, Mulin E, Noda A, Le Duff F, Kennedy Q, et al. Lack of association between COMT polymorphisms and apathy in Alzheimer's disease. J Alzheimers Dis. 2011;27(1):155–61.

83. Ruthirakuhan MT, Herrmann N, Abraham EH, Chan S, Lanctôt KL. Pharmacological interventions for apathy in Alzheimer's disease. Cochrane Database Syst Rev. 2018;5:CD012197.

84. Padala PR, Burke WJ, Bhatia SC. Modafinil therapy for apathy in an elderly patient. Ann Pharmacother. 2007;41(2):346–9.

85. Frakey LL, Salloway S, Buelow M, Malloy P. A randomized, double-blind, placebo-controlled trial of modafinil for the treatment of apathy in individuals with mild-to-moderate Alzheimer's disease. J Clin Psychiatry. 2012;73(6):796–801.

86. Padala PR, Padala KP, Lensing SY, Ramirez D, Monga V, Bopp MM, et al. Methylphenidate for apathy in community-dwelling older veterans with mild Alzheimer's disease: a double-blind, randomized, placebo-controlled trial. Am J Psychiatry. 2018;175(2):159–68.

87. Herrmann N, Rothenburg LS, Black SE, Ryan M, Liu BA, Busto UE, et al. Methylphenidate for the treatment of apathy in Alzheimer disease: prediction of response using dextroamphetamine challenge. J Clin Psychopharmacol. 2008;28(3):296–301.

88. Rosenberg PB, Lanctôt KL, Drye LT, Herrmann N, Scherer RW, Bachman DL, et al. Safety and efficacy of methylphenidate for apathy in Alzheimer's disease: a randomized, placebo-controlled trial. J Clin Psychiatry. 2013;74(8):810–6.

89. Scherer RW, Drye L, Mintzer J, Lanctôt K, Rosenberg P, Herrmann N, et al. The Apathy in Dementia Methylphenidate Trial 2 (ADMET 2): study protocol for a randomized controlled trial. Trials. 2018;19(1):46.

90. Waldemar G, Gauthier S, Jones R, Wilkinson D, Cummings J, Lopez O, et al. Effect of donepezil on emergence of apathy in mild to moderate Alzheimer's disease. Int J Geriatr Psychiatry. 2011;26(2):150–7.

91. Herrmann N, Rabheru K, Wang J, Binder C. Galantamine treatment of problematic behavior in Alzheimer disease: post-hoc analysis of pooled data from three large trials. Am J Geriatr Psychiatry. 2005;13(6):527–34.

92. Gauthier S, Feldman H, Hecker J, Vellas B, Ames D, Subbiah P, et al. Efficacy of donepezil on behavioral symptoms in patients with moderate to severe Alzheimer's disease. Int Psychogeriatr. 2002;14(4):389–404.

93. Kaufer D. Beyond the cholinergic hypothesis: the effect of metrifonate and other cholinesterase inhibitors on neuropsychiatric symptoms in Alzheimer's disease. Dement Geriatr Cogn Disord. 1998;(9 Suppl 2):8–14.

94. Cummings JL, Koumaras B, Chen M, Mirski D. Effects of rivastigmine treatment on the neuropsychiatric and behavioral disturbances of nursing home residents with moderate to severe probable Alzheimer's disease: a 26-week, multicenter, open-label study. Am J Geriatr Pharmacother. 2005;3(3):137–48.

95. Siddique H, Hynan LS, Weiner MF. Effect of a serotonin reuptake inhibitor on irritability, apathy, and psychotic symptoms in patients with Alzheimer's disease. J Clin Psychiatry. 2009;70(6):915–8.

96. Treusch Y, Majic T, Page J, Gutzmann H, Heinz A, Rapp MA. Apathy in nursing home residents with dementia: results from a cluster-randomized controlled trial. Eur Psychiatry. 2015;30(2):251–7.

97. Ferrero-Arias J, Goni-Imizcoz M, Gonzalez-Bernal J, Lara-Ortega F, da Silva-Gonzalez A, Diez-Lopez M. The efficacy of nonpharmacological treatment for dementia-related apathy. Alzheimer Dis Assoc Disord. 2011;25(3):213–9.

98. Lam LC, Lui VW, Luk DN, Chau R, So C, Poon V, et al. Effectiveness of an individualized functional training program on affective disturbances and functional skills in mild and moderate dementia—a randomized control trial. Int J Geriatr Psychiatry. 2010;25(2):133–41.

99. Suemoto CK, Apolinario D, Nakamura-Palacios EM, Lopes L, Leite RE, Sales MC, et al. Effects of a non-focal plasticity protocol on apathy in moderate Alzheimer's disease: a randomized, double-blind, sham-controlled trial. Brain Stimul. 2014;7(2):308–13.

100. Nguyen JP, Boutoleau-Bretonniere C, Lefaucheur JP, Suarez A, Gaillard H, Chapelet G, et al. Efficacy of transcranial direct current stimulation combined with cognitive training in the treatment of apathy in patients with Alzheimer's disease: study protocol for a randomized trial. Rev Recent Clin Trials. 2018;13(4):319–27.

101. Nguyen JP, Suarez A, Kemoun G, Meignier M, Le Saout E, Damier P, et al. Repetitive transcranial magnetic stimulation combined with cognitive training for the treatment of Alzheimer's disease. Neurophysiol Clin. 2017;47(1):47–53.

4

Apathy in Movement Disorders (Parkinson's Disease, Huntington's Disease)

Gabriella Santangelo

Introduction

Movement disorders are common conditions, with clinical presentations that can be so heterogeneous and complex as to make the diagnosis difficult. Generally, two main categories of movement disorders can be distinguished: the first includes akinetic–rigid disorders such as Parkinson's disease (PD), the second includes hyperkinetic disorders such as Huntington's disease (HD), which are usually perceived as being more difficult to diagnose correctly (1). PD represents the second most common degenerative disease of the central nervous system and is characterized by bradykinesia, tremor, rigidity, and postural instability. The disease affects 1–2 per 1000 of the population at any time; it usually occurs at an age of 65–70 years (2) and is slightly more frequent in men than women. Neuropathologically, the marker of PD is loss of dopaminergic neurons and alpha-synuclein-containing Lewy bodies in the substantia nigra, manifesting as reduced facilitation of voluntary movements (3). With the progression of PD, Lewy body pathology spreads to neocortical and cortical regions leading to the onset of several non-motor symptoms such as cognitive deficits, apathy, depression, anxiety, and psychosis.

The hyperkinetic disorder HD is the most common monogenic neurodegenerative disease, caused by an autosomal dominantly inherited CAG trinucleotide repeat expansion in the huntingtin (*HTT*) gene on chromosome 4. The prevalence of HD in Western populations is 10.6–13.7 individuals per 100,000; phenomenologically, chorea is one of the most prominent symptoms in HD and occurs early in the disease. Neuropathologically, early macroscopic changes occur in the striatum with involvement of the cortex as the disease progresses. Therefore, HD is characterized by cognitive and psychiatric disturbances which become more severe with the progression of the disease (4). The cognitive disturbances have a subcortical pattern, including deficit of emotion recognition, processing speed, and visuospatial and executive functions. The psychiatric disturbances include apathy, irritability, anxiety, depression, obsessive–compulsive behaviour, and psychosis.

Apathy in Parkinson's Disease

Prevalence of Apathy in Parkinson's Disease

Apathy is a neuropsychiatric symptom of PD, with reported estimates of the prevalence ranging from 13.9% to 70% (5). Several factors contribute to the wide variability of apathy prevalence rates, including different recruitment criteria (i.e. inclusion or exclusion of apathetic patients with comorbid depression and/or dementia), differences in population characteristics studied (i.e. patients recruited from the community versus ones from movement disorders units), and different diagnostic/screening instruments used to assess apathy (i.e. self-reported version versus caregiver- or clinician-reported version or diagnostic criteria). More recently, to obtain a reliable estimate of the prevalence of apathy, den Brok and colleagues performed a meta-analytic study (6) on 23 primary studies by adopting restrictive inclusion/exclusion criteria. The meta-analysis revealed a prevalence of apathy in PD of 39.8%, with a high heterogeneity across primary studies. However, sensitivity and subgroup analyses regarding measurement source, assessment tool, cut-off used, exclusion of cognitive deficits, outpatient versus inpatient population, mean disease duration, performance on Mini-Mental State Examination, and stage of PD did not substantially reduce the high value of the heterogeneity across the studies. On the other hand, depression and severity of motor symptoms evaluated by part III of the Unified Parkinson's Disease Rating Scale (UPDRS) did affect apathy rate. However, the meta-analysis also revealed that in almost half of PD patients (42.8%) apathy occurred without concomitant depression or cognitive impairment, supporting the idea that apathy in PD also occurs as a separate symptom, which could be defined as 'pure apathy'.

Longitudinal studies revealed that apathy occurred in 14.5% of the patients in a 2-year-follow-up study (7) and in 49.4% in a 4-year-follow-up study (8), suggesting that apathy is a non-motor symptom of PD which occurs from the early stages of disease, and increases in frequency as the disease progresses. Moreover, apathy seems to be a persistent behavioural feature of PD since in previous longitudinal studies a subgroup of patients showed apathy at both baseline and follow-up evaluations (7, 8).

Assessment and Phenomenology of Apathy in Parkinson's Disease

Apathy is an under-recognized and underestimated neuropsychiatric disturbance for people with chronic neurological disorders and also in PD. To diagnose the presence of apathy, diagnostic criteria were developed by a task force during the European

Psychiatric Association congress in 2008 and published in 2009 (9) and then were validated in PD patients (10). According to the diagnostic criteria, clinically significant apathy occurs when a patient meets four criteria (A–D). Criterion A specifies the presence of a loss of (or diminished) motivation in comparison to the person's previous level of functioning, which is not consistent with his age or culture (the change in motivation may be reported by the patient himself or by the observations of others). Criterion B specifies the presence of symptoms (which can be detected either in self-initiated or environment-stimulated activities) in at least two of three domains (behaviour, cognition, and emotion) for a period of at least 4 weeks and present most of the time. Criterion C specifies that the symptoms (A–B) must cause clinically significant impairment in personal, social, occupational domains, or other important areas of functioning. Finally, Criterion D specifies that the symptoms (A–B) should not be exclusively explained or due to physical or motor disabilities, to diminished level of consciousness, or to the direct physiological effects of a substance. These diagnostic criteria for apathy are now widely used in clinical and research practice; however, in response to some criticisms, a task force in 2018 revised the diagnostic criteria for apathy, proposing some modifications (11): in Criterion A, the term motivation was replaced by goal-directed behaviour which is easier to observe and to describe compared to motivation; in Criterion B, 'social interaction' was added as a separate dimension (B3), whereas behavioural and cognitive domains were included in one category (B1). The new version of the criteria could provide a clinical and scientific framework to improve the validity and the clinical construct of the apathy. However, the revised diagnostic criteria for apathy have not yet been validated in PD patients. Table 4.1 describes both original and modified versions of the diagnostic criteria for apathy, which is useful for a direct comparison between the two versions.

Several instruments are available to screen for and measure the severity of apathy in PD patients; in detail, item 4 of part I of the UPDRS allows apathetic patients and non-apathetic patients to be screened and, therefore, it should be considered for screening only followed by assessment with a longer apathy scale in order to assess and monitor the severity of apathy. Some scales specifically developed for measuring the severity of apathy have been validated in PD, demonstrating good psychometric properties. For example, the Apathy Evaluation Scale (AES) was not developed specifically for PD patients but it was validated in PD, showing good internal consistency, criterion validity, and discriminant validity. The scale is able to identify apathetic patients with an optimal cut-off score of 37 (12) and it has a high level of sensitivity and specificity (both 90%) (13). In contrast, the Lille Apathy Rating Scale (LARS (14)) and the Starkstein Apathy Scale (AS (15)) (which is an abbreviated version of the AES) were developed for PD patients and showed good psychometric properties such as reliability and validity. In particular, the AS showed an acceptable internal consistency in PD and questionable internal consistency in early PD, but it is reported to be a valid tool in assessing apathy in early PD, with a high level of specificity (100%) (13). As for clinimetric properties, the AS is clinically valid when used either to exclude the presence of symptoms of apathy or to evaluate the side effects of medications (16).

Table 4.1 Diagnostic criteria for apathy: original version and revisited version

Diagnostic criteria for apathy, original version (2009)	Diagnostic criteria for apathy, revisited version (2018)
Criterion A Loss of or diminished motivation in comparison to the patient's previous level of functioning and which is not consistent with his age or culture. These changes in motivation may be reported by the patient himself or by the observations of others	**Criterion A** A quantitative reduction of goal-directed activity either in behavioural, cognitive, emotional, or social dimensions in comparison to the patient's previous level of functioning in these areas. These changes may be reported by the patient himself/herself or by observation of others
Criterion B Presence of at least one symptom in at least two of the three following domains for a period of at least 4 weeks and present most of the time	**Criterion B** The presence of at least two of the three following dimensions for a period of at least 4 weeks and present most of the time
Domain B1 Loss of, or diminished, goal-directed behaviour as evidenced by at least one of the following: • Loss of self-initiated behaviour • Loss of environment-stimulated behaviour	*Domain B1. Behaviour and cognition* Loss of, or diminished, goal-directed behaviour or cognitive activity as evidenced by at least one of the following: • General level of activity • Persistence of activity • Making choices • Interest in external issue • Personal well-being
Domain B2 Loss of, or diminished, goal-directed cognitive activity as evidenced by at least one of the following: • Loss of spontaneous ideas and curiosity for routine and new events • Loss of environment-stimulated ideas and curiosity for routine and new events	*Domain B1. Emotion* Loss of, or diminished, emotion as evidenced by at least one of the following: • Spontaneous emotions • Emotional reactions to environment • Impact on others • Empathy • Verbal or physical expressions
Domain B3 Loss of, or diminished, emotion as evidenced by at least one of the following: • Loss of spontaneous emotion, observed or self-reported • Loss of emotional responsiveness to positive or negative stimuli or events	*Domain B3. Social interaction* Loss of, or diminished engagement in social interaction as evidenced by at least one of the following: • Spontaneous social initiative • Environmentally stimulated social interaction • Relationship with family members • Verbal interaction • Homebound
Criterion C These symptoms (A and B) cause clinically significant impairment in personal, social, occupational, or other important areas of functioning	**Criterion C** These symptoms (A–B) cause clinically significant impairment in personal, social, occupational, or other important areas of functioning

Table 4.1 *Continued*

Diagnostic criteria for apathy, original version (2009)	Diagnostic criteria for apathy, revisited version (2018)
Criterion D The symptoms (A and B) are not exclusively explained or due to physical disabilities (e.g. blindness and loss of hearing), to motor disabilities, to diminished level of consciousness, or to the direct physiological effects of a substance (e.g. drug of abuse, a medication)	**Criterion D** The symptoms (A–B) are not exclusively explained or due to physical disabilities (e.g. blindness and loss of hearing), to motor disabilities, to a diminished level of consciousness, to the direct physiological effects of a substance (e.g. drug of abuse, medication), or to major changes in the patient's environment

The LARS (14) evaluates the following nine domains: reduction in everyday productivity, lack of interest, lack of initiative, extinction of novelty seeking and motivation, blunting of emotional responses, lack of concern, poor social life, and extinction of self-awareness. The self-rated and informant-rated versions of the LARS were shown to be reliable and valid tools for assessing apathy in PD patients. Subsequently, as the original has a lengthy administration time, a short form of the LARS was developed to evaluate seven domains (i.e. reduction in everyday productivity, lack of interest, lack of initiative, extinction of novelty seeking and motivation, blunting of emotional responses, and poor social life). Until quite recently, only the LARS and AES allow assessment of multiple dimensions of apathy: cognitive, behavioural, and emotive. However, considering the above-mentioned Criterion D, and as PD is mainly characterized by disabling motor symptoms which may cause or contribute to exogenous apathy, the available scales (i.e. AES and LARS) do not allow apathy to be assessed while avoiding the possible confounding effect of motor impairments and thus do not satisfy the diagnostic Criterion D. Thus, in 2014, the Dimensional Apathy Scale (DAS (17)) was developed to assess apathy while minimizing the effect of motor dysfunctions in patients with amyotrophic lateral sclerosis. The DAS allows the three subtypes of apathy to be evaluated in relation to the Levy and Dubois model (18). It consists of three subscales: (i) an executive subscale assessing apathetic impairments associated with planning, attention, or organization; (ii) an emotional subscale assessing apathy associated with altered emotion integration; and (iii) a behavioural/cognitive initiation subscale assessing apathy associated with loss of self-generation of behaviours or cognition. Psychometric properties of the DAS have been investigated in PD patients in validation studies showing that the DAS is a reliable and valid assessment tool for apathy in PD (19, 20). PD patients were reported to show significantly higher scores on executive and initiation apathy subscales of self-rated DAS compared to healthy subjects, whereas they were perceived as having only more severe executive apathy by their caregivers. Thus, it is conceivable that executive apathy appears to be the most reliable subtype impairment in PD patients (19). Another study determined a specific apathy profile in PD patients as compared to healthy subjects, evidencing that the score on behavioural/cognitive initiation and emotional subscales of the DAS was higher in PD patients than in healthy controls. The findings suggested that reduced initiation of thought and behaviour and emotional blunting characterized PD patients, without confounding effects of motor disability (20). The two above-mentioned studies underlined the multidimensional character of apathy in PD, independently of severity of motor symptoms, and suggested the clinical relevance of identifying the subtype of the apathy by a valid and reliable tool such as the DAS in order to adequately manage the apathetic symptom by an individualized treatment approach.

Demographic, Clinical, Neuropsychological, and Neural Correlates of Apathy in Parkinson's Disease

A few studies have reported that apathy occurs more frequently in male than in female PD patients (21, 22). Though the explanation for such a sex difference is unclear, the possibility of a role of testosterone in the pathophysiology of apathy in males could be considered (23). On the other hand, the relationship between apathy and male sex might suggest that female caregivers tend to attribute negative affective symptoms more frequently than male caregivers (22). Of note, other studies failed to confirm a relationship between male sex and apathy (24, 25), and this thus deserves further investigation.

Apathy has been reported to be associated with older age and lower education (26); moreover, as for clinical correlates, apathy has been related to use of higher daily levodopa doses, longer disease duration, and more severe parkinsonism (21, 22, 24, 26, 27), although some studies did not confirm these relationships (22, 23, 28). Although apathy is associated with more severe motor symptoms, it occurs both in early and advanced stages of PD and also as a prodrome of disease, before the development of relevant motor disability (22).

As for cognitive correlates, apathy is related to deficits of selective cognitive domains in patients with PD; however, recent neuropsychological studies showed mixed results within each cognitive domain. Some studies revealed that apathy did not affect memory functions (29–33) while other studies reported poorer performance in apathetic PD patients than in non-apathetic ones (15, 21, 34–36). As for the executive function domain, although an association between apathy and frontal deficits has been reported (7, 12, 29, 31, 32, 34–38), some studies failed to confirm this (25, 33, 39, 40). Regarding processing speed/attention/working memory domains, many studies revealed that patients with apathy scored lower in cognitive tasks assessing these domains (7, 15, 25, 29–31, 35, 40, 41); however, three studies failed to confirm the relationship between apathy and poor performance in attentional tasks (32, 36). As for visuospatial abilities, some studies revealed no difference between apathetic and non-apathetic patients (29, 31, 32), while only one study (7) found a significant difference between the two groups of patients. In addition, apathy seems to influence language abilities (31, 38, 40) although the relationship was not confirmed by more recent studies (33, 34).

The inconsistency in findings about the association between apathy and cognitive deficits (memory and frontal dysfunctions) may be accounted for by methodological differences among the studies such as the use of different measures to assess apathy or cognitive functions and different inclusion and exclusion criteria (i.e. inclusion or exclusion of depressed or demented patients). In order to overcome the methodological differences across the studies and to better investigate the effect of 'pure apathy' on cognitive domains, D'Iorio and colleagues (42) performed a meta-analysis which revealed a moderate relationship between 'pure apathy' and poor performance on tasks assessing global cognitive functioning, long-term verbal memory, processing speed/attention/working memory, visuospatial ability, and selective executive functions (i.e. abstraction ability/concept formation, generativity, and inhibition) in patients with PD (42). Indirectly, the identification of impaired cognitive processes underlining apathy in PD suggests that apathy is related to structural and/or functional abnormalities of prefrontal cortex and subcortical structures which are connected by fronto-striatal circuits. To date, although apathy is among the major neuropsychiatric features of PD, only a limited number of magnetic resonance imaging and functional studies have explored neural correlates of apathy in PD. These few studies with structural magnetic resonance imaging have found mixed results: whereas some studies did not report structural differences between apathetic and non-apathetic patients (20, 43, 44), other studies revealed that patients with apathy had lower grey matter volumes in several brain areas such as the insula (29, 45, 46), the inferior/middle/medial frontal gyrus (29, 45, 48), the superior frontal gyrus (49), the anterior cingulate (29), the superior temporal gyrus (29), the precentral gyrus (45, 47), the post-central gyrus (48), the superior and inferior parietal gyrus (45, 48), the (posterior) cingulate gyrus (45), the precuneus (45, 46), the cerebellar vermis (46), the nucleus accumbens (48), and the supplementary motor area (48). Moreover, positron emission tomography studies revealed that the presence of apathy in PD was associated with changes in glucose metabolism in the ventral striatum (49, 50), the frontal middle gyrus (51–53), the inferior frontal gyrus (51–54), the posterior cingulate gyrus (51, 54), the anterior cingulate cortex (55), the orbitofrontal lobe (55), the medial frontal lobe (51), the right cuneus (52), the right anterior insula (52), the cerebellum (52), and the temporoparietal association cortex (55).

Neuroimaging studies with functional magnetic resonance imaging revealed that reductions of resting-state functional connectivity affecting fronto-striatal circuits play a relevant role in PD-related apathy. More specifically, apathetic PD patients have been reported to show reduced functional connectivity when compared with healthy subjects and with non-apathetic patients, mainly in left-sided circuits, and predominantly involving limbic striatal and frontal territories (43). Zhang and colleagues reported that white matter change is associated with apathy in PD patients and suggested that it could be a promising marker to predict the severity of apathy (56).

The role of altered dopaminergic neurotransmission in the striatum in the occurrence of apathy in PD patients was revealed by a study performed on untreated PD patients in Italy (41). However, another study on PD patients in Korea failed to find the same results, but it was characterized by some limitations such as a long delay between dopamine transporter and apathy evaluation (57). Moreover, a study in 2016 showed that an alteration of serotoninergic neurotransmission in the ventral striatum, in the dorsal and the subgenual parts of the anterior cingulate cortices, bilaterally, as well as in the right-sided caudate nucleus and the right-sided orbitofrontal cortex (58) was associated with the occurrence of apathy in PD patients, suggesting that altered serotoninergic neurotransmission in cortical and subcortical regions might be responsible for onset of apathy. A description of structural and functional imaging studies exploring neural correlates of apathy in patients affected by PD is shown in Table 4.2.

In conclusion, apathy in PD has been considered to be a consequence of functional deficits of prefrontal-subcortical circuitry associated with dopaminergic nigrostriatal and mesocortical dopamine depletion in the putamen and caudate nucleus, respectively. Recently, serotoninergic mechanism signalling was also identified as likely to be of importance in the pathophysiology of the apathy in PD.

Since understanding the pathophysiology of apathy is very relevant for efficient therapeutic strategies, further studies should better elucidate neuropsychological and neural correlates of apathy in PD patients.

Pharmacological and Non-Pharmacological Treatment of Apathy in Parkinson's Disease

As mentioned previously, the results of several studies have suggested that apathy is related mainly to dopaminergic nigrostriatal and mesocortical dopamine depletion and, therefore, dopaminergic treatments are considered a main therapeutic strategy. Some studies have attempted to use dopamine to manage patients with apathy to provide evidence of efficacy in reducing the severity of apathy (59–65). However, these studies tended to be small, unblinded, uncontrolled, and only used self-report scales.

As for dopaminergic treatment for reducing apathy, preliminary evidence indicated that levodopa (59) and dopaminergic agonists such as pramipexole, ropinirole, and piribedil may improve apathy associated with PD (60–64). In open-label studies, pramipexole and rotigotine have shown significant improvements in the motivational items of the UPDRS-I and the Nonmotor Symptoms Scale (62, 63). A study in 2015 compared the neuropsychiatric effects of levodopa, pramipexole, and ropinirole in 515 non-demented PD patients, with apathy measured by the Neuropsychiatric Inventory (64). The results indicated that the frequency and the severity of apathy were reduced with pramipexole rather than with either ropinirole or levodopa, suggesting the efficacy of D_3 receptor agonists in the treatment of apathy.

Table 4.2 Description of structural and functional imaging studies on neural correlates of apathy in patients affected by Parkinson's disease

Authors	Type of technique	Sample	Apathy scale	Results
Isella et al., 2002 (101)	MRI	26 PD patients	Apathy Scale	No correlation between any specific measure of frontotemporal atrophy and severity of apathy
Remy et al., 2005 (49)	PET	8 PD patients with episodes of major depression based on DSM-IV criteria and 12 PD patients without depression	Apathy Evaluation Scale	Apathy score was related to lower dopamine and noradrenaline transporter binding in the ventral striatum bilaterally
Le Jeune et al., 2009 (51)	PET	12 PD patients	Apathy Evaluation Scale	Variation of apathy scores positively correlated with changes in glucose metabolism in the right frontal middle gyrus and right inferior frontal gyrus. Variation of apathy scores negatively correlated with changes in glucose metabolism in the right posterior cingulate gyrus and left medial frontal lobe
Reijnders et al., 2010 (45)	3 T MRI	55 PD patients	Informant-Apathy Evaluation Scale, Lille Apathy Rating Scale	Apathy scores correlated with low grey matter density in the right posterior cingulate gyrus, and the bilateral inferior frontal gyrus. High apathy scores were correlated with low grey matter density values in the bilateral precentral gyrus, the bilateral inferior parietal gyrus, the bilateral inferior frontal gyrus, the bilateral insula, the right (posterior) cingulate gyrus, and the right precuneus
Skidmore et al., 2013 (102)	Resting fMRI	15 PD patients	Caregiver and self-report Lille Apathy Rating Scale	Association between more severity of apathy and increased normalized ALFF signal in the right middle orbital gyrus and in the subgenual cingulated bilaterally and decreased activity in the left supplementary motor region, left inferior parietal lobule and in the left fusiform gyrus. Decreased ALFF activity in the supplementary motor cortex and increased activity in the right orbitofrontal cortex, and the right middle frontal gyrus predicts apathy score

Continued

Table 4.2 *Continued*

Authors	Type of technique	Sample	Apathy scale	Results
Robert et al., 2012 (39)	PET	45 PD patients without dementia or depression	Apathy Evaluation Scale	Positive correlation between apathy score and metabolism in the right inferior frontal gyrus, right middle frontal gyrus, right cuneus, and right anterior insula was found. Negative correlation was found between apathy and cerebellar metabolism
Alzahrani et al., 2016 (29)	Structural MRI	65 PD patients and 24 healthy controls	Neuro-psychiatric Inventory	Apathy was associated with lower grey matter volume in the left insula, left inferior/middle/medial frontal gyrus, right anterior cingulate, and the left superior temporal gyrus
Baggio et al., 2015 (43)	MRI, fMRI	31 healthy controls and 62 age-, sex-, and education-matched PD	Apathy Scale	Apathy scores correlated negatively with the functional connectivity between both limbic and executive divisions of the left striatum and the left frontal lobe; between the limbic region of the left frontal lobe and the left striatum; and between the caudal and rostral frontal lobe and right striatum. Apathy scores correlated negatively with the functional connectivity between the different subdivisions of the left frontal lobe
Auffret et al., 2017 (54)	PET	12 patients with PD	Patient-rated and informant-based Lille Apathy Rating Scale	Changes in apathy score were correlated with metabolic changes in the cingulate gyrus or the inferior frontal cortex
Huang et al., 2013 (55)	PET	26 PD subjects and 12 control subjects	Apathy Evaluation Scale	Apathy scores correlated with increased metabolism in the anterior cingulate and orbitofrontal lobe and decreased metabolism in the temporoparietal association cortex
Robert et al., 2014 (50)	PET	44 PD patients	Apathy Evaluation Scale	Apathy change correlated with decreased metabolism within the right ventral striatum
Robert et al., 2014 (53)	PET	36 PD patients	Apathy Evaluation Scale	Correlation between increased metabolism within the bilateral frontal gyri, right premotor cortex and left posterior cingulate and higher apathy scores was found

Table 4.2 *Continued*

Authors	Type of technique	Sample	Apathy scale	Results
Thobois et al., 2010 (103)	PET	12 PD patients	Apathy Scale	Apathy score was related to lower dopamine transporter binding bilaterally in the orbitofrontal, dorsolateral prefrontal, posterior cingulate and temporal cortices, left striatum, and right amygdala
Terada et al., 2018 (47)	MRI	40 PD patients	Frontal Systems Behavior Scale	Apathy score correlated negatively with right precentral volume
Shen et al., 2018 (104)	fMRI	20 PD patients with apathy and 22 PD patients without apathy	Apathy Scale	Apathetic patients showed more decreased ALFF in left orbital middle frontal gyrus and bilateral superior frontal gyrus than patients without apathy. ALFF values in right superior frontal gyrus and apathy score were correlated negatively between them
Shin et al., 2017 (46)	PET, MRI	10 PD patients without apathy and 12 PD patients with apathy	Apathy Scale	Apathy was associated with atrophy and hypometabolism in precuneus in patients with isolated apathy. Apathy severity was also positively correlated with grey matter volume in the superior frontal gyrus and cerebellar vermis, and with metabolism in the medial frontal and anterior cingulate regions
Zhang et al., 2018 (56)	DTI	18 PD patients with apathy, 21 PD patients without apathy	Lille Apathy Rating Scale	Apathetic patients had more reduced FA values in the genu and body of corpus callosum, bilateral anterior corona radiata, left superior corona radiata, and left cingulum than non-apathetic patients. FA values were negatively correlated with apathy score in apathetic patients
Martínez-Horta et al., 2017 (48)	MRI	18 PD patients with apathy, and 18 PD patients without apathy	Diagnostic criteria for apathy; item 4 of part I of the Unified Parkinson's Disease Rating Sale	Apathetic patients showed grey matter volume loss in inferior parietal lobule, post-central gyrus, pars opercularis, nucleus accumbens, supplementary motor area, inferior orbital prefrontal cortex, and superior parietal gyrus

Continued

Table 4.2 *Continued*

Authors	Type of technique	Sample	Apathy scale	Results
Carriere et al., 2014 (44)	MRI (SPHARM-PDM analysis)	10 PD patients with apathy, 10 PD patients without apathy	Diagnostic criteria for apathy, Lille Apathy Rating Scale	Apathy was associated with atrophy of the left nucleus accumbens. The SPHARM-PDM analysis highlighted (i) a positive correlation between the severity of apathy and atrophy of the left nucleus accumbens; (ii) greater atrophy of the dorsolateral head of the left caudate in apathetic patient
Santangelo et al., 2015 (41)	DAT	15 PD patients with apathy and 15 PD patients without apathy	Apathy Evaluation Scale	Apathetic PD patients showed lower DAT levels in the striatum than non-apathetic patients
Chung et al., 2016 (57)	DAT	108 PD patients	Apathy Evaluation Scale	No correlation between DAT level and apathy score
Maillet et al., 2016 (58)	PET	15 PD patients with apathy and 15 PD patients without apathy	Lille Apathy Rating Scale	Apathetic patients showed greater serotonergic alteration in the ventral striatum, the dorsal and the subgenual parts of the anterior cingulate cortices, bilaterally, as well as in the right-sided caudate nucleus and the right-sided orbitofrontal cortex

ALFF, amplitude of low-frequency fluctuation; DAT, dopamine transporter; DSM-IV, *Diagnostic and Statistical Manual of Mental Disorders*, fourth edition; DTI, diffusion tensor imaging; FA, fractional anisotropy; fMRI, MRI, magnetic resonance imaging; PD, Parkinson's disease; PET, positron emission tomography; MRI, functional magnetic resonance imaging; SPHARM-PDM, spherical harmonic parameterization and sampling in a three-dimensional point distribution model.

Among dopaminergic drugs, methylphenidate is a stimulant chemically related to amphetamine, which stimulates dopamine release (65). The efficacy of methylphenidate in reducing apathy in PD has been reported in a single case (66). No significant change in apathy was found after treatment with atomoxetine in a randomized controlled trial (67).

Monoamine oxidase B inhibitors, such as selegiline and rasagiline, are most often used in the treatment of PD and selectively target the isoform of the monoamine oxidase enzyme engaged in the metabolic breakdown of dopamine in the brain (68). A retrospective review of 181 PD patients found that patients on selegiline or rasagiline showed lower scores on the AS than those taking other antiparkinsonian agents (69).

Amantadine, a glutamatergic antagonist, has been used to stimulate the release of dopamine and delay dopamine reuptake. Most reports of a beneficial effect of amantadine in improving apathy have involved small cohorts (70).

As for the possible efficacy of the acetylcholinesterase inhibitors in improving apathy, a double-blind, placebo-controlled study of 31 non-demented and non-depressed PD patients with moderate to severe apathy revealed a significant improvement of apathy after 6 months of treatment with rivastigmine (71). However, a longitudinal study failed to find a prolonged effect after 1 year of follow-up (72).

Among the antidepressants, selective serotonin reuptake inhibitors have not been found to be effective in the management of apathy in PD (69, 70); moreover, bupropion (norepinephrine–dopamine reuptake inhibitor) was not associated with greater apathy (69).

The efficacy of deep brain stimulation in reducing apathy has been evaluated in some studies (73, 74). However, those studies revealed that apathy may arise or worsen after subthalamic deep brain stimulation, when dopaminergic medication tapering is rapid (73, 75–78). An increase of apathy in terms of severity and frequency in some PD patients is probably due to discontinuation of dopaminergic treatment after surgery.

Among non-pharmacological treatments of apathy, the application of repetitive transcranial magnetic stimulation over the supplementary motor area for 5 days led to a short-term significant improvement of apathy in a case series (79).

Apathy in Huntington's Disease

Prevalence of Apathy in Huntington's Disease

HD is characterized by motor abnormalities, cognitive deficits, and behavioural symptoms. Among these neuropsychiatric disturbances of HD, apathy is a debilitating symptom that manifests before motor diagnosis. Therefore, it could be considered as an excellent therapeutic target in the preclinical phase of HD. Apathy occurs in 50% of HD patients and appears to be intrinsic to the evolution and progression of HD (80). In the REGISTRY study, apathy was observed in 47.4% of patients; this value increased as disease progressed (54.6% at stage 4–5) (81). More recently, Martínez-Horta and colleagues showed that apathy was already present in 32% of premanifest far-from motor-based disease onset and increased to 62% of early symptomatic HD patients (82). The probability of presenting apathetic symptoms was 15–88 times higher in premanifest far-from and close-to motor-based disease onset respectively than in healthy subjects. These findings suggested that HD mutation carriers are characterized by the highest probability to develop apathy, with an increasing prevalence along disease stages (82).

Since apathy is a common neuropsychiatric symptom which occurs in premanifest HD patients and is a risk factor for suicidal ideation in manifest HD patients (83), an early identification of apathy seems to be clinically relevant in order to manage the neuropsychiatric symptom adequately and to improve patients' and caregivers' quality of life.

Assessment and Phenomenology of Apathy in Huntington's Disease

Apathy has been reported to be a risk factor for suicidal ideation (83), and it affects the patients' and caregivers' quality of life; for these reasons, the evaluation of apathy in HD patients should be based on rating scales which are characterized by good psychometric properties (i.e. validity and reliability). To evaluate the apathy in HD, a committee on Rating Scales Development of the Movement Disorders Society evaluated the psychometric properties of several scales evaluating behavioural disturbances related to HD (84). The Committee identified and evaluated three scales for the evaluation of the apathy: one of these, the AS, has been used in some studies to assess apathy in premanifest and manifest HD patients. The score on the AS does not correlate with hypokinesia but is significantly associated with the *Diagnostic and Statistical Manual of Mental Disorders*, fourth edition, diagnosis of depression (84). The Committee of the Movement Disorders Society evaluated the AS as 'suggested' for screening of apathy only and, moreover, indicated that the association of the AS with the diagnosis of depression 'requires further characterization' (84).

The Apathy Subscale of the Frontal Systems Behavior Scale has been employed in observational and imaging studies (i.e. PREDICT-HD and IMAGE-HD) in premanifest and manifest HD patients (85, 86). To date, psychometric properties of the scale have not been evaluated specifically in HD patients. The Committee of the Movement Disorders Society proposed the scale as 'suggested' for assessing severity of apathy (84). The AES consists of three versions: self-reported (AES-S), clinician reported (AES-C), and informant reported (AES-I). The AES-C has showed a good construct validity. The Committee proposed the AES as a tool 'suggested' for assessing severity of apathy (84). The AES-C should be favoured in light of the risk of lack of insight by HD patients (84).

Demographic, Clinical, Neuropsychological, and Neural Correlates of Apathy in Huntington's Disease

Apathy in HD is associated with older age, male sex, previous suicide attempt, depression, obsessive–compulsive behaviours, unemployment, lower total functional capacity, and poorer patient-reported health-related quality of life (87, 88). Among clinical aspects related to HD, apathy is strongly correlated with disease duration and severity (89) indicating that apathy occurs at several stages of disease and its severity increases with the progression of disease (90).

Apathy is linked to a poor performance on some neuropsychological tests assessing memory, attention, and executive functions (89, 90): HD patients with apathy show poorer performance when compared to HD patients without apathy. Since executive functions and apathy are mediated by prefrontal-subcortical circuitries, the relationship between apathy and deficit of attention, executive functions, and retrieval ability in HD patients would indicate that apathy is a consequence of neurodegeneration of basal ganglia and consequent frontal deafferentation, and not a direct result of depression (91). Indeed, some recent studies revealed that caudate and putamen volumes were significantly related to apathy scores even after controlling for depression (91) in HD patients. Baake and colleagues performed a longitudinal study to evaluate the relationship between volume loss of subcortical structures and apathy in HD and the occurrence of possible changes over time (92). The study revealed that at baseline, smaller volume of the thalamus was related to apathy score in HD gene carriers; moreover, after 2 years, no association between atrophy of any subcortical structures and change in degree of apathy was found. The results suggested that apathy occurs in early stages of HD and is associated with atrophy of the thalamus in HD gene carriers. Moreover, the absence of an association between atrophy of the subcortical brain structures and change in the severity of apathy over a time period of 2-year follow-up might have been due to the fact that the time period (i.e. 2 years) was too short to identify a significant increase in apathy in premanifest and early HD patients. Evidence from a recent positron emission tomography study suggests that, besides striatal atrophy, altered activity in prefrontal cortex is related to apathy in premanifest HD (93). Moreover, Martínez-Horta and colleagues investigated both structural and metabolic brain changes associated with the severity of apathy in patients with HD, finding a strong association between decreased grey matter within a cortico-subcortical network, and alteration of bilateral amygdala and temporal cortex. The finding of the study suggests that apathy in HD is not only associated with altered basal ganglia but also frontal-executive alterations, supporting the notion that the prefrontal cortex–basal ganglia circuit is involved in apathy in HD (94).

To date, only one study has used diffusion tensor imaging, to investigate structural connectivity between brain regions and any putative microstructural changes associated with apathy in HD. That study revealed a significant association between severity of apathy and white matter changes (95).

Although neuroanatomical and neurochemical substrates have been explored in some studies, they are still largely unknown and deserve to be better clarified.

Treatment of Apathy in Huntington's Disease

Apathy is a debilitating symptom occurring frequently in premanifest HD and leads to a significant decrease in day-to-day activities and social interactions, negatively impacting patients' and caregivers' quality of life; for these reasons, apathy should be considered a potential target for treatment in HD. However, only recently has an international core committee of 11 multidisciplinary experts been constituted to develop clinical practice guidelines for apathy in HD (96). The guidelines are based on a modified Institute of Medicine guideline process. The panel of experts recommends: (i) to differentiate apathy from impaired ability to perform motor or cognitive tasks; (ii) to consider dose reductions of medications for other symptoms which might contribute to apathy; and (iii) to treat coexisting depression which might be associated with apathy. In addition, the panel proposes behavioural recommendations, such as to encourage the regular scheduling of both social and physical activities adapted to the subject, and some pharmacological recommendations, such as (i) the prescription of antidepressants as the preferred pharmacological option when differentiating between apathy as a behavioural disturbance and apathy as a symptom of depression in HD is difficult; (ii) the prescription of an activating antidepressant or stimulant drug as a pharmacological option for the subject without depression; and (iii) giving a warning about potential worsening of irritability and sleep disturbance when prescribing an activating antidepressant or a stimulant drug.

Moreover, before starting a new drug treatment, psychoeducation about both the behavioural manifestations of HD and information about the drug treatment should be provided to the patient and caregivers to improve drug adherence.

Until now, bupropion was considered as a potential pharmacological treatment for apathy in HD, but its efficacy is questionable since a double-blind, 10-week, multicentre, placebo-controlled trial conducted on 40 HD patients revealed that apathy scores improved in both the bupropion-treated (given at 150–300 mg per day for 10 weeks) and placebo-treated patients (97).

Similarly, although cholinesterase inhibitors are frequently used for apathy in neurodegenerative diseases, no studies have reported their effect on apathy in HD. Among psychostimulants, in a crossover study, HD patients perceived themselves as less apathetic after treatment with modafinil; however, no difference was found on overall ratings of apathy under drug and placebo conditions (98). The effect of methylphenidate was described in an 8-year-old boy with juvenile HD and attention deficit hyperactivity disorder; the use of methylphenidate might have contributed to an increase of motor symptoms (99). A controlled crossover study showed no efficacy of atomoxetine in reducing apathy in 20 HD patients compared to placebo (100).

Conclusion

In PD and in HD, apathy and its subtypes should be evaluated with validated tools in order to identify apathy and its profile and to manage it by individually tailored pharmacological and non-pharmacological interventions. A combination of pharmacological and psychosocial treatments might yield optimal results in reducing apathy and should be evaluated by randomized clinical trials.

References

1. Abdo WF, van de Warrenburg BP, Burn DJ, Quinn NP, Bloem BR. The clinical approach to movement disorders. Nat Rev Neurol. 2010;6(1):29–37.
2. Tysnes OB, Storstein A. Epidemiology of Parkinson's disease. J Neural Transm (Vienna). 2017;124(8):901–5.
3. Braak H, Del Tredici K, Rub U, de Vos RA, Jansen Steur EN, Braak E. Staging of brain pathology related to sporadic Parkinson's disease. Neurobiol Aging. 2003;24(2):197–211.

4. McColgan P, Tabrizi SJ. Huntington's disease: a clinical review. Eur J Neurol. 2018;25(1):24–34.
5. Santangelo G, Trojano L, Barone P, Errico D, Grossi D, Vitale C. Apathy in Parkinson's disease: diagnosis, neuropsychological correlates, pathophysiology and treatment. Behav Neurol. 2013;27(4):501–13.
6. den Brok MG, van Dalen JW, van Gool WA, Moll van Charante EP, de Bie RM, Richard E. Apathy in Parkinson's disease: a systematic review and meta-analysis. Mov Disord. 2015;30(6):759–69.
7. Santangelo G, Vitale C, Trojano L, Picillo M, Moccia M, Pisano G, et al. Relationship between apathy and cognitive dysfunctions in de novo untreated Parkinson's disease: a prospective longitudinal study. Eur J Neurol. 2015;22(2):253–60.
8. Pedersen KF, Alves G, Aarsland D, Larsen JP. Occurrence and risk factors for apathy in Parkinson disease: a 4-year prospective longitudinal study. J Neurol Neurosurg Psychiatry. 2009;80(11):1279–82.
9. Robert P, Onyike CU, Leentjens AF, Dujardin K, Aalten P, Starkstein S, et al. Proposed diagnostic criteria for apathy in Alzheimer's disease and other neuropsychiatric disorders. Eur Psychiatry. 2009;24(2):98–104.
10. Drijgers RL, Dujardin K, Reijnders JS, Defebvre L, Leentjens AF. Validation of diagnostic criteria for apathy in Parkinson's disease. Parkinsonism Relat Disord. 2010;16(10):656–60.
11. Robert P, Lanctôt KL, Agüera-Ortiz L, Aalten P, Bremond F, Defrancesco M, et al. Is it time to revise the diagnostic criteria for apathy in brain disorders? The 2018 international consensus group. Eur Psychiatry. 2018;54:71–6.
12. Santangelo G, Barone P, Cuoco S, Raimo S, Pezzella D, Picillo M, et al. Apathy in untreated, de novo patients with Parkinson's disease: validation study of Apathy Evaluation Scale. J Neurol. 2014;261(12):2319–28.
13. Mele B, Merrikh D, Ismail Z, Goodarzi Z. Detecting apathy in individuals with Parkinson's disease: a systematic review. J Parkinsons Dis. 2019;9(4):653–64.
14. Sockeel P, Dujardin K, Devos D, Deneve C, Destee A, Defebvre L. The Lille Apathy Rating Scale (LARS), a new instrument for detecting and quantifying apathy: validation in Parkinson's disease. J Neurol Neurosurg Psych. 2006;77(5):579–84.
15. Starkstein SE, Mayberg HS, Preziosi TJ, Andrezejewski P, Leiguarda R, Robinson RG. Reliability, validity, and clinical correlates of apathy in Parkinson's disease. J Neuropsych Clin Neurosci. 1992;4(2):134–9.
16. Carrozzino D. Clinimetric approach to rating scales for the assessment of apathy in Parkinson's disease: a systematic review. Prog Neuropsychopharmacol Biol Psychiatry. 2019;94:109641.
17. Radakovic R, Abrahams S. Developing a new apathy measurement scale: Dimensional Apathy Scale. Psychiatry Res. 2014;219(3):658–63.
18. Levy R, Dubois B. Apathy and the functional anatomy of the prefrontal cortex–basal ganglia circuits. Cereb Cortex. 2006;16:916–28.
19. Radakovic R, Davenport R, Starr JM, Abrahams S. Apathy dimensions in Parkinson's disease. Int J Geriatr Psychiatry. 2018;33(1):151–8.
20. Santangelo G, D'Iorio A, Piscopo F, Cuoco S, Longo K, Amboni M, et al. Assessment of apathy minimising the effect of motor dysfunctions in Parkinson's disease: a validation study of the dimensional apathy scale. Qual Life Res. 2017;26(9):2533–40.
21. Dujardin K, Sockeel P, Devos D, Delliaux M, Krystkowiak P, Destee A, et al. Characteristics of apathy in Parkinson's disease. Mov Disord. 2007;22(6):778–84.
22. Pedersen KF, Alves G, Brønnick K, Aarsland D, Tysnes OB, Larsen JP. Apathy in drug-naïve patients with incident Parkinson's disease: the Norwegian ParkWest study. J Neurol. 2010;257(2):217–23.

23. Ready RE, Friedman J, Grace J, Fernandez H. Testosterone deficiency and apathy in Parkinson's disease: a pilot study. J Neurol Neurosurg Psychiatry. 2004;75(9):1323–6.
24. Ziropadja LJ, Stefanova E, Petrovic M, Stojkovic T, Kostic VS. Apathy and depression in Parkinson's disease: the Belgrade PD study report. Parkinsonism Relat Disord. 2012;18(4):339–42.
25. Dujardin K, Sockeel P, Delliaux M, Destee A, Defebvre L. Apathy may herald cognitive decline and dementia in Parkinson's disease. Mov Disord. 2009;24(16):2391–7.
26. Cubo E, Benito-Leon J, Coronell C, Armesto D, ANIMO Study Group. Clinical correlates of apathy in patients recently diagnosed with Parkinson's disease: the ANIMO study. Neuroepidemiology. 2012;38(1):48–55.
27. Benito-Leon J, Cubo E, Coronell C; ANIMO Study Group. Impact of apathy on health-related quality of life in recently diagnosed Parkinson's disease: the ANIMO study. Mov Disord. 2012;27(2):211–8.
28. Kirsch-Darrow L, Marsiske M, Okun MS, Bauer R, Bowers D. Apathy and depression: separate factors in Parkinson's disease. J Int Neuropsychol Soc. 2011;17(6):1058–66.
29. Alzahrani H, Antonini A, Venneri A. Apathy in mild Parkinson's disease: neuropsychological and neuroimaging evidence. J Parkinsons Dis. 2016;6(4):821–32.
30. Cohen ML, Aita S, Mari Z, Brandt J. The unique and combined effects of apathy and depression on cognition in Parkinson's disease. J Parkinsons Dis. 2015;5(2):351–9.
31. Grossi D, Santangelo G, Barbarulo AM, Vitale C, Castaldo G, Proto MG, et al. Apathy and related executive syndromes in dementia associated with Parkinson's disease and in Alzheimer's disease. Behav Neurol. 2013;27(4):515–22.
32. Santangelo G, D'Iorio A, Maggi G, Cuoco S, Pellecchia MT, Amboni M, et al. Cognitive correlates of "pure apathy" in Parkinson's disease. Parkinsonism Relat Disord. 2018;53:101–4.
33. Szymkowicz SM, Dotson VM, Jones JD, Okun MS, Bowers D. Symptom dimensions of depression and apathy and their relationship with cognition in Parkinson's disease. J Int Neuropsychol Soc. 2018;24(3):269–82.
34. Butterfield LC, Cimino CR, Oelke LE, Hauser RA, Sanchez-Ramos J. The independent influence of apathy and depression on cognitive functioning in Parkinson's disease. Neuropsychology. 2010;24(6):721–30.
35. Martínez-Horta S, Pagonabarraga J, Fernandez de Bobadilla R, Garcia-Sanchez C, Kulisevsky J. Apathy in Parkinson's disease: more than just executive dysfunction. J Int Neuropsychol Soc. 2013;19(5):571–82.
36. Varanese S, Perfetti B, Ghilardi MF, Di Rocco A. Apathy, but not depression, reflects inefficient cognitive strategies in Parkinson's disease. PLoS One. 2011;6(3):e17846.
37. Liu H, Ou R, Wei Q, Hou Y, Zhang L, Cao B, et al. Apathy in drug-naïve patients with Parkinson's disease. Parkinsonism Relat Disord. 2017;44:28–32.
38. Meyer A, Zimmermann R, Gschwandtner U, Hatz F, Bousleiman H, Schwarz N, et al. Apathy in Parkinson's disease is related to executive function, gender and age but not to depression. Front Aging Neurosci. 2015;6:350.
39. Robert G, Le Jeune F, Lozachmeur C, Drapier S, Dondaine T, Péron J, et al. Apathy in patients with Parkinson disease without dementia or depression: a PET study. Neurology. 2012;79(11):1155–60.
40. Zgaljardic DJ, Borod JC, Foldi NS, Rocco M, Mattis PJ, Gordon MF, et al. Relationship between self-reported apathy and executive dysfunction in nondemented patients with Parkinson disease. Cogn Behav Neurol. 2007;20(3):184–92.
41. Santangelo G, Vitale C, Picillo M, Cuoco S, Moccia M, Pezzella D, et al. Apathy and striatal dopamine transporter levels in de-novo, untreated Parkinson's disease patients. Parkinsonism Relat Disord. 2015;21(5):489–93.

42. D'Iorio A, Maggi G, Vitale C, Trojano L, Santangelo G. "Pure apathy" and cognitive dysfunctions in Parkinson's disease: a meta-analytic study. Neurosci Biobehav Rev. 2018;94:1–10.

43. Baggio HC, Segura B, Garrido-Millan JL, et al. Resting-state frontostriatal functional connectivity in Parkinson's disease-related apathy. Mov Disord. 2015;30(5):671–9.

44. Carriere N, Besson P, Dujardin K, Duhamel A, Defebvre L, Delmaire C, et al. Apathy in Parkinson's disease is associated with nucleus accumbens atrophy: a magnetic resonance imaging shape analysis. Mov Disord. 2014;29(7):897–903.

45. Reijnders JS, Scholtissen B, Weber WE, Aalten P, Verhey FR, Leentjens AF. Neuroanatomical correlates of apathy in Parkinson's disease: a magnetic resonance imaging study using voxel-based morphometry. Mov Disord. 2010;25(14):2318–25.

46. Shin JH, Shin SA, Lee JY, Nam H, Lim JS, Kim YK. Precuneus degeneration and isolated apathy in patients with Parkinson's disease. Neurosci Lett. 2017;653:250–7.

47. Terada T, Miyata J, Obi T, Kubota M, Yoshizumi M, Murai T. Reduced gray matter volume is correlated with frontal cognitive and behavioral impairments in Parkinson's disease. J Neurol Sci. 2018;390:231–8.

48. Martínez-Horta S, Sampedro F, Pagonabarraga J, Fernandez-Bobadilla R, Marin-Lahoz J, Riba J, et al. Non-demented Parkinson's disease patients with apathy show decreased grey matter volume in key executive and reward-related nodes. Brain Imaging Behav. 2017;11(5):1334–42.

49. Remy P, Doder M, Lees A, Turjanski N, Brooks D. Depression in Parkinson's disease: loss of dopamine and noradrenaline innervation in the limbic system. Brain. 2005;128(6):1314–22.

50. Robert GH, Le Jeune F, Lozachmeur C, Drapier S, Dondaine T, Péron J, et al. Preoperative factors of apathy in subthalamic stimulated Parkinson disease: a PET study. Neurology. 2014;83(18):1620–6.

51. Le Jeune F, Drapier D, Bourguignon A, Péron J, Mesbah H, Drapier S, et al. Subthalamic nucleus stimulation in Parkinson disease induces apathy: a PET study. Neurology. 2009;73(21):1746–51.

52. Robert G, Le Jeune F, Lozachmeur C, Drapier S, Dondaine T, Péron J, et al. Apathy in patients with Parkinson disease without dementia or depression: a PET study. Neurology. 2012;79(11):1155–60.

53. Robert G, Le Jeune F, Dondaine T, Drapier S, Péron J, Lozachmeur C, et al. Apathy and impaired emotional facial recognition networks overlap in Parkinson's disease: a PET study with conjunction analyses. J Neurol Neurosurg Psychiatry. 2014;85(10):1153–8.

54. Auffret M, Le Jeune F, Maurus A, Drapier S, Houvenaghel JF, Robert GH, et al. Apomorphine pump in advanced Parkinson's disease: effects on motor and nonmotor symptoms with brain metabolism correlations. J Neurol Sci. 2017;372:279–87.

55. Huang C, Ravdin LD, Nirenberg MJ, Piboolnurak P, Severt L, Maniscalco JS, et al. Neuroimaging markers of motor and nonmotor features of Parkinson's disease: an 18f fluorodeoxyglucose positron emission computed tomography study. Dement Geriatr Cogn Disord. 2013;35(3–4):183–96.

56. Zhang Y, Wu J, Wu W, Liu R, Pang L, Guan D, et al. Reduction of white matter integrity correlates with apathy in Parkinson's disease. Int J Neurosci. 2018;128(1):25–31.

57. Chung SJ, Lee JJ, Ham JH, Lee PH, Sohn YH. Apathy and striatal dopamine defects in non-demented patients with Parkinson's disease. Parkinsonism Relat Disord. 2016;23:62–5.

58. Maillet A, Krack P, Lhommée E, Météreau E, Klinger H, Favre E, et al. The prominent role of serotonergic degeneration in apathy, anxiety and depression in de novo Parkinson's disease. Brain. 2016;139(Pt 9):2486–502.

59. Czernecki V, Pillon B, Houeto JL, Pochon JB, Levy R, Dubois B. Motivation, reward, and Parkinson's disease: influence of dopatherapy. Neuropsychologia. 2002;40(13):2257–67.

60. Rektorova I, Balaz M, Svatova J, Zarubova K, Honig I, Dostal V, et al. Effects of ropinirole on nonmotor symptoms of Parkinson disease: a prospective multicenter study. Clin Neuropharmacol. 2008;31(5):261–6.

61. Thobois S, Lhommée E, Klinger H, Ardouin C, Schmitt E, Bichon A, et al. Parkinsonian apathy responds to dopaminergic stimulation of D2/D3 receptors with piribedil. Brain. 2013;136(Pt 5):1568–77.

62. Leentjens AF, Koester J, Fruh B, Shephard DT, Barone P, Houben JJ. The effect of pramipexole on mood and motivational symptoms in Parkinson's disease: a meta-analysis of placebo-controlled studies. Clin Ther. 2009;31(1):89–98. Erratum in: Clin Ther. 2009;31(3):677.

63. Ray Chaudhuri K, Martínez-Martin P, Antonini A, Brown RG, Friedman JH, Onofrj M, et al. Rotigotine and specific non-motor symptoms of Parkinson's disease: post hoc analysis of RECOVER. Parkinsonism Relat Disord. 2013;19(7):660–5.

64. Pérez-Pérez J, Pagonabarraga J, Martínez-Horta S, Fernández-Bobadilla R, Sierra S, Pascual-Sedano B, et al. Head-to-head comparison of the neuropsychiatric effect of dopamine agonists in Parkinson's disease: a prospective, cross-sectional study in non-demented patients. Drugs Aging. 2015;32(5):401–7.

65. Seeman P, Madras B. Methylphenidate elevates resting dopamine which lowers the impulse-triggered release of dopamine: a hypothesis. Behav Brain Res. 2002;130(1–2):79–83.

66. Chatterjee A, Fahn S. Methylphenidate treats apathy in Parkinson's disease. J Neuropsychiatry Clin Neurosci. 2002;14(4):461–2.

67. Weintraub D, Mavandadi S, Mamikonyan E, Siderowf AD, Duda JE, Hurtig HI, et al. Atomoxetine for depression and other neuropsychiatric symptoms in Parkinson disease. Neurology. 2010;75(5):448–55.

68. Fernandez HH, Chen JJ. Monoamine oxidase-B inhibition in the treatment of Parkinson's disease. Pharmacotherapy. 2007;27(12 Pt 2):174S–85S.

69. Zahodne LB, Bernal-Pacheco O, Bowers D, Ward H, Oyama G, Limotai N, et al. Are selective serotonin reuptake inhibitors associated with greater apathy in Parkinson's disease? J Neuropsychiatry Clin Neurosci. 2012;24(3):326–30.

70. Kaji Y, Hirata K. Apathy and anhedonia in Parkinson's disease. ISRN Neurol. 2011;2011:219427.

71. Devos D, Moreau C, Maltete D, Lefaucheur R, Kreisler A, Eusebio A, et al. Rivastigmine in apathetic but dementia and depression-free patients with Parkinson's disease: a double-blind, placebo-controlled, randomised clinical trial. J Neurol Neurosurg Psychiatry. 2014;85(6):668–74.

72. Moretti R, Caruso P, Dal Ben M. Rivastigmine as a symptomatic treatment for apathy in Parkinson's dementia complex: new aspects for this riddle. Parkinsons Dis. 2017;2017:6219851.

73. Atkinson-Clement C, Cavazzini É, Zénon A, Witjas T, Fluchère F, Azulay JP, et al. Effects of subthalamic nucleus stimulation and levodopa on decision-making in Parkinson's disease. Mov Disord. 2019;34(3):377–85.

74. Hindle Fisher I, Pall HS, Mitchell RD, Kausar J, Cavanna AE. Apathy in patients with Parkinson's disease following deep brain stimulation of the subthalamic nucleus. CNS Spectr. 2016;21(3):258–64.

75. Rossi M, Bruno V, Arena J, Cammarota Á, Merello M. Challenges in PD patient management after DBS: a pragmatic review. Mov Disord Clin Pract. 201828;5(3):246–54.

76. Abbes M, Lhommée E, Thobois S, Klinger H, Schmitt E, Bichon A, et al. Subthalamic stimulation and neuropsychiatric symptoms in Parkinson's disease: results from a long-term follow-up cohort study. J Neurol Neurosurg Psychiatry. 2018;89(8):836–43.

77. Lhommée E, Boyer F, Wack M, Pélissier P, Klinger H, Schmitt E, et al. Personality, dopamine, and Parkinson's disease: insights from subthalamic stimulation. Mov Disord. 2017;32(8):1191–200.

78. Maier F, Lewis CJ, Horstkoetter N, Eggers C, Dembek TA, Visser-Vandewalle V, et al. Subjective perceived outcome of subthalamic deep brain stimulation in Parkinson's disease one year after surgery. Parkinsonism Relat Disord. 2016;24:41–7.

79. Oguro H, Nakagawa T, Mitaki S, Ishihara M, Onoda K, Yamaguchi S. Randomized trial of repetitive transcranial magnetic stimulation for apathy and depression in Parkinson's disease. J Neurol Neurophysiol. 2014;5(6):1000242.

80. Thompson JC, Harris J, Sollom AC, Stopford CL, Howard E, Snowden JS, et al. Longitudinal evaluation of neuropsychiatric symptoms in Huntington's disease. J Neuropsychiatry Clin Neurosci. 2012;24(1):53–60.

81. van Duijn E, Craufurd D, Hubers AA, Giltay EJ, Bonelli R, Rickards H, et al. Neuropsychiatric symptoms in a European Huntington's disease cohort (REGISTRY). J Neurol Neurosurg Psychiatry. 2014;85(12):1411–8.

82. Martínez-Horta S, Perez-Perez J, van Duijn E, Fernandez-Bobadilla R, Carceller M, Pagonabarraga J, et al. Neuropsychiatric symptoms are very common in premanifest and early stage Huntington's disease. Parkinsonism Relat Disord. 2016;25:58–64.

83. Honrath P, Dogan I, Wudarczyk O, Görlich KS, Votinov M, Werner CJ, et al. Risk factors of suicidal ideation in Huntington's disease: literature review and data from Enroll-HD. J Neurol. 2018;265(11):2548–61.

84. Mestre TA, van Duijn E, Davis AM, Bachoud-Lévi AC, Busse M, Anderson KE, et al. Rating scales for behavioral symptoms in Huntington's disease: critique and recommendations. Mov Disord. 2016;31(10):1466–78.

85. Paulsen JS, Long JD, Ross CA, Harrington DL, Erwin CJ, Williams JK, et al. Prediction of manifest Huntington's disease with clinical and imaging measures: a prospective observational study. Lancet Neurol. 2014;13(12):1193–201.

86. Poudel GR, Egan GF, Churchyard A, Chua P, Stout JC, Georgiou-Karistianis N. Abnormal synchrony of resting state networks in premanifest and symptomatic Huntington disease: the IMAGE-HD study. J Psychiatry Neurosci. 2014;39:87–96.

87. Jacobs M, Hart EP, Roos RAC. Cognitive performance and apathy predict unemployment in Huntington's disease mutation carriers. J Neuropsychiatry Clin Neurosci. 2018;30(3):188–93.

88. Fritz NE, Boileau NR, Stout JC, Ready R, Perlmutter JS, Paulsen JS, et al. Relationships among apathy, health-related quality of life, and function in Huntington's disease. J Neuropsychiatry Clin Neurosci. 2018;30(3):194–201.

89. Sousa M, Moreira F, Jesus-Ribeiro J, Marques I, Cunha F, Canário N, et al. Apathy profile in Parkinson's and Huntington's disease: a comparative cross-sectional study. Eur Neurol. 2018;79(1–2):13–20.

90. Baudic S, Maison P, Dolbeau G, Boissé MF, Bartolomeo P, Dalla Barba G, et al. Cognitive impairment related to apathy in early Huntington's disease. Dement Geriatr Cogn Disord. 2006;21(5–6):316–21.

91. Misiura MB, Ciarochi J, Vaidya J, Bockholt J, Johnson HJ, Calhoun VD, et al. Apathy is related to cognitive control and striatum volumes in prodromal Huntington's disease. J Int Neuropsychol Soc. 2019;25(5):462–9.

92. Baake V, Coppen EM, van Duijn E, Dumas EM, van den Bogaard SJA, Scahill RI, et al. Apathy and atrophy of subcortical brain structures in Huntington's disease: a two-year follow-up study. Neuroimage Clin. 2018;27;19:66–70.

93. Ceccarini J, Ahmad R, Van de Vliet L, Casteels C, Vandenbulcke M, Vandenberghe W, et al. Behavioral symptoms in premanifest Huntington disease correlate with reduced frontal CB(1)R levels. J Nucl Med. 2019;60(1):115–21.

94. Martínez-Horta S, Perez-Perez J, Sampedro F, Pagonabarraga J, Horta-Barba A, Carceller-Sindreu M, et al. Structural and metabolic brain correlates of apathy in Huntington's disease. Mov Disord. 2018;33(7):1151–9.

95. Gregory S, Scahill RI, Seunarine KK, Stopford C, Zhang H, Zhang J, et al. Neuropsychiatry and white matter microstructure in Huntington's disease. J Huntingtons Dis. 2015;4(3):239–49.

96. Anderson KE, van Duijn E, Craufurd D, Drazinic C, Edmondson M, Goodman N, et al. Clinical management of neuropsychiatric symptoms of Huntington disease: expert-based consensus guidelines on agitation, anxiety, apathy, psychosis and sleep disorders. J Huntingtons Dis. 2018;7(3):355–66.

97. Gelderblom H, Wüstenberg T, McLean T, Mütze L, Fischer W, Saft C, et al. Bupropion for the treatment of apathy in Huntington's disease: a multicenter, randomised, double-blind, placebo-controlled, prospective crossover trial. PLoS One. 2017;12(3):e0173872.

98. Blackwell AD, Paterson NS, Barker RA, Robbins TW, Sahakian BJ. The effects of modafinil on mood and cognition in Huntington's disease. Psychopharmacology (Berl). 2008;199(1):29–36.

99. Waugh JL, Miller VS, Chudnow RS, Dowling MM. Juvenile Huntington disease exacerbated by methylphenidate: case report. J Child Neurol. 2008;23(7):807–9.

100. Beglinger LJ, Adams WH, Paulson H, Fiedorowicz JG, Langbehn DR, Duff K, et al. Randomized controlled trial of atomoxetine for cognitive dysfunction in early Huntington disease. J Clin Psychopharmacol. 2009;29(5):484–7.

101. Isella V, Melzi P, Grimaldi M, Iurlaro S, Piolti R, Ferrarese C, Frattola L, Appollonio I. Clinical, neuropsychological, and morphometric correlates of apathy in Parkinson's disease. Mov Disord. 2002;17(2):366–71.

102. Skidmore FM, Yang M, Baxter L, von Deneen K, Collingwood J, He G, Tandon R, Korenkevych D, Savenkov A, Heilman KM, Gold M, Liu Y. Apathy, depression, and motor symptoms have distinct and separable resting activity patterns in idiopathic Parkinson disease. Neuroimage. 2013;81:484–95. doi:10.1016/j.neuroimage.2011.07.012

103. Thobois S, Ardouin C, Lhommée E, Klinger H, Lagrange C, Xie J, Fraix V, Coelho Braga MC, Hassani R, Kistner A, Juphard A, Seigneuret E, Chabardes S, Mertens P, Polo G, Reilhac A, Costes N, LeBars D, Savasta M, Tremblay L, Quesada JL, Bosson JL, Benabid AL, Broussolle E, Pollak P, Krack P. Non-motor dopamine withdrawal syndrome after surgery for Parkinson's disease: predictors and underlying mesolimbic denervation. Brain. 2010;133(Pt 4):1111–27. doi:10.1093/brain/awq032

104. Shen YT, Li JY, Yuan YS, Wang XX, Wang M, Wang JW, Zhang H, Zhu L, Zhang KZ. Disrupted amplitude of low-frequency fluctuations and causal connectivity in Parkinson's disease with apathy. Neurosci Lett. 2018;683:75–81. doi:10.1016/j.neulet.2018.06.043

5
Apathy in Mild Behavioural Impairment

Zahinoor Ismail, Bria Mele, Zahra Goodarzi,
Jayna Holroyd-Leduc, and Moyra Mortby

Introduction

Apathy is increasingly recognized as not only a common and debilitating symptom in neurodegenerative diseases such as Parkinson's disease and Huntington's disease, but also as a significant symptom in preclinical and prodromal dementia (1, 2). Individuals experiencing apathy in preclinical and prodromal dementia may experience losses of interest, motivation, and drive (3). Progression to dementia, as well as severity of dementia, may in part be related to the presence of apathy in preclinical and prodromal dementia. Given this possible predictive relationship, it is important to understand the link between apathy and dementia states (4, 5).

As much of the research on apathy in dementia populations is focused on later stages of dementia, this chapter aims to provide an overview of apathy in preclinical and prodromal phases of dementia. Specifically, this chapter focuses on emergence, diagnosis, epidemiology, treatment, and mechanisms associated with apathy as it presents in preclinical and prodromal dementia.

Emergence of Behavioural Symptoms and Risk of Dementia

It is well established that neuropsychiatric symptoms (NPS) are a common feature of dementia syndromes irrespective of disease aetiology and stage (6). NPS are recognized as a core clinical manifestation of dementia, affecting between 31–50% of individuals with mild cognitive impairment (MCI) (7–9) and 61–97% of individuals with dementia (10, 11). NPS are among the most challenging and costly aspects of neurocognitive disorders and, if left untreated, are linked to hastened disease progression, greater functional impairment, higher burden of dementia-related neuropathological markers, poorer quality of life, increased healthcare utilization, greater caregiver burden, accelerated placement in residential care, and increased mortality risk (4, 12–15).

Longitudinal cohort studies have provided an abundance of evidence demonstrating comorbid presentation of NPS in MCI to be associated with a greater risk of dementia than MCI without NPS (7, 16–19). Similarly, research has shown an increased risk of cognitive impairment in cognitively healthy older adults with NPS. For instance, among cognitively healthy older adults aged 70 years or greater, with or without NPS, the presence of NPS (especially agitation, apathy, anxiety, irritability, and depression) was linked to a higher risk of developing MCI when compared to those without NPS (20). Furthermore, a population-based study in 2017 showed that the presence of NPS increased the risk of cognitive impairment across the cognitive spectrum from cognitively normal to dementia (21).

Recent advances and a growing evidence base have identified later-life emergent and persistent NPS, also referred to as mild behavioural impairment (MBI), as an intrinsic aspect of prodromal dementia and an early marker of cognitive decline (22). MBI is a neurobehavioural syndrome, characterized by later-life acquired, sustained NPS (23). Considered an at-risk state for cognitive decline and dementia, MBI may reflect an early neurodegenerative disease manifestation that precedes cognitive impairment (18, 23, 24).

In an effort to standardize research into early non-cognitive markers of dementia, the NPS Professional Interest Area of the International Society to Advance Alzheimer Research and Treatment (ISTAART), a subgroup of the Alzheimer's Association (AA), published research diagnostic criteria for MBI (23). The ISTAART-AA MBI criteria stipulate the emergence of later-life symptoms, sustained for a minimum duration of 6 months, in order to minimize false positives due to reactive symptomatology or medical comorbidity. These symptoms must reflect a clear change from the person's usual behaviour or personality and have been observed by the patient, informant, or clinician (23). Importantly, the criteria explicitly state that MBI (considered the neurobehavioural axis) can precede, co-occur with, or emerge after subjective cognitive decline or MCI (considered the neurocognitive axis). A diagnosis of MBI requires at least minimal impairment in interpersonal relationships, social functioning, or occupational ability as a result of the NPS, rather than cognitive symptoms (23).

According to the ISTAART-AA MBI criteria, later-life emergent NPS cluster into five core domains: (i) impaired drive and motivation (apathy) (25); (ii) affective/emotional dysregulation (mood and anxiety symptoms) (26, 27); (iii) impulse dyscontrol/agitation/abnormal reward salience (changes in response inhibition and self-regulation) (28); (iv) social inappropriateness (impaired social cognition) (29); and (v) abnormal thoughts/perceptions (psychotic symptoms) (30). Changes must be evident in at least one of the five domains (23).

The assessment of MBI has been operationalized through the development of the Mild Behavioural Impairment Checklist (MBI-C) (3). The MBI-C has specifically been developed as a case ascertainment tool for MBI in preclinical and prodromal dementia. It is a general psychopathology scale and is available in multiple languages (freely available at https://mbitest.org/). The MBI-C consists of 34 questions that reflect the five MBI domains (decreased motivation, affective dysregulation, impulse dyscontrol, social inappropriateness, and abnormal perception or thought content).

The 'decreased motivation' (i.e. apathy) domain focuses on the cognitive, behavioural, and emotional aspects of apathy. Each apathy aspect is assessed by two questions. The 'affective dysregulation' domain is assessed through four items that measure aspects of depression (i.e. sad mood, anhedonia, hopelessness, and feelings of guilt) and two items focusing on aspects of anxiety and panic. The 'impulse dyscontrol' domain is the largest section, consisting of 12 questions that assess agitation, aggression, impulsivity, eating dyscontrol, dangerous behaviour, and alteration of the reward system. The 'social inappropriateness' domain consists of five items that investigate social grace, empathy, and tact. Finally, the 'abnormal perceptions or thought content' domain is assessed using five items that explore suspiciousness, grandiosity, and visual and auditory hallucinations. In accordance with the ISTAART-AA MBI criteria, the MBI-C also requires symptoms to be of later-life onset and to have been persistent for at least 6 months (3). The MBI-C therefore provides a new and specific measure to ascertain apathy in preclinical and prodromal states, including normal cognition, subjective cognitive decline, and MCI.

Apathy as Part of Mild Behavioural Impairment

Apathy is one of the most common, stable, and persistent NPS observed in dementia, and is linked to more disability, poorer health, higher levels of caregiver stress and burden, as well as a higher likelihood of mortality (4, 5). While much of the research on apathy has been driven by dementia research (13), it is also a common preclinical symptom (1). The ISTAART-AA MBI criteria recognize the importance of NPS, including apathy, as early non-cognitive markers of preclinical and prodromal dementia (23). With the development of the MBI-C, research is now in a better position to investigate the role of NPS such as apathy in preclinical and prodromal states.

Diagnosing Apathy in Preclinical and Prodromal Dementia

The identification of valid measures to diagnose apathy in preclinical and prodromal populations is crucial when considering it as a marker of dementia risk. To date, the majority of measures (e.g. Neuropsychiatric Inventory (NPI), Apathy Evaluation Scale (AES), and Apathy Index) used to ascertain apathy in preclinical and prodromal dementia have been developed for use in other clinical populations, and not necessarily as dementia prognosticators. While these measures have been proven to be valuable within the context of MCI and dementia, their value as an apathy ascertainment tool in the context of preclinical and prodromal dementia needs further investigation. Furthermore, with the development of the ISTAART-AA MBI criteria, which require the presence of symptoms for at least 6 months before a diagnosis can be made, the utility of traditional apathy measures may be less specific given the short reference timeframes (commonly 2–4 weeks) used.

The MBI-C (3) has specifically been developed as a case ascertainment tool for MBI in preclinical and prodromal dementia. Apathy is one of the five MBI domains assessed in the MBI-C, with questions reflecting the cognitive (interest), behavioural (initiative), and emotional domains of apathy. Each apathy domain is assessed by two questions. Future research will need to evaluate the efficacy of the MBI-C apathy domain against existing apathy scales (e.g. Dimensional Apathy Scale (31), Apathy Motivation Index (32)) developed for apathy ascertainment in healthy people.

Epidemiology of Apathy in Preclinical and Prodromal Dementia

Apathy in preclinical and prodromal dementia populations, such as those with MBI and MCI, is recognized as an indicator of more rapid progression to dementia (5, 33). Apathy in pre-dementia populations has also been linked to greater cognitive decline, poorer functional performance, reduced daytime activity, greater weight loss, and higher levels of caregiver burden (25).

Individuals with MCI and apathy have an increased risk of developing dementia, ranging from a 42% to 60% greater rate of conversion to dementia (34, 35). Specifically, individuals with MCI and apathy have a 52% higher risk of dementia compared to MCI patients with depression, a 41% higher risk of dementia compared to MCI patients with both depression and apathy, and a 36% higher risk of dementia compared to MCI patients without apathy or depression (34) (Fig. 5.1). As apathy

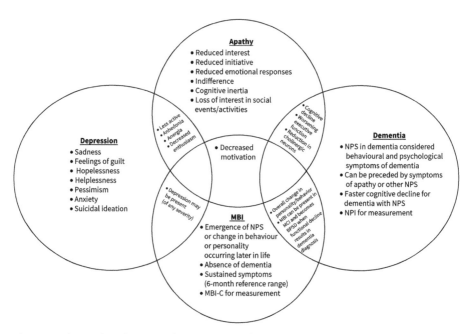

Fig. 5.1 Relationships between dementia, MBI, depression, and apathy.

may precede or be a specific phenotype of MCI and dementia, it is important to understand the prevalence and distribution of apathy among those with preclinical dementia (36).

Similarly, research has also shown that MBI, defined more broadly, confers a 43% higher risk of conversion to dementia compared to MCI (37) in a specialty clinic population. It has been proposed that apathy may be a driving factor underpinning this difference, with apathy reported in 29.4% of patients with MBI compared to only 11.7% of those with MCI (37). Similarly, in cognitively healthy older adults aged 70 years and greater, NPS (especially agitation, apathy, anxiety, irritability, and depression) were linked to an increased risk of developing MCI when compared to cognitively healthy older adults without NPS (20). These findings highlight the importance of apathy as a risk factor for cognitive impairment and dementia.

Despite the growing body of literature suggesting the predictive role apathy plays in progression from pre-dementia to dementia, there is limited research on the prevalence of apathy in preclinical dementia populations. This may in part be due to the fact that many available apathy detection scales were designed for use in populations with more severe impairment and/or dementia (3). The Mild Behavioural Impairment Checklist (MBI-C) offers a scale specific to the assessment of neuropsychiatric symptoms, including apathy, in pre-dementia states (3). The development of such a scale may allow for more detailed understandings of the epidemiology of apathy within preclinical dementia populations.

While the MBI-C has been used to ascertain NPS prevalence in preclinical and prodromal states (38–40), data on apathy prevalence as determined by the MBI-C are sparse. Mean MBI-C apathy domain scores have been reported in the Spanish MBI-C validation studies in primary care patients. In subjective cognitive decline, the mean apathy score was 0.55 (range 0–6) (38). In MCI, the mean apathy score was 1.27 (range 0–11) (39). This suggests that later-life sustained and emergent apathy does occur in these populations, increasing with greater cognitive decline. Research using the operationalized ISTAART-AA MBI criteria (specifically an approximation of Criterion 1, measured with the NPI) in a population-based study has reported prevalence estimates for apathy in 3.1% of cognitively healthy adults, 8.3% of cognitively normal but at-risk adults, and 9% of adults with MCI (41). Higher prevalence estimates of apathy using the same operationalized criteria (using the Neuropsychiatric Inventory Questionnaire (NPI-Q) for measurement) have also been reported for a cognitive neurology clinical sample of subjective cognitive decline (apathy in 38.8%) and MCI (apathy in 49.1%) (42). These estimates are similar to previously reported prevalences of apathy in preclinical and prodromal dementia populations, specifically 39.2% in MBI populations and 3–50.5% in MCI populations (43–45). Apathy levels are also higher in those with premanifest MCI versus those with no cognitive impairment (NCI) (36). Of note, these prevalence estimates are likely inflated and less specific than those with the MBI-C, given the shorter reference range of the ascertainment instrument of 1 month. Certainly, more MBI-C data are required to clarify this issue.

Risk Factors for Apathy in Preclinical and Prodromal Dementia

Apathy in preclinical dementia populations has been largely conceptualized as a subcomponent of depression (2). However, depression is primarily characterized by feelings of self-dislike, guilt, sadness, and worthlessness in contrast to lack of emotion, effort, and initiation observed in those with apathy (46–50). Research also suggests apathy is a stronger predictor of progression from MCI to dementia than depression (34). Interestingly, motivational components of the Beck Depression Inventory are more accurate predictors of progression from preclinical dementia to dementia compared to the somatic and mood components (51).

Some research has suggested age of onset of NPS may influence risk of presenting with apathy versus depression, with older individuals experiencing more apathetic than depressive symptoms (52). Apathy can be misdiagnosed as depression in older adults, especially when it presents as a dementia prodrome (26). Further, ample evidence from longitudinal studies suggests that age of onset of depressive symptoms is an important feature of distinguishing between late-life depression as a classic psychiatric syndrome, and depressive symptoms (some of which may in fact be apathy) as markers of prodromal dementia (27, 53–55). Overall, however, there is a limited understanding of the specific risk factors for the development of apathy in preclinical and prodromal dementia populations.

Treatment and Management of Apathy in Preclinical and Prodromal Dementia

There is limited evidence regarding how to treat apathy in preclinical dementia, both with pharmacological and non-pharmacological interventions (25). This is in part due to inconsistency in how apathy is defined, as well as the lack of a standardized and universally applied scale to assess apathy within preclinical dementia-specific populations (2, 25). However, the development of the aforementioned MBI-C may facilitate preclinical dementia-specific clinical trials (2). Confounding factors such as depression presenting with apathy may also affect understanding of how to specifically target apathy in preclinical dementia populations (2). Relevant to this issue of differentiating apathy from depression, recent factor analyses of the MBI-C in community and clinical samples have demonstrated the stability of a five-factor model, consistent with the five MBI domains. In both groups, the anhedonia affective item loaded onto the apathy factor (56, 57). These findings may suggest that anhedonia in older adults is an element of apathy, in contrast to the conventional major depression construct in which anhedonia is a cardinal symptom, along with depressed mood. Further confirmatory studies are required to explore this interesting finding, and its relevance for treatment. Evidence that does exist for treating apathy in preclinical dementia populations addresses apathy in MCI populations, with no studies investigating treatment of apathy in MBI (25).

Pharmacological

The effects of rivastigmine, an acetylcholinesterase inhibitor frequently used to treat dementia, were evaluated in persons with MCI to slow progression to dementia (33, 58). As a secondary outcome, apathy levels were also assessed. However, no significant difference was seen between placebo and treatment groups in this double-blinded randomized control trial (33). Galantamine (also an acetylcholinesterase inhibitor) and risperidone (an atypical antipsychotic) were used in an open-label randomized control trial in persons with MCI and probable dementia (59–61). Overall, both drugs decreased apathy levels non-significantly, although risperidone was suggested for use to manage only irritability and agitation (25, 61). It is, however, important to note that apathy levels were not a primary outcome of this study (61). Overall, there are limited pharmacological therapies that have been investigated specifically in preclinical dementia populations. Future research should investigate pharmacotherapies such as donepezil, which has yielded improvements in apathy levels in those with mild Alzheimer's Disease (AD) (62, 63). Methylphenidate, a psychostimulant used in those with attention deficit disorder, has also been observed to improve apathy in those with AD (64, 65). Recent studies suggest the investigation of antidepressants to manage apathy in neurodegenerative diseases, such as Parkinson's disease; however, there is limited understanding of the effect of antidepressants in pre-dementia populations, thus further research is warranted (66).

Non-Pharmacological

Repetitive transcranial magnetic stimulation has been found to improve apathy levels in those with MCI (67). Specifically, repetitive transcranial magnetic stimulation significantly decreased apathy levels in the treatment group compared to the control group, among those with MCI (67). Chapter 15 discusses brain stimulation approaches in more detail.

Virtual reality tasks have also been found to improve interest among persons with apathy and MCI, compared to paper-based tasks and the interest expressed by non-apathetic persons with MCI (68). Similarly, engagement and satisfaction levels of those with apathy and MCI mimicked those without apathy and MCI when playing a tablet game. The game was focused on kitchen and cooking tasks and played as much as participants wanted over 4 weeks (69).

Mechanisms of Apathy in Preclinical and Prodromal Dementia

Much of the imaging and biomarker evidence for apathy in pre-dementia comes from MCI or prodromal AD. One of the earliest studies assessing apathy in pre-dementia used structural imaging. From a longitudinal study of 369 participants in an AD research centre, Duara and colleagues described a group of 'pre-MCI' participants who presented with symptomatic cognitive and subtle functional impairment on history, but without neuropsychological testing confirmation of deficits (36). Current nosology might consider these participants as having subjective cognitive decline and preclinical dementia. Compared to those with NCI, there were higher apathy scores and lower left hippocampal volumes in those with pre-MCI. Over 2–3 years, 28.6% of pre-MCI subjects and less than 5% of NCI subjects progressed to MCI or dementia. Apathy was measured as a symptom with the NPI, rather than a syndromic description of apathy. Nonetheless, this suggests that the hippocampus may be associated with preclinical apathy. A small study by Marshall and colleagues supports the notion of apathy as a pre-dementia manifestation (70). In 24 participants with MCI, apathy (measured by the AES) was associated with greater amyloid burden based on Pittsburgh B Compound uptake. A magnetic resonance imaging study of a mixed population of NCI (n = 19) and MCI (n = 47) found that inferior temporal cortex thinning was predictive of AES-measured apathy, suggesting apathy-specific structural changes in pre-dementia (71).

With respect to functional neuroimaging, two Alzheimer's Disease Neuroimaging Initiative (ADNI) studies provide insight. Delrieu and colleagues assessed 65 ADNI-1 participants with MCI, 11 of whom had apathy as measured by the NPI-Q (72). There were no differences between groups in neuropsychological testing, or global and hippocampal volumetric analysis. However, the apathy group revealed a significant decrease of glucose cerebral metabolism over the posterior cingulum. Again, apathy was measured as a symptom, rather than a syndrome, but the study provides some compelling evidence for apathy as a prodromal symptom. These are important findings given that the earliest fluorodeoxyglucose-positron emission tomography (FDG-PET) manifestations of AD are often posterior cingulate hypometabolism, which may emerge in advance of clear structural changes. Gatchel and colleagues analysed FDG-PET data in 402 ADNI participants with NCI (n = 104), amnestic MCI (n = 203), and mild AD dementia (n = 95) (73). Consistent with the findings of Delrieu and colleagues, they determined that cross-sectionally, posterior cingulate hypometabolism was associated with higher apathy scores (measured by the NPI-Q). Longitudinally, there was an interaction between posterior cingulate and supramarginal gyrus hypometabolism and higher apathy scores across time. Together these findings suggest an association of apathy with metabolic changes in parietal regions, usually associated with early-stage AD, in contrast to medial frontal regions often implicated in later-stage AD.

Exploratory imaging studies have also assessed the role of tau in MCI and early AD. Marshall and colleagues used PET flortaucipir in a small sample (24 MCI, 16 AD dementia) of participants, with apathy syndromically measured using the AES informant report (74). Using whole-brain analysis, apathy was associated with tau in small clusters within the right anterior cingulate and dorsolateral prefrontal cortices, which were more pronounced in individuals with greater amyloid. However, it is un-clear to what extent the AD participants drove the results and if information can be generalized to other pre-dementia participants.

Proton magnetic resonance spectroscopy has also been used to assess the neural sig-natures of apathy. In a clinically diagnosed sample with amnestic MCI ($n = 28$) versus controls ($n = 20$), Tumati and colleagues determined that apathy in amnestic MCI pa-tients was associated with neurometabolite changes indicative of altered membranal integrity and glial function in the right temporoparietal cortex (75). Apathy was measured using the AES, and depression, measured with the Geriatric Depression Scale, was controlled for. Importantly, this study suggested that in amnestic MCI, ap-athy symptoms may be suggestive of neural changes that are distinct from amnestic MCI without apathy, emphasizing the utility of assessing apathy in MCI.

Functional connectivity studies may help in the integration of the structural and functional neuroimaging findings. Joo and colleagues used functional magnetic res-onance imaging to assess 50 NCI participants and 50 participants with amnestic MCI (76). Apathy was syndromically measured using the Apathy Inventory. In the MCI group, total apathy score was negatively correlated with functional connectivity of the anterior and posterior cingulate within the default mode network. In contrast, apathy was positively correlated with functional connectivity of the middle frontal, inferior frontal, and supramarginal gyrus within the central executive network. In sum, these findings suggest that there may be circuitry changes in pre-dementia that are associ-ated with apathy, with the default mode network playing a central role. Theoretically, disruption of any node in the circuit could be associated with apathy. As better evi-dence in preclinical dementia emerges, with improved mechanisms to detect early phase disease, this circuitry will become clearer.

The Role of Apathy in Mild Behavioural Impairment and Understanding Preclinical and Prodromal Dementia

With the evolution of research into apathy, it is becoming clear that there is public health significance and clinical utility in identifying apathy. In pre-dementia states, an underappreciation of apathy can result in delays in seeking clinical care, and a pas-sive acceptance to the 'mellowing out' of older adults. This acquiescence stems from a lack of understanding about the role of apathy in incident cognitive decline and de-mentia. A systematic review and meta-analysis by van Dalen and colleagues assessed

16 studies comprising 7365 participants (1470 with apathy) from prospective cohorts in the general population and in memory clinics (5). The authors suggested, 'Apathy is a relevant, non-invasive, cheap, and easily implementable prognostic factor prodromal to dementia'. It was felt that findings were generalizable to memory clinics but less so to a general population. The question remains, then, regarding how to reliably detect apathy in advance of MCI or prodromal dementia, in a specific and reliable way in order to identify those at risk. Measurement was a source of bias, and apathy definition contributed to study heterogeneity.

As described previously, MBI is a validated syndrome that describes the neurobehavioural axis of dementia risk, as a complement to the neurocognitive axis represented by subjective cognitive decline and MCI. Apathy is a prominent domain (domain one) in MBI, and the MBI-C is the case ascertainment tool developed specifically to capture MBI criteria, including the mandated symptom duration of 6 months and emergence in later life. The sustained duration of symptoms in the criteria were included to decrease false positives, increasing the specificity of the criteria. Importantly, apathy, as represented in the MBI-C, is a syndromic rather than symptomatic measurement of apathy. In the MBI-C there are six questions about apathy, two each mapping onto interest (cognitive apathy), initiative (behavioural apathy), and emotion (emotional apathy). The a priori development of the MBI-C was to capture apathy syndromically and allow abstraction of each of the three apathy domains for subsequent research and clinical prognostication.

Outcomes and Future Directions

In order to improve outcomes of apathy in those with preclinical and prodromal dementia, future research must focus on further investigation into the use of detection tools suitable for those populations, such as the MBI-C. It is anticipated there will be clinical utility in early detection and subsequent treatment of NPS, such as apathy in preclinical and prodromal dementia populations (40). Overall, apathy in preclinical and prodromal dementia is at the early stages of understanding. Researchers hypothesize that improved early detection of NPS such as apathy will offer an efficient and cost-effective means to increase early detection of dementia (40). Further understandings surrounding the mechanistic underpinnings of apathy may also help expand the number of available and understood treatment options for those with preclinical and prodromal dementia.

References

1. Lanctôt KL, Agüera-Ortiz L, Brodaty H, Francis PT, Geda YE, Ismail Z, et al. Apathy associated with neurocognitive disorders: recent progress and future directions. Alzheimers Dement. 2017;13(1):84–100.

2. Cummings J, Friedman JH, Garibaldi G, Jones M, Macfadden W, Marsh L, et al. Apathy in neurodegenerative diseases: recommendations on the design of clinical trials. J Geriatr Psychiatry Neurol. 2015;28(3):159–73.

3. Ismail Z, Agüera-Ortiz L, Brodaty H, Cieslak A, Cummings J, Fischer CE, et al. The mild behavioral impairment checklist (MBI-C): a rating scale for neuropsychiatric symptoms in pre-dementia populations. J Alzheimers Dis. 2017;56(3):929–38.

4. van der Linde RM, Matthews FE, Dening T, Brayne C. Patterns and persistence of behavioural and psychological symptoms in those with cognitive impairment: the importance of apathy. Int J Geriatr Psychiatry. 2017;32(3):306–15.

5. van Dalen JW, van Wanrooij LL, Moll van Charante EP, Brayne C, van Gool WA, Richard E. Association of apathy with risk of incident dementia: a systematic review and meta-analysis. JAMA Psychiatry. 2018;75(10):1012–21.

6. Lyketsos CG, Carrillo MC, Ryan JM, Khachaturian AS, Trzepacz P, Amatniek J, et al. Neuropsychiatric symptoms in Alzheimer's disease. Alzheimers Dementia. 2011;7(5):532–9.

7. Peters ME, Rosenberg PB, Steinberg M, Tschanz JT, Norton MC, Welsh-Bohmer KA, et al. Prevalence of neuropsychiatric symptoms in CIND and its subtypes: the Cache County Study. Am J Geriatr Psychiatry. 2012;20(5):416–24.

8. Geda YE, Roberts RO, Knopman DS, Petersen RC, Christianson TJ, Pankratz VS, et al. Prevalence of neuropsychiatric symptoms in mild cognitive impairment and normal cognitive aging: population-based study. Arch Gen Psychiatry. 2008;65(10):1193–8.

9. Ismail Z, Elbayoumi H, Smith EE, Fischer CE, Schweizer TA, Millikin C, et al. A systematic review and meta-analysis for the prevalence of depression in mild cognitive impairment. JAMA Psychiatry. 2017;74(1):58–67.

10. Steinberg M, Shao H, Zandi P, Lyketsos CG, Welsh-Bohmer KA, Norton MC, et al. Point and 5-year period prevalence of neuropsychiatric symptoms in dementia: the Cache County Study. Int J Geriatr Psychiatry. 2008;23(2):170–7.

11. Lyketsos CG, Lopez O, Jones B, Fitzpatrick AL, Breitner J, DeKosky S. Prevalence of neuropsychiatric symptoms in dementia and mild cognitive impairment: results from the cardiovascular health study. JAMA. 2002;288(12):1475–83.

12. Gitlin LN, Piersol CV, Hodgson N, Marx K, Roth DL, Johnston D, et al. Reducing neuropsychiatric symptoms in persons with dementia and associated burden in family caregivers using tailored activities: design and methods of a randomized clinical trial. Contemp Clin Trials. 2016;49:92–102.

13. Lanctot KL, Amatniek J, Ancoli-Israel S, Arnold SE, Ballard C, Cohen-Mansfield J, et al. Neuropsychiatric signs and symptoms of Alzheimer's disease: new treatment paradigms. Alzheimers Dement (N Y). 2017;3(3):440–9.

14. Fischer CE, Ismail Z, Schweizer TA. Delusions increase functional impairment in Alzheimer's disease. Dement Geriatr Cogn Disord. 2012;33(6):393–9.

15. Fischer CE, Ismail Z, Schweizer TA. Impact of neuropsychiatric symptoms on caregiver burden in patients with Alzheimer's disease. Neurodegener Dis Manag. 2012;2(3):269–77.

16. Pink A, Stokin GB, Bartley MM, Roberts RO, Sochor O, Machulda MM, et al. Neuropsychiatric symptoms, APOE epsilon4, and the risk of incident dementia: a population-based study. Neurology. 2015;84(9):935–43.

17. Rosenberg PB, Mielke MM, Appleby BS, Oh ES, Geda YE, Lyketsos CG. The association of neuropsychiatric symptoms in MCI with incident dementia and Alzheimer disease. Am J Geriatr Psychiatry. 2013;21(7):685–95.

18. Taragano FE, Allegri RF, Heisecke SL, Martelli MI, Feldman ML, Sanchez V, et al. Risk of conversion to dementia in a mild behavioral impairment group compared to a psychiatric group and to a mild cognitive impairment group. J Alzheimers Dis. 2018;62(1):227–38.

19. Forrester SN, Gallo JJ, Smith GS, Leoutsakos JM. Patterns of neuropsychiatric symptoms in mild cognitive impairment and risk of dementia. Am J Geriatr Psychiatry. 2016;24(2):117–25.
20. Geda YE, Roberts RO, Mielke MM, Knopman DS, Christianson TJ, Pankratz VS, et al. Baseline neuropsychiatric symptoms and the risk of incident mild cognitive impairment: a population-based study. Am J Psychiatry. 2014;171(5):572–81.
21. Mortby ME, Burns R, Eramudugolla R, Ismail Z, Anstey KJ. Neuropsychiatric symptoms and cognitive impairment: understanding the importance of co-morbid symptoms. J Alzheimers Dis. 2017;59(1):141–53.
22. Mortby ME, Lyketsos CG, Geda YE, Ismail Z. Special Issue on mild behavioral impairment and non-cognitive prodromes to dementia. Int Psychogeriatr. 2018;30(2):167–9.
23. Ismail Z, Smith EE, Geda Y, Sultzer D, Brodaty H, Smith G, et al. Neuropsychiatric symptoms as early manifestations of emergent dementia: provisional diagnostic criteria for mild behavioral impairment. Alzheimers Dement. 2016;12(2):195–202.
24. Matsuoka T, Ismail Z, Narumoto J. Prevalence of mild behavioral impairment and risk of dementia in a psychiatric outpatient clinic. J Alzheimers Dis. 2019;70(2):505–13.
25. Sherman C, Liu CS, Herrmann N, Lanctôt KL. Prevalence, neurobiology, and treatments for apathy in prodromal dementia. Int Psychogeriatr. 2018;30(2):177–84.
26. Cieslak A, Smith EE, Lysack J, Ismail Z. Case series of mild behavioral impairment: toward an understanding of the early stages of neurodegenerative diseases affecting behavior and cognition. Int Psychogeriatr. 2018;30(2):273–80.
27. Ismail Z, Gatchel J, Bateman DR, Barcelos-Ferreira R, Cantillon M, Jaeger J, et al. Affective and emotional dysregulation as pre-dementia risk markers: exploring the mild behavioral impairment symptoms of depression, anxiety, irritability, and euphoria. Int Psychogeriatr. 2018;30(2):185–96.
28. Nagata T, Kobayashi N, Shinagawa S, Yamada H, Kondo K, Nakayama K. Plasma BDNF levels are correlated with aggressiveness in patients with amnestic mild cognitive impairment or Alzheimer disease. J Neural Transm. 2014;121(4):433–41.
29. Desmarais P, Lanctot KL, Masellis M, Black SE, Herrmann N. Social inappropriateness in neurodegenerative disorders. Int Psychogeriatr. 2018;30(2):197–207.
30. Fischer CE, Agüera-Ortiz L. Psychosis and dementia: risk factor, prodrome, or cause? Int Psychogeriatr. 2018;30(2):209–19.
31. Radakovic R, Abrahams S. Developing a new apathy measurement scale: Dimensional Apathy Scale. Psychiatry Res. 2014;219(3):658–63.
32. Ang YS, Lockwood P, Apps MA, Muhammed K, Husain M. Distinct subtypes of apathy revealed by the apathy motivation index. PLoS One. 2017;12(1):e0169938.
33. Feldman HH, Ferris S, Winblad B, Sfikas N, Mancione L, He Y, et al. Effect of rivastigmine on delay to diagnosis of Alzheimer's disease from mild cognitive impairment: the InDDEx study. Lancet Neurol. 2007;6(6):501–12.
34. Vicini Chilovi B, Conti M, Zanetti M, Mazzu I, Rozzini L, Padovani A. Differential impact of apathy and depression in the development of dementia in mild cognitive impairment patients. Dement Geriatr Cogn Disord. 2009;27(4):390–8.
35. Richard E, Schmand B, Eikelenboom P, Yang SC, Ligthart SA, Charante EPM van, et al. Symptoms of apathy are associated with progression from mild cognitive impairment to Alzheimer's disease in non-depressed subjects. Dement Geriatr Cogn Disord. 2012;33(2–3):204–9.
36. Duara R, Loewenstein DA, Potter E, Barker W, Raj A, Schoenberg M, et al. Pre-MCI and MCI: neuropsychological, clinical, and imaging features and progression rates. Am J Geriatr Psychiatry. 2011;19(11):951–60.

37. Taragano FE, Allegri RF, Krupitzki H, Sarasola DR, Serrano CM, Lon L, et al. Mild behavioral impairment and risk of dementia: a prospective cohort study of 358 patients. J Clin Psychiatry. 2009;70(4):584–92.

38. Mallo SC, Ismail Z, Pereiro AX, Facal D, Lojo-Seoane C, Campos-Magdaleno M, et al. Assessing mild behavioral impairment with the mild behavioral impairment checklist in people with subjective cognitive decline. Int Psychogeriatr. 2019;31(2):231–9.

39. Mallo SC, Ismail Z, Pereiro AX, Facal D, Lojo-Seoane C, Campos-Magdaleno M, et al. Assessing mild behavioral impairment with the Mild Behavioral Impairment-Checklist in people with mild cognitive impairment. J Alzheimers Dis. 2018;66(1):83–95.

40. Creese B, Brooker H, Ismail Z, Wesnes K, Hampshire A, Khan Z, et al. Mild behavioral impairment as a marker of cognitive decline in cognitively normal older adults. Am J Geriatr Psychiatry. 2019;27(8):823–34.

41. Mortby ME, Ismail Z, Anstey KJ. Prevalence estimates of mild behavioral impairment in a population-based sample of pre-dementia states and cognitively healthy older adults. Int Psychogeriatr. 2018;30(2):221–32.

42. Sheikh F, Ismail Z, Mortby ME, Barber P, Cieslak A, Fischer K, et al. Prevalence of mild behavioral impairment in mild cognitive impairment and subjective cognitive decline, and its association with caregiver burden. Int Psychogeriatr. 2018;30(2):233–44.

43. Barcelos-Ferreira R, Folquitto JC, Tascone LDS, Bottino CMC. Mild behavioral impairment associated to higher prevalence of dementia in community-dwelling elderly subjects. Alzheimers Dement. 2015;11(7):P521.

44. Onyike CU, Sheppard JME, Tschanz JT, Norton MC, Green RC, Steinberg M, et al. Epidemiology of apathy in older adults: the Cache County Study. Am J Geriatr Psychiatry. 2007;15(5):365–75.

45. Fernández-Martínez M, Molano A, Castro J, Zarranz JJ. Prevalence of neuropsychiatric symptoms in mild cognitive impairment and Alzheimer's disease, and its relationship with cognitive impairment. Curr Alzheimer Res. 2010;7(6):517–26.

46. Kirsch-Darrow L, Marsiske M, Okun MS, Bauer R, Bowers D. Apathy and depression: separate factors in Parkinson's disease. J Int Neuropsychol Soc. 2011;17(6):1058–66.

47. Kirsch-Darrow L, Fernandez HF, Marsiske M, Okun MS, Bowers D. Dissociating apathy and depression in Parkinson disease. Neurology. 2006;67(1):33–8.

48. Alzahrani H, Venneri A. Cognitive and neuroanatomical correlates of neuropsychiatric symptoms in Parkinson's disease: a systematic review. J Neurol Sci. 2015;356(1–2):32–44.

49. Oguru M, Tachibana H, Toda K, Okuda B, Oka N. Apathy and depression in Parkinson's disease. J Geriatr Psychiatry Neurol. 2010;23(1):35–41.

50. Levy ML, Cummings JL, Fairbanks LA, Masterman D, Miller BL, Craig AH, et al. Apathy is not depression. J Neuropsychiatry Clin Neurosci. 1998;10(3):314–9.

51. Bartolini M, Coccia M, Luzzi S, Provinciali L, Ceravolo MG. Motivational symptoms of depression mask preclinical Alzheimer's disease in elderly subjects. Dement Geriatr Cogn Disord. 2005;19(1):31–6.

52. Mehta M, Whyte E, Lenze E, Hardy S, Roumani Y, Subashan P, et al. Depressive symptoms in late life: associations with apathy, resilience and disability vary between young-old and old-old. Int J Geriatr Psychiatry. 2008;23(3):238–43.

53. Singh-Manoux A, Dugravot A, Fournier A, Abell J, Ebmeier K, Kivimäki M, et al. Trajectories of depressive symptoms before diagnosis of dementia: a 28-year follow-up study. JAMA Psychiatry. 2017;74(7):712–8.

54. Tapiainen V, Hartikainen S, Taipale H, Tiihonen J, Tolppanen AM. Hospital-treated mental and behavioral disorders and risk of Alzheimer's disease: a nationwide nested case-control study. Eur Psychiatry. 2017;43:92–8.

55. Almeida OP, Hankey GJ, Yeap BB, Golledge J, Flicker L. Depression as a modifiable factor to decrease the risk of dementia. Transl Psychiatry. 2017;7(5):e1117.

56. Hu S. Validation of the mild behavioral impairment-checklist in subjective cognitive decline, mild cognitive impairment and dementia (Unpublished master's thesis). University of Calgary, Calgary, AB, Canada. 2019. Available at: https://prism.ucalgary.ca/handle/1880/110515.

57. Creese B, Griffiths A, Brooker H, Corbett A, Aarsland D, Ballard C, et al. Profile of mild behavioral impairment and factor structure of the mild behavioral impairment checklist in cognitively normal older adults. Int Psychogeriatr. 2020;32(6):705–17.

58. Khoury R, Rajamanickam J, Grossberg GT. An update on the safety of current therapies for Alzheimer's disease: focus on rivastigmine. Ther Adv Drug Saf. 2018;9(3):171–8.

59. Scott LJ, Goa KL. Galantamine. Drugs. 2000;60(5):1095–122.

60. Grant S, Fitton A. Risperidone. Drugs. 1994;48(2):253–73.

61. Freund-Levi Y, Jedenius E, Tysen-Bäckström AC, Lärksäter M, Wahlund LO, Eriksdotter M. Galantamine versus risperidone treatment of neuropsychiatric symptoms in patients with probable dementia: an open randomized trial. Am J Geriatr Psychiatry. 2014;22(4):341–8.

62. Cacabelos R. Donepezil in Alzheimer's disease: from conventional trials to pharmacogenetics. Neuropsychiatr Dis Treat. 2007;3(3):303–33.

63. Drijgers RL, Aalten P, Winogrodzka A, Verhey FRJ, Leentjens AFG. Pharmacological treatment of apathy in neurodegenerative diseases: a systematic review. Dement Geriatr Cogn Disord. 2009;28(1):13–22.

64. Rosenberg PB, Lanctôt KL, Drye LT, Herrmann N, Scherer RW, Bachman DL, et al. Safety and efficacy of methylphenidate for apathy in Alzheimer's disease: a randomized, placebo-controlled trial. J Clin Psychiatry. 2013;74(8):810–6.

65. Lanctôt KL, Chau SA, Herrmann N, Drye LT, Rosenberg PB, Scherer RW, et al. Effect of methylphenidate on attention in apathetic AD patients in a randomized, placebo-controlled trial. Int Psychogeriatr. 2014;26(2):239–46.

66. Takahashi M, Tabu H, Ozaki A, Hamano T, Takeshima T, Group for the R study. Antidepressants for depression, apathy, and gait instability in Parkinson's disease: a multicenter randomized study. Intern Med. 2019;58(3):361–8.

67. Padala PR, Padala KP, Lensing SY, Jackson AN, Hunter CR, Parkes CM, et al. Repetitive transcranial magnetic stimulation for apathy in mild cognitive impairment: a double-blind, randomized, sham-controlled, cross-over pilot study. Psychiatry Res. 2018;261:312–8.

68. Manera V, Chapoulie E, Bourgeois J, Guerchouche R, David R, Ondrej J, et al. A feasibility study with image-based rendered virtual reality in patients with mild cognitive impairment and dementia. PLoS One. 2016;11(3):e0151487.

69. Manera V, Petit PD, Derreumaux A, Orvieto I, Romagnoli M, Lyttle G, et al. 'Kitchen and cooking,' a serious game for mild cognitive impairment and Alzheimer's disease: a pilot study. Front Aging Neurosci. 2015;7:24.

70. Marshall GA, Donovan NJ, Lorius N, Gidicsin CM, Maye J, Pepin LC, et al. Apathy is associated with increased amyloid burden in mild cognitive impairment. J Neuropsychiatry Clin Neurosci. 2013;25(4):302–7.

71. Guercio BJ, Donovan NJ, Ward A, Schultz A, Lorius N, Amariglio RE, et al. Apathy is associated with lower inferior temporal cortical thickness in mild cognitive impairment and normal elderly individuals. J Neuropsychiatry Clin Neurosci. 2015;27(1):e22–7.

72. Delrieu J, Desmidt T, Camus V, Sourdet S, Boutoleau-Bretonnière C, Mullin E, et al. Apathy as a feature of prodromal Alzheimer's disease: an FDG-PET ADNI study. Int J Geriatr Psychiatry. 2015;30(5):470–7.

73. Gatchel JR, Donovan NJ, Locascio JJ, Becker JA, Rentz DM, Sperling RA, et al. Regional 18F-fluorodeoxyglucose hypometabolism is associated with higher apathy scores over time in early Alzheimer disease. Am J Geriatr Psychiatry. 2017;25(7):683–93.

74. Marshall GA, Gatchel JR, Donovan NJ, Muniz MC, Schultz AP, Becker JA, et al. Regional tau correlates of instrumental activities of daily living and apathy in mild cognitive impairment and Alzheimer's disease dementia. J Alzheimers Dis. 2019;67(2):757–68.

75. Tumati S, Opmeer EM, Marsman JC, Martens S, Reesink FE, De Deyn PP, et al. Lower choline and myo-inositol in temporo-parietal cortex is associated with apathy in amnestic MCI. Front Aging Neurosci. 2018;10:106.

76. Joo SH, Lee CU, Lim HK. Apathy and intrinsic functional connectivity networks in amnestic mild cognitive impairment. Neuropsychiatr Dis Treat. 2017;13:61–7.

6

Apathy in Cerebrovascular Disorders

Sergio Starkstein and Bradleigh Hayhow

Introduction

Apathy is defined as a pervasive neuropsychiatric syndrome characterized by a lack of motivation that persists over time and which causes identifiable functional impairment (1). In one of the first studies to examine the frequency and correlates of apathy in stroke, Starkstein et al. (2) assessed a consecutive series of 80 patients in the acute stage post stroke using a scale to measure the severity of apathy and reported that 11% had apathy in the absence of depression. Since this review publication, a number of other studies have examined the frequency, clinical correlates, mechanism, and treatment of post-stroke apathy.

We begin this chapter by reviewing the phenomenology and diagnosis of apathy in stroke. This is followed by a review of the frequency, comorbidities, mechanism, and treatment of this condition. We finish by addressing the limitations to the study of post-stroke apathy, and by providing suggestions for future studies.

Phenomenology and Diagnosis of Post-Stroke Apathy

In 1991, Robert Marin formulated a concept of apathy as an independent neuro-psychiatric syndrome characterized by deficits in goal-directed behaviours as manifested by the simultaneous diminution in the cognitive, behavioural, and emotional concomitants of motivation (3). Marin described reduced goal-directed behaviour as manifested by lack of effort, initiative, and productivity. Finally, reduced goal-directed cognition is manifested by decreased interests, lack of plans and goals, and lack of concern about one's own health and functional status, and reduced emotional state as manifested by flat affect, emotional indifference, and restricted responses to important life events (3). Later, Marin and Wilkosz conceptualized apathy as a psychological syndrome of reduced motivation manifested as behavioural changes (4). In contrast, Levy and Dubois conceptualized apathy as a pure behavioural syndrome and suggested that apathy should not be defined as lack of motivation (5). They considered apathy to be an observable behavioural syndrome comprising a reduction of self-generated voluntary and purposeful behaviours, stressing that the behavioural change should occur in the absence of contextual or physical changes, and should be reversed by external stimulation.

Besides this conceptual discrepancy, an empirical problem is how to separate apathy from depression, given the overlap of symptoms such as diminished interest and pleasure, loss of energy, poor concentration, and diminished motor activity. Given this overlap, it is not surprising that several studies have reported a significant association between depression and apathy in stroke (2, 6), although this was not replicated in other studies (7, 8). It is likely that this discrepancy is related to the different strategies and instruments used to assess apathy in stroke. One of the main limitations is that there are no valid and reliable structured interviews for apathy in neurological conditions, and standardized criteria for the diagnosis of apathy are in the process of validation and replication (1) (Box 6.1).

Ideally, any psychiatric disorder should be diagnosed using a structured interview and standardized diagnostic criteria. Marin and Wilkosz suggested that the assessment of apathy should include the individual's social and physical environment, and further stressed the importance of taking into consideration the great variability in each individual's goals, interests, emotional displays, and activities, which are all influenced by life experience, education, social status, and age cohort (4). Marin also suggested that apathy should not be diagnosed in the context of poor attention, moderate or severe cognitive deficits, or marked emotional distress (9). Nevertheless, apathy is a frequent finding among individuals with some degree of cognitive impairment, and cognitive deficits are not sufficient to produce apathy, since individuals with similar cognitive deficits may show major differences in apathy levels (10). Whether the syndrome of apathy associated with cognitive deficits has a different phenomenology than the syndrome of apathy in other neurological conditions such as cerebrovascular disease has yet to be empirically examined.

Assessing for apathy in neurological conditions is still a complex undertaking. A semi-structured interview for apathy has been validated for use in Alzheimer's disease (11), but such an instrument for stroke patients is still lacking. A set of standardized diagnostic criteria to diagnose apathy have been validated for use in Parkinson's disease but not yet among stroke patients (12).

An extensive revision for preliminary diagnostic criteria for apathy has recently been published (1). This revision was based on recommendations from a Delphi panel based on empirical findings. These criteria are yet to be validated in cerebrovascular disorders (13). Apathy scales should be used to measure the severity of this condition, although in research studies cut-off scores on these instruments are usually used for diagnostic purposes.

The apathy rating scales most commonly used in stroke are the apathy section of the Neuropsychiatric Inventory (NPI) (14), the Apathy Evaluation Scale (AES) (15), and the Apathy Scale (AS) (2). The AES is an 18-item instrument with three versions to be rated by the patient, the clinician, or the caregiver. The AS is a 14-item scale rated by the patient which is based on the AES. The NPI is a multidimensional instrument that

Box 6.1 Diagnostic criteria for apathy

Criterion A A quantitative reduction of behavioural, cognitive, or emotional goal-directed activity as compared to previous level of functioning.

Criterion B The presence of symptoms in at least two of the following three syndromes for at least 4 weeks:

B1. *Behaviour and cognition*:
  - *General level of activity*: reduced activity in daily life activities, with less effort and needs to be prompted.
  - *Persistence of activity*: decreased persistence in communication and in finding solutions to obstacles.
  - *Making choices*: loss of interest in choosing activities.
  - *Interest in external issues*: decreased reactivity to daily events or in starting new activities.
  - *Personal well-being*: less interest in one's own health and appearance.

B2. *Emotion*:
  - *Spontaneous emotions*: diminished emotions about own affairs.
  - *Emotional reactions to environment*: diminished emotions about external events.
  - *Impact on others*: diminished concern about the influence of own actions on others.
  - *Empathy*: less interest in the emotions or needs of others.
  - *Verbal or physical expressions*: reduced expressions demonstrating a reduced emotional state.

B3. *Social interaction*:
  - *Spontaneous social initiative*: loss of initiative in social activities.
  - *Environmentally stimulated social interaction*: less participation and indifference to social activities.
  - *Relationship with family members*: loss of interest in arranging or participating in family activities.
  - *Verbal interaction*: decreased conversations and/or withdrawing from verbal interaction.

Criterion C Symptoms A and B cause significant impairment in social and working areas of functioning.

Criterion D Apathy symptoms are not exclusively explained due to physical disabilities, motor, or attentional problems, the use of substances that may produce symptoms of apathy, or major changes in the individual's environment.

is administered to caregivers, and apathy is assessed together with nine other behavioural and emotional domains. It has been empirically demonstrated that using the NPI and the AS on the same sample results in different rates of apathy (16). Therefore, the type of instrument used should be carefully considered when reviewing the frequency of apathy in stroke.

Starkstein et al. (11) validated a structured interview to diagnose apathy in dementia based on clinical criteria proposed by Starkstein and Leentjens (13). The structured interview includes questions assessing the domains of lack of motivation relative to the individual's previous level of functioning, lack of effort to perform everyday activities, dependency on others to structure activity, lack of interest in learning new things or in new experiences, lack of concern about one's own personal problems, unchanging or flat affect, and lack of emotional response to positive or negative personal events.

In conclusion, the nosological position of apathy in stroke is still unclear. Apathy is not listed in either the *Diagnostic and Statistical Manual of Mental Disorders*, fifth edition (DSM-5) (17) or in the International Classification of Diseases, tenth revision (ICD-10) (18). This could change given the high prevalence of this syndrome in neuropsychiatric disorders. Nevertheless, it has yet to be established what the necessary and sufficient symptoms are for a reliable diagnosis of apathy, and whether apathy should be considered as a symptom or a syndrome.

Prevalence of Apathy in Stroke

Several cross-sectional and longitudinal studies have examined the prevalence of apathy in stroke. The first study in stroke was carried out by Starkstein and colleagues who reported a frequency of apathy in the absence of depression of 11% (2). Later studies reported higher frequencies. Angelelli et al. (6) administered the NPI to a group of 124 individuals at different intervals since stroke and to 61 healthy controls. Apathy was significantly more frequent among stroke patients (27% of the sample), and was more frequent in the chronic phase after the stroke. Brodaty et al. (19) examined the frequency of apathy in 135 patients 3–6 months after an acute ischaemic stroke and in 109 control subjects matched for sex and age. Apathy was diagnosed in 27% of stroke patients and in 5% of age-comparable healthy controls. Using the NPI, Hama et al. (20) diagnosed apathy in 19% of 237 patients with acute stroke. Within a period of 3 months after stroke, Santa et al. (21) diagnosed apathy in 21% of 14 patients using the AS.

The Mikami et al. (22) study examined the frequency of apathy after excluding stroke patients with both major and minor depression. Patients with an acute stroke were assessed for apathy using the Robert criteria (1) at 3, 6, 9, and 12 months based on the modified AS. The authors found that 23 patients (41% of the sample) had apathy at one or more of the assessments during the 12-month follow-up, and apathy was most frequent during the first months after stroke. About one-third of the patients with apathy also developed major depression, as compared to only 9% of the non-apathy group, suggesting that post-stroke apathy may lead to depression.

Kennedy et al. (23) carried out an important study examining the frequency of apathy among patients with aphasia. The study included inpatients for acute rehabilitation, and the main finding was that apathy was present in 53% of patients with aphasia as compared to 22% among patients without aphasia. Patients with apathy were more likely to be discharged from the rehabilitation unit to a nursing home rather than to their homes. In contrast, Carota et al. (8) did not find significant differences in the frequency of apathy between individuals with or without aphasia. This discrepancy could be related to the implicit difficulty in measuring apathy among individuals with aphasia given the lack of a valid instrument for this population.

Caeiro et al. (24) carried out a systematic review and meta-analysis of the frequency of apathy that included 26 publications from 19 stroke samples. The pooled rate of apathy was 36% (95% confidence interval (CI) 30–43%) with a range of 15–71%. This wide range may be explained by the fact that some studies included patients with depression, which may have increased the frequency of apathy. The frequency of apathy during the acute stage was estimated at 39.5% (95% CI 29–51%), and 34% for the post-acute stage (95% CI 28–41%).

In one of the few longitudinal studies, Caeiro et al. (25) reported that 41% of stroke patients with baseline apathy remained apathetic 12 months later. When only the frequency of apathy without depression was estimated, the pooled estimate declined to 21% (95% CI 15–29%). The Caeiro et al. (24) meta-analysis only included two longitudinal studies of apathy in stroke, with 55% of patients with apathy remaining apathetic at 15-month follow-up in one study (26), with similar findings reported by the second study (50% of patients with apathy remained apathetic 12 months later) (27). In another longitudinal study, Brodaty et al. (28) examined the course of apathy during a 5-year period. They found that the frequency of apathy increased steadily over this timeframe from 27% to 39%. The high attrition rate was an important limitation of the study, which may have underrated the 5-year frequency of post-stroke apathy.

Lohner et al. (29) examined the frequency of apathy among patients with systematic lacunar strokes as compared to age-comparable healthy controls. The authors used subitems of the Geriatric Depression Scale (GDS) to diagnose apathy such as 'prefer to stay at home', 'avoid social gatherings', dropped activities and interests', 'find life very exciting', 'hard to start new projects', and 'full of energy'. Whereas there is a clear conceptual overlap between these items and questions for apathy, the authors confirmed their approach with a factor analysis. They found that 16% of patients had apathy only, 12% had apathy and depression, and 1% had depression only, an unusual finding given the well-replicated high frequency of depression among individuals with subcortical strokes. Hollocks et al. (30) examined the frequency of apathy and depression among individuals with small vessel disease (SVD), produced by pathology in small perforating arteries leading to white matter lesions and lacunar infarcts. This study compared 121 individuals with SVD and 398 healthy controls. The main finding was that whereas 18% of SVD individuals had apathy alone, 34% had apathy and depression. Unfortunately, the frequency of apathy in controls was not reported.

Van Dalen et al. (16) carried out another systematic review and meta-analysis that included 35 publications (24 on the prevalence of apathy and 11 on treatment). These authors reported a frequency of apathy of 30% regardless of time since stroke, with 40% of patients with apathy having comorbid depression. Among age-comparable healthy volunteers, the frequency of apathy was 6% at baseline and 16% 5 years later. The authors stressed that the use of the NPI resulted in lower estimates of apathy (e.g. 19% of participants diagnosed with apathy based on the NPI as compared to 41% based on the AS) (20).

Of note, a study in the community showed that about a quarter of non-demented community dwelling elderly individuals also have apathy (31, 32). In a study by Caeiro et al. (25) in a sample of 94 patients assessed immediately after stroke, 38% had apathy as compared to 24% of acute admissions to a coronary unit, although the difference was not significant.

In conclusion, about one-third of stroke patients will show apathy in the acute phase after stroke. There are few longitudinal studies on apathy in stroke, and the frequency of apathy is usually confounded by coexistent depression or cognitive impairments.

Clinical Impact

The impact of apathy on the recovery process from stroke is still unclear. Hama et al. (7) and Caeiro et al. (25) found a significant correlation between higher apathy scores and less functional recovery. On the other hand, a systematic review (24) found no significant association between apathy and functional outcome.

Jorge et al. (33) reported no overlap between apathy and depression during the acute stage post stroke, but there was a significant overlap 12 months later. Caeiro et al. (25) found no association between apathy and depression, although 25% of patients with apathy also had depression. In the meta-analysis study, Caeiro et al. (24) reported depression to be more frequent among patients with apathy as compared to those without apathy (odds ratio (OR) 2.29; 95% CI 1.41–3.72).

Several studies found that apathy was associated with cognitive deficits, most often executive dysfunction, but also with deficits in concentration and information processing and speed (19–21, 26, 27). Lohner et al. (29) reported a significant association between apathy and executive dysfunction among individuals with symptomatic lacunar strokes and deficits in executive functions, memory, and orientation, and similar findings were reported in a systematic review (16). In an exploratory longitudinal study, Caeiro et al. (25) found a significant association between apathy and increased cognitive deficits (mainly verbal abstract reasoning), and this association was confirmed in one meta-analysis (24) (OR 2.90; 95% CI 1.09–7.72). More recently, Fishman et al. reported that apathy, but not depression, is related to worse verbal memory performance (34) and is a significant predictor of semantic and phonemic fluency after stroke (35). Finally, another meta-analysis (16) found a significant association between apathy and worse cognitive function.

Mayo et al. (27) reported that low functional status, poor cognition, and high physical comorbidity were significant predictors of post-stroke apathy. On the other hand, high apathy scores had a negative impact on physical functioning, participation in social activities, health perception, and physical health. The systematic review and meta-analysis by Caeiro et al. (24) which included 26 publications from 19 study samples found that older age, decreased functioning, and increased cognitive deficits were significant predictors of apathy. Significant associations between post-stroke apathy and increased age, reduced cognitive function, and increased depression and disability were reported in the meta-analysis by van Dalen et al. (16). Finally, Douven et al. (36) examined whether personality profile may explain the development of apathy and depression after stroke. They examined a cohort of 250 stroke patients to assess the development and course of apathy and depression over 12 months post stroke, and found a significant association between post-stroke depression and neuroticism, as well as a negative relation between post-stroke apathy and extroversion. The relevance of this finding will have to be determined in future studies.

In conclusion, apathy is significantly associated with worse functional outcomes and increased cognitive deficits. On the other hand, the association between apathy and depression is less consistent, with some studies showing a small overlap and others showing a large one.

Neurobiology

The mechanism of apathy after stroke has been associated with damage to subcortical regions (33). Starkstein et al. (2) reported a significant association between post-stroke apathy and lesions in the posterior limb of the internal capsule, and stressed the association between lesions in the pallidal output and loss of motivation. This finding is in agreement with a previous study by Bhatia and Marsden (37) who reported abulia (a syndrome resembling apathy) in 13% of 240 patients with stroke lesions affecting the caudate and lenticular nuclei. More recently, Murakami et al. (38) assessed 149 stroke patients with the modified AS and found a significant association between higher scores and lesions in the brainstem and bilateral striatum. An association between apathy and brainstem lesions was reported by Tang et al. (39) in a study that included 185 patients with acute stroke, 11% of whom had apathy. The frequency of pontine infarcts was 35% in patients with apathy, as compared to 11% among those with no apathy. Pontine lesions may affect the pedunculopontine nucleus which has a relevant role in activating behaviours towards rewards (40).

Whereas the anterior cingulate cortex (ACC) has been considered an important component of a putative motivation circuit (41), only one study demonstrated significant changes in the cingulate cortex among patients with post-stroke apathy. Matsuoka et al. (42) reported that stroke patients showed a significant association between increased apathy scores and a decreased volume of the anterior part of the posterior cingulate cortex 6 months post stroke as compared to a healthy control sample. The authors suggested that the cingulate cortex may work as a hub connecting regions relevant to goal-oriented behaviours.

Finally, Yang et al. (43) assessed 80 individuals with an acute stroke using the AES and diffusion tensor imaging to examine the presence of specific white matter tracts related to post-stroke apathy. They found no association between apathy and lesion location, but reported an association between higher apathy scores and 'decreased global efficiency' in networks including the limbic system, the frontal, parietal, temporal, and occipital lobes, the basal ganglia, and the insula. Based on these findings, Yang et al. (43) suggested that post-stroke apathy results from disconnection of a 'complex' subnetwork of brain regions. In a second publication (44), these investigators reported a significant reduction in the fraction of anisotropy at the genu and splenium of the corpus callosum, left corona radiata, and right frontal white matter, associated with higher apathy scores. They suggested that these abnormal findings may relate to subtypes of apathy. Thus, 'emotional apathy' may result from damage to the orbitofrontal cortex and the inferior frontal lobe, 'cognitive apathy' may result from damage to the dorsolateral prefrontal cortex, and 'behavioural apathy' may result from damage to the genu and splenium of the corpus callosum. As we suggested in a recent publication (41), one problem with this analysis is that lesions in any brain region may seem to result in apathy, and furthermore, the subtypes of apathy, while conceptually sound, are in need of empirical validation. Furthermore, several studies were unable to find a significant association between lesion location and post-stroke apathy. Using diffusion tensor imaging to examine pathology among 121 individuals with SVD, Hollocks et al. (31) reported that SVD was associated with apathy but not with depression, and pathological findings associated with apathy included the ACC, fornix, uncinate fasciculus, and the corpus callosum. The authors suggested that disruption of frontal-striatal circuits, which select and initiate goal-directed behaviour based on reward information, may explain post-stroke apathy.

The anterior cingulate, nucleus accumbens, ventral pallidum, and the ventral tegmental area are considered as core structures of a putative motivation circuit (38). Post-stroke apathy has been related to the disruption of networks connecting the anterior cingulate gyrus, the dorsomedial frontal cortex, and the frontal pole with the ventral caudate, globus pallidus, and the thalamic nuclei mentioned previously (45). Nevertheless, empirical studies confirming this hypothesis are still lacking.

A meta-analysis by van Dalen (16) showed no association between post-stroke apathy and lesion location, but suggested that basal ganglia lesions are the most consistent finding underlying post-stroke apathy. Brodaty et al. (19) examined 167 stroke patients with the AES and found no association between apathy and the location and volume of stroke.

Tang and colleagues stressed that the pedunculopontine nucleus and the raphe nuclei are central components in a circuit regulating motivation and reward (39). Since the pedunculopontine nucleus is connected to multiple basal ganglia structures, providing an excitatory input to midbrain dopaminergic cells, this structure may play an important role in the autonomic and locomotor outputs of this circuit. Other studies (46) highlight dysfunction of the prefrontal cortex in the production of apathy, including (i) the orbitomedial prefrontal cortex, responsible for emotional-affective processing; (ii) the dorsolateral prefrontal cortex, responsible for cognitive processing; and (iii) the dorsal anterior cingulate, responsible for 'auto-activation'.

In conclusion, there is still a lack of consistent association between post-stroke apathy and lesion variables. Different techniques have been used, including computed tomography, magnetic resonance imaging, single-photon emission computed tomography, and diffusion tensor imaging. Whereas some studies found significant associations between lesion location or dysfunction of white matter tracts and apathy, findings are quite heterogeneous and no validation has been provided that damage to a putative 'anterior cingulate circuit' results in apathy. Thus, damage to this circuit may be sufficient to produce apathy, but may not be necessary, since lesions in other brain areas, with no clear connection to the ACC, may also produce apathy.

Treatment

In spite of the frequency and impact of post-stroke apathy, only two randomized controlled trials (RCTs) have been conducted in relation to its treatment (47, 48). The first was a double-blind, placebo-controlled study using the nootropic nefiracetam as a treatment for post-stroke depression, with apathy as a secondary outcome (45). Patients were randomized to either 600 or 900 mg/day of nefiracetam or identical placebo. A secondary analysis showed that nefiracetam 900 mg/day significantly decreased apathy scores, with good tolerability.

Based on these findings, Starkstein et al. (48) conducted a parallel-group, randomized, placebo-controlled, double-blind, two-centre trial in patients with acute stroke and apathy. Participants were randomized to receive placebo or nefiracetam 900 mg/day after 8 weeks post stroke, given that this is the stage when rehabilitation or readjustment to home environment may be compromised by apathy. The authors also screened for pre-stroke apathy and excluded those patients who scored positive. The main outcome measure was the 14-item AS, and efficacy was examined during a 3-month period. There were a total of 2514 admissions to two stroke centres during a 3-year period, but only 15% of patients were considered eligible. Of these, 61% declined further participation, and of the remaining 39%, only 13 patients underwent randomization. Six patients were allocated to nefiracetam and seven to placebo. An intention-to-treat analysis showed no significant between-group differences for AS scores, either adjusted or unadjusted for baseline scores. The low recruitment rate was not explained by a potential low rate of apathy given that 19% of the sample assessed for potential randomization had apathy. Perhaps the main consequence of this study is that future trials for post-stroke apathy will need to recruit very large samples in the context of multicentre studies.

A number of small treatment case series or case reports have been published among patients with neuropsychiatric disorders, suggesting good response upon treatment with methylphenidate (49), the anticholinesterase inhibitor donepezil (50), amantadine, bromocriptine, selegiline, and zolpidem (51). Recently, Aragona et al. (52) used bupropion 150 mg daily on a patient with post-stroke apathy, who experienced full remission. The authors proposed that bupropion may improve apathy by acting upon dopaminergic pathways. This anecdotal evidence should be considered against a multicentre, randomized, double-blind, placebo-controlled prospective trial (53) using bupropion as the active component in a study that included patients with Huntington's disease with apathy but no depression, which showed no benefits in terms of improving apathy.

Another study examined repetitive transcranial magnetic stimulation (rTMS) to the frontal cortex in 13 patients with chronic stroke and apathy (46). Seven patients were randomized to five sessions of rTMS on consecutive days, and six patients were allocated to placebo rTMS. Parameters used for the active arm were high frequency and 80% of resting motor threshold. The authors found a significant improvement on apathy scores in the rTMS arm but not in the placebo group.

Psychotherapy has also been investigated as a treatment for post-stroke apathy. Problem-solving therapy (PST) proved to be effective to prevent apathy in a single study (33). PST includes goal-setting and planning, self-evaluation and self-monitoring of behaviour, and activity-based training in problem-solving skills (22). Another study compared strategy training versus attention control intervention. This was a single-blind, phase II study examining strategy training among adults with cognitive impairments after stroke (54). After adjusting for executive dysfunction and depression, strategy training resulted in a significant decrease in the levels of post-stroke apathy as compared to the control intervention during the first 6 months after stroke. The authors concluded that strategy training may prevent rather than treat apathy and considered that by focusing on goal-setting, planning, self-monitoring, and problem-solving, strategy training may address the main symptoms of apathy. One limitation of the study was that patients had sub-syndromal apathy, and only two patients scored higher than the cut-off score for apathy on the AES.

An interesting question is whether psychoactive medication could prevent post-stroke apathy. Mikami et al. (22) reviewed the results of a 1-year RCT to prevent post-stroke depression, which used the antidepressant escitalopram or PST. Patients were excluded if they met DSM-IV criteria for depression, but participants were not screened for the presence of pre-stroke apathy. The reanalysis showed that over the first year following an acute stroke, the development of apathy was almost four times higher among patients given placebo than escitalopram, and almost two times more likely among patients given placebo than PST. If confirmed, these findings suggest that both antidepressants and psychotherapy may help to reduce the rate of post-stroke apathy.

More recently, Chan et al. (55) examined the efficacy of the Motor Relearning Programme to treat apathy. This programme places emphasis on active participation in training activities rather than being passive. The authors carried out a RCT comparing the Motor Relearning Programme to Bobath therapy and found the Motor Relearning Programme to have a significantly higher efficacy. This is a preliminary study that requires replication.

In conclusion, no RCT has demonstrated that pharmacotherapy improves apathy. On the other hand, several studies suggest that both pharmacological and non-pharmacological interventions have the potential to prevent post-stroke apathy.

Conclusion

Apathy is a frequent behavioural problem in stroke, affecting about one-third of patients. Apathy may persist for at least 6 months after stroke, but frequencies due to new cases of apathy are still elevated years after stroke. The main comorbid condition of post-stroke apathy is depression. Of note, there is a considerable empirical overlap between both apathy and depression given the commonality of some symptoms. Apathy has also been associated with cognitive deficits, especially executive dysfunction. This is not surprising since cognitive deficits may limit patients' performance of usual hobbies and pastimes. Finally, several studies demonstrated a significant association between apathy and low functioning. The mechanism of post-stroke apathy remains unknown, although dysfunction of the ACC seems to play a central role. There is still no evidence-based treatment for post-stroke apathy. Promising compounds such as the nootropic nefiracetam did not showed significant efficacy on a very small RCT. Challenges for the future include developing instruments to specifically diagnose and measure the severity of apathy after stroke, examining the prevalence and incidence of apathy in longitudinal studies, examining the overlap between apathy, depression, and cognitive deficits in more detail, and carrying out large multicentre studies to examine the efficacy of pharmacological and behavioural interventions.

References

1. Robert P, Lanctot KL, Aguera-Ortiz L, Aalten P, Bremond F, Defrancesco M, et al. Is it time to revise the diagnostic criteria for apathy in brain disorders? The 2018 international consensus group. Eur Psychiatry. 2018;54:71–6.
2. Starkstein SE, Fedoroff JP, Price TR, Leiguarda R, Robinson RG. Apathy following cerebrovascular lesions. Stroke. 1993;24(11):1625–30.
3. Marin RS. Apathy: a neuropsychiatric syndrome. J Neuropsychiatry Clin Neurosci. 1991;3(3):243–54.
4. Marin RS, Wilkosz PA. Disorders of diminished motivation. J Head Trauma Rehabil. 2005;20(4):377–88.
5. Levy R, Dubois B. Apathy and the functional anatomy of the prefrontal cortex-basal ganglia circuits. Cereb Cortex. 2006;16:916–28.

6. Angelelli P, Paolucci S, Bivona U, Piccardi L, Ciurli P, Cantagallo A, et al. Development of neuropsychiatric symptoms in poststroke patients: a cross-sectional study. Acta Psychiatr Scand. 2004;110(1):55–63.
7. Hama S, Yamashita H, Yamawaki S, Kurisu K. Post-stroke depression and apathy: interactions between functional recovery, lesion location, and emotional response. Psychogeriatrics. 2011;11(1):68–76.
8. Carota A, Berney A, Aybek S, Iaria G, Staub F, Ghika-Schmid F, et al. A prospective study of predictors of poststroke depression. Neurology. 2005;64(3):428–33.
9. Marin RS. Differential diagnosis and classification of apathy. Am J Psychiatry. 1990;147(1):22–30.
10. Starkstein SE, Migliorelli R, Manes F, Teson A, Petracca G, Chemerinski E, et al. The prevalence and clinical correlates of apathy and irritability in Alzheimer's disease. Eur J Neurol. 1995;2:540–6.
11. Starkstein SE, Ingram L, Garau ML, Mizrahi R. On the overlap between apathy and depression in dementia. J Neurol Neurosurg Psychiatry. 2005;76(8):1070–4.
12. Drijgers RL, Dujardin K, Reijnders JS, Defebvre L, Leentjens AF. Validation of diagnostic criteria for apathy in Parkinson's disease. Parkinsonism Relat Disord. 2010;16(10):656–60.
13. Starkstein S, Leentjens AF. The nosological position of apathy in clinical practice. J Neurol Neurosurg Psychiatry. 2008;79:1088–92.
14. Cummings JL, Mega M, Gray K, Rosenberg-Thompson S, Carusi DA, Gornbein J. The Neuropsychiatric Inventory: comprehensive assessment of psychopathology in dementia. Neurology. 1994;44(12):2308–14.
15. Marin RS, Biedrzycki RC, Firinciogullari S. Reliability and validity of the Apathy Evaluation Scale. Psychiatry Res. 1991;38(2):143–62.
16. van Dalen JW, Moll van Charante EP, Nederkoorn PJ, van Gool WA, Richard E. Poststroke apathy. Stroke. 2013;44(3):851–60.
17. American Psychiatric Association. Diagnostic and Statistical Manual of Mental Disorders, Fifth Edition. Arlington, VA: American Psychiatric Association; 2013.
18. World Health Organization. The ICD-10 Classification of Mental and Behavioural Disorders. Geneva: World Health Organization; 1993.
19. Brodaty H, Sachdev PS, Withall A, Altendorf A, Valenzuela MJ, Lorentz L. Frequency and clinical, neuropsychological and neuroimaging correlates of apathy following stroke – the Sydney Stroke Study. Psychol Med. 2005;35(12):1707–16.
20. Hama S, Yamashita H, Shigenobu M, Watanabe A, Hiramoto K, Kurisu K, et al. Depression or apathy and functional recovery after stroke. Int J Geriatr Psychiatry. 2007;22(10):1046–51.
21. Santa N, Sugimori H, Kusuda K, Yamashita Y, Ibayashi S, Lida M. Apathy and functional recovery following first-ever stroke. Int J Rehabil Res. 2008;31:321–6.
22. Mikami K, Jorge RE, Moser DJ, Jang M, Robinson RG. Incident apathy during the first year after stroke and its effect on physical and cognitive recovery. Am J Geriatr Psychiatry. 2013;21(9):848–54.
23. Kennedy JM, Granato DA, Goldfine AM. Natural history of poststroke apathy during acute rehabilitation. J Neuropsychiatry Clin Neurosci. 2015;27(4):333–8.
24. Caeiro L, Ferro JM, Costa J. Apathy secondary to stroke: a systematic review and meta-analysis. Cerebrovasc Dis. 2013;35(1):23–39.
25. Caeiro L, Ferro JM, Pinho EMT, Canhao P, Figueira ML. Post-stroke apathy: an exploratory longitudinal study. Cerebrovasc Dis. 2013;35(6):507–13.
26. Withall A, Brodaty H, Altendorf A, Sachdev PS. A longitudinal study examining the independence of apathy and depression after stroke: the Sydney Stroke Study. Int Psychogeriatr. 2011;23(2):264–73.

27. Mayo NE, Fellows LK, Scott SC, Cameron J, Wood-Dauphinee S. A longitudinal view of apathy and its impact after stroke. Stroke. 2009;40(10):3299–307.

28. Brodaty H, Liu Z, Withall A, Sachdev PS. The longitudinal course of post-stroke apathy over five years. J Neuropsychiatry Clin Neurosci. 2013;25(4):283–91.

29. Lohner V, Brookes RL, Hollocks MJ, Morris RG, Markus HS. Apathy, but not depression, is associated with executive dysfunction in cerebral small vessel disease. PLoS One. 2017;12(5):e0176943.

30. Hollocks MJ, Lawrence AJ, Brookes RL, Barrick TR, Morris RG, Husain M, et al. Differential relationships between apathy and depression with white matter microstructural changes and functional outcomes. Brain. 2015;138(Pt 12):3803–15.

31. Ligthart SA, Richard E, Fransen NL, Eurelings LS, Beem L, Eikelenboom P, et al. Association of vascular factors with apathy in community-dwelling elderly individuals. Arch Gen Psychiatry. 2012;69(6):636–42.

32. van der Mast RC, Vinkers DJ, Stek ML, Bek MC, Westendorp RG, Gussekloo J, et al. Vascular disease and apathy in old age. The Leiden 85-Plus Study. Int J Geriatr Psychiatry. 2008;23(3):266–71.

33. Jorge RE, Starkstein SE, Robinson RG. Apathy following stroke. Can J Psychiatry. 2010;55(6):350–4.

34. Fishman KN, Ashbaugh AR, Lanctot KL, Cayley ML, Herrmann N, Murray BJ, et al. Apathy, not depressive symptoms, as a predictor of semantic and phonemic fluency task performance in stroke and transient ischemic attack. J Clin Exp Neuropsychol. 2018;40(5):449–61.

35. Fishman KN, Ashbaugh AR, Lanctot KL, Cayley ML, Herrmann N, Murray BJ, et al. The role of apathy and depression on verbal learning and memory performance after stroke. Arch Clin Neuropsychol. 2019;34(3):327–36.

36. Douven E, Staals J, Schievink SHJ, van Oostenbrugge RJ, Verhey FRJ, Wetzels-Meertens S, et al. Personality traits and course of symptoms of depression and apathy after stroke: results of the CASPER study. J Psychosom Res. 2018;111:69–75.

37. Bhatia KP, Marsden CD. The behavioural and motor consequences of focal lesions of the basal ganglia in man. Brain. 1994;117(Pt 4):859–76.

38. Murakami T, Hama S, Yamashita H, Onoda K, Kobayashi M, Kanazawa J, et al. Neuroanatomic pathways associated with poststroke affective and apathetic depression. Am J Geriatr Psychiatry. 2013;21(9):840–7.

39. Tang WK, Chen YK, Liang HJ, Chu WC, Mok VC, Ungvari GS, et al. Location of infarcts and apathy in ischemic stroke. Cerebrovasc Dis. 2013;35(6):566–71.

40. Haber SN, Knutson B. The reward circuit: linking primate anatomy and human imaging. Neuropsychopharmacology. 2010;35(1):4–26.

41. Starkstein SE, Brockman S. The neuroimaging basis of apathy: empirical findings and conceptual challenges. Neuropsychologia. 2018;118(Pt B):48–53.

42. Matsuoka K, Yasuno F, Taguchi A, Yamamoto A, Kajimoto K, Kazui H, et al. Delayed atrophy in posterior cingulate cortex and apathy after stroke. Int J Geriatr Psychiatry. 2015;30(6):566–72.

43. Yang S, Hua P, Shang X, Cui Z, Zhong S, Gong G, et al. Deficiency of brain structural subnetwork underlying post-ischaemic stroke apathy. Eur J Neurol. 2015;22(2):341–7.

44. Yang SR, Shang XY, Tao J, Liu JY, Hua P. Voxel-based analysis of fractional anisotropy in post-stroke apathy. PLoS One. 2015;10(1):e116168.

45. Chong TT, Husain M. The role of dopamine in the pathophysiology and treatment of apathy. Prog Brain Res. 2016;229:389–426.

46. Sasaki N, Hara T, Yamada N, Niimi M, Kakuda W, Abo M. The efficacy of high-frequency repetitive transcranial magnetic stimulation for improving apathy in chronic stroke patients. Eur Neurol. 2017;78(1–2):28–32.

47. Robinson RG, Jorge RE, Clarence-Smith K, Starkstein S. Double-blind treatment of apathy in patients with poststroke depression using nefiracetam. J Neuropsychiatry Clin Neurosci. 2009;21(2):144–51.
48. Starkstein SE, Brockman S, Hatch KK, Bruce DG, Almeida OP, Davis WA, et al. A randomized, placebo-controlled, double-blind efficacy study of nefiracetam to treat poststroke apathy. J Stroke Cerebrovasc Dis. 2016;25(5):1119–27.
49. Galynker I, Ieronimo C, Miner C, Rosenblum J, Vilkas N, Rosenthal R. Methylphenidate treatment of negative symptoms in patients with dementia. J Neuropsychiatry Clin Neurosci. 1997;9(2):231–9.
50. Deb S, Crownshaw T. The role of pharmacotherapy in the management of behaviour disorders in traumatic brain injury patients. Brain Inj. 2004;18(1):1–31.
51. Autret K, Arnould A, Mathieu S, Azouvi P. Transient improvement of poststroke apathy with zolpidem: a single-case, placebo-controlled double-blind study. BMJ Case Rep. 2013;2013:bcr2012007816.
52. Aragona B, De Luca R, Piccolo A, Le Cause M, Destro M, Casella C, et al. Is bupropion useful in the treatment of post-stroke thalamic apathy? A case report and considerations. Funct Neurol. 2018;33(4):213–6.
53. Gelderblom H, Wustenberg T, McLean T, Mutze L, Fischer W, Saft C, et al. Bupropion for the treatment of apathy in Huntington's disease: a multicenter, randomised, double-blind, placebo-controlled, prospective crossover trial. PLoS One. 2017;12(3):e0173872.
54. Skidmore ER, Whyte EM, Butters MA, Terhorst L, Reynolds CF, 3rd. Strategy training during inpatient rehabilitation may prevent apathy symptoms after acute stroke. PM R. 2015;7(6):562–70.
55. Chen L, Xiong S, Liu Y, Lin M, Zhu L, Zhong R, et al. Comparison of Motor Relearning Program versus Bobath approach for prevention of poststroke apathy: a randomized controlled trial. J Stroke Cerebrovasc Dis. 2019;28(3):655–64.

7
Apathy and Schizophrenia

Ann Faerden and André Aleman

Introduction

Apathy is considered to be a core feature of schizophrenia that contributes to the functional disability and its presence is still a major challenge for effective treatment, remission, and recovery of this often-debilitating disorder (1, 2). The importance of apathy has been acknowledged for more than a decade, but only recently has apathy been a separate target of investigation. We are therefore still short of a sound understanding of the underlying mechanisms of apathy in schizophrenia that can contribute to effective treatments. However, recent research findings are emerging that contribute to an enhanced understanding of this debilitating condition. This chapter will try to summarize the current knowledge and give suggestions for future work.

Apathy is a common state most people are familiar with and have experienced. Apathy and motivation are considered opposites along a continuum. This opposing relationship is reflected in the words used to describe the symptom of apathy in schizophrenia and psychotic disorders where apathy, apathy/avolition, avolition, amotivation, and motivational deficits are used as synonymous when the state of apathy is described or studied (3).

The clinical presentation of apathy in patients with schizophrenia or psychosis is described as a person who lacks initiative, seems content with sitting at home, and who may have some general goals but has difficulties maintaining them and translating them into actions. Patients may seem enlightened here and now when talking about something but cannot use it for realizing future goals. Planning for the future is often unrealistic and they have difficulties in planning for the next day or accomplishing daily tasks. The person is often quiet, can be overseen by the staff, and has difficulties in seeking help. It is not surprising that this functional disability has a significant impact on studies, and leads to difficulties in independent living and maintaining a paid job. Schizophrenia affects young people at the start of their adult life, and the functional disabilities interfere with normal development. The state of apathy can be hard for the family to understand and they often do everything they can to motivate, but often in vain and with the consequence of despair and feeling of inadequacy, feelings that also apply to professional helpers. This underscores how important it is to find better treatments for the state of apathy in people with psychosis.

Apathy was described by Kraepelin as a core feature of schizophrenia and the state and origin of apathy challenged the minds of both Kraepelin and Bleuler—Kraepelin focusing on the loss of volition and Bleuler on the affective indifference (4, 5). The current knowledge of schizophrenia is in agreement with both Kraepelin and Bleuler in their understanding of what is central to the disorder and especially what contributes to the poor functional outcome (1). Despite having this knowledge for more than a century, research into the state of apathy in psychotic disorders has only taken place during the last 15 years. This is due to different reasons which are linked to the history of the understanding of the human mental state, the challenge of classification of mental disorders (6), agreement of diagnostic criteria for schizophrenia (7), if schizophrenia symptoms reflect one or several underlying processes (8), and difficulties in defining motivation and apathy (9).

The understanding of the human mind and functioning of the brain develops in parallel with our understanding of mental disorders. Despite Kraepelin's early description of apathy and loss of volition, it is only recently that these research areas can support each other with the common goal of understanding disorders of motivation (10, 11). Schizophrenia represents heterogeneity in clinical presentation, which has challenged the understanding, description, and diagnostic criteria up to the present day (7). There have been many attempts to organize the different symptoms on both sides of the Atlantic during the first half of the last century, but the introduction of the negative–positive dichotomy by Strauss and Carpenter in the 1970s, later refined by Nancy Andreasen, has been proven to be robust and meaningful (12). Indeed, it is a common distinction used in the clinic and in the research community (13, 14). The term has its origin from two neurologists, Russell Reynolds and Hughlings Jackson, who in the 1860s used these two terms to describe excess and negations of vital properties (15). In schizophrenia research and clinical practice, positive symptoms primarily refer to hallucinations and delusions, whereas negative symptoms primarily refer to social withdrawal, lack of initiative, and anhedonia.

The study of apathy is closely linked to the study of negative symptoms. The introduction of negative symptoms was the start of studies on apathy in schizophrenia, since apathy/avolition was one of five sub-symptoms described by Andreasen that encompass the negative symptom domain (16), the other being anhedonia, affective flattening, alogia, and asociality. But despite the introduction of apathy as one of the negative symptoms in the 1980s, negative symptoms were mostly studied as one complex for the next 30 years. The introduction of the negative symptom complex and the development of scales for assessment inspired a large body of research. This research confirmed that there was a strong association between negative symptoms and functional disability (1), but this knowledge did not give rise to more effective treatments and outcomes did not improve. This was the background for the National Institute of Mental Health (NIMH) Consensus Statement on Negative Symptoms, published in 2006 (1), which together with different research groups suggested that studies at the sub-symptom level, especially apathy/avolition, had the prospect of reaching new insight that would benefit patients (17). The focus on apathy and motivation was also one of five domains suggested by the NIMH as research domain criteria for mental disorders (18). Indeed, since 2005, and even more so since 2009 with establishment of research domain criteria, studies on apathy and motivation in schizophrenia have increased substantially (Table 7.1).

Apathy reflects a complicated process of the brain involving dysfunction in affective and cognitive systems, comprising motivation and the reward system, as well as agency and motor functions. The understanding of the normal process of motivation has also paved the way for more sophisticated assessment of apathy in schizophrenia. New assessments have been taken into use such as new symptoms scales, paradigms from experimental psychology, and functional neuroimaging. In the following sections, we briefly review studies of apathy in schizophrenia, with a focus on assessment, cognitive and neural investigations, and treatment approaches.

Assessment of Apathy

Clinical Assessment of Apathy in Schizophrenia

Apathy originates from old Greek, meaning lack of emotions, interest, and passivity. Despite the common use, apathy has been hard to define for the field of medicine and it was not clearly defined until 1991 by Robert S. Marin (19). Marin defined apathy as a lack of goal-directed activity not due to depression, intellectual deficit, and diminished level of consciousness. This definition is now used across different medical fields in the study of apathy and represented in much the same way in different scales (20). Based on his definition of apathy, Marin developed the Apathy Evaluation Scale (AES), which is one of the most used scales in different medical disorders, mainly neurology (21–24), but also in the study of apathy in schizophrenia and psychotic disorders (25).

The assessment of apathy in schizophrenia has developed along three lines; one is the use of the apathy/amotivation subscales from the different negative scales in use, another is by factor analysis of the negative symptoms scale, and the third is by the use of a specific apathy scale such as the AES. As can be seen in Table 7.2 and Table 7.3, there is no consensus on the definition of apathy in schizophrenia and the scales score different items including degree of initiative, interests, pleasure, anhedonia, and social interest in a global score of apathy.

When Nancy Andreasen defined the negative symptoms, she also developed the first scale for their assessment, the Scale for the Assessment of Negative Symptoms (SANS), where all the five sub-symptoms are represented with a subscale, the avolition/apathy subscale that includes three items regarding interest in daily hygiene, impersistence at work, and physical inertia (Table 7.3). At about the same time, the Positive and Negative Symptoms Scale (PANSS) was developed (26). Both are the two most used assessment scales of negative symptoms, but the two differ in how they assess apathy in that the PANSS does not have a subscale for the different

Table 7.1 Major studies on apathy in schizophrenia: 2003–2019

2019	Chang WC, et al.	Effort-based decision-making impairment in patients with clinically-stabilized first-episode psychosis and its relationship with amotivation and psychosocial functioning. Eur Neuropsychopharmacol. 2019;29(5):629–42
2019	Chang WC, et al.	Executive dysfunctions differentially predict amotivation in first-episode schizophrenia-spectrum disorder: a prospective 1-year follow-up study. Eur Arch Psychiatry Clin Neurosci. 2019;269(8):887–96
2019	Dondaine T, et al.	Apathy alters emotional arousal in chronic schizophrenia. J Psychiatry Neurosci. 2019;44(1):54–61
2019	Favrod J, et al.	Improving pleasure and motivation in schizophrenia: a randomized controlled clinical trial. Psychother Psychosom. 2019;88(2):84–95
2019	Kirschner M, et al.	Shared and dissociable features of apathy and reward system dysfunction in bipolar I disorder and schizophrenia. Psychol Med. 2019:1–12
2019	Luther L, et al.	Clarifying the overlap between motivation and negative symptom measures in schizophrenia research: a meta-analysis. Schizophr Res. 2019;206:27–36
2019	Raffard S, et al.	The cognitive, affective motivational and clinical longitudinal determinants of apathy in schizophrenia. Eur Arch Psychiatry Clin Neurosci. 2019;269(8):911–20
2019	Schneider K, et al.	Cerebral blood flow in striatal regions is associated with apathy in patients with schizophrenia. J Psychiatry Neurosci. 2019;44(2):102–10
2019	Servaas MN, et al.	Rigidity in motor behavior and brain functioning in patients with schizophrenia and high levels of apathy. Schizophr Bull. 2019; 45(3):542–51
2019	Xu P, et al.	Intrinsic mesocorticolimbic connectivity is negatively associated with social amotivation in people with schizophrenia. Schizophr Res. 2019;208:353–9
2018	Amodio A, et al.	Avolition-apathy and white matter connectivity in schizophrenia: reduced fractional anisotropy between amygdala and insular cortex. Clin EEG Neurosci. 2018;49(1):55–65
2018	Beck AT, et al.	What accounts for poor functioning in people with schizophrenia: a re-evaluation of the contributions of neurocognitive v. attitudinal and motivational factors. Psychol Med. 2018;48(16):2776–85
2018	Bortolon C, et al.	Apathy in schizophrenia: A review of neuropsychological and neuroanatomical studies. Neuropsychologia. 2018;118(Pt B):22–33

Continued

Table 7.1 *Continued*

2018	Caravaggio F, et al.	Amotivation is associated with smaller ventral striatum volumes in older patients with schizophrenia. Int J Geriatr Psychiatry. 2018;33(3):523–30
2018	Caravaggio F, et al.	The neural correlates of apathy in schizophrenia: an exploratory investigation. Neuropsychologia. 2018;118(Pt B):34–9
2018	Dondaine T, et al.	Apathy alters emotional arousal in chronic schizophrenia. J Psychiatry Neurosci. 2018;43(6):170172
2018	Faerden A, et al.	Reliability and validity of the self-report version of the apathy evaluation scale in first-episode psychosis: concordance with the clinical version at baseline and 12 months follow-up. Psychiatry Res. 2018;267:140–7
2018	Fervaha G, et al.	Achievement motivation in early schizophrenia: relationship with symptoms, cognition and functional outcome. Early Interv Psychiatry. 2018;12(6):1038–44.
2018	Giordano GM, et al.	Neurophysiological correlates of avolition-apathy in schizophrenia: a resting-EEG microstates study. Neuroimage Clin. 2018;20:627–36
2018	Kluge A, et al.	Combining actigraphy, ecological momentary assessment and neuroimaging to study apathy in patients with schizophrenia. Schizophr Res. 2018;195:176–82
2018	Luther L, et al.	A meta-analytic review of self-reported, clinician-rated, and performance-based motivation measures in schizophrenia: are we measuring the same 'stuff'? Clin Psychol Rev. 2018;61:24–37
2018	Lyngstad SH, et al.	Consequences of persistent depression and apathy in first-episode psychosis—a one-year follow-up study. Compr Psychiatry. 2018; 86:60–6
2018	Najs-Garcia A, et al.	The relationship of motivation and neurocognition with functionality in schizophrenia: a meta-analytic review. Community Ment Health J. 2018;54(7):1019–49
2018	Ringen PA, et al.	Using motivational techniques to reduce cardiometabolic risk factors in long term psychiatric inpatients: a naturalistic interventional study. BMC Psychiatry. 2018;18(1):255
2018	Schlosser DA, et al.	Efficacy of PRIME, a mobile app intervention designed to improve motivation in young people with schizophrenia. Schizophr Bull. 2018;44(5):1010–20
2018	Suri G, et al.	An investigation into the drivers of avolition in schizophrenia. Psychiatry Res. 2018;261:225–31
2018	Vignapiano A, et al.	Impact of reward and loss anticipation on cognitive control: an event-related potential study in subjects with schizophrenia and healthy controls. Clin EEG Neurosci. 2018;49(1):46–54

Table 7.1 *Continued*

2017	Chang WC, et al.	Prediction of motivational impairment: 12-month follow-up of the randomized-controlled trial on extended early intervention for first-episode psychosis. Eur Psychiatry. 2017;41:37–41
2017	Da Silva S, et al.	Investigating consummatory and anticipatory pleasure across motivation deficits in schizophrenia and healthy controls. Psychiatry Res. 2017;254:112–7
2017	Park IH, et al.	Effort-based reinforcement processing and functional connectivity underlying amotivation in medicated. patients with depression and schizophrenia. J Neurosci. 2017;37(16):4370–80
2016	Barch DM, et al.	Mechanisms underlying motivational deficits in psychopathology: similarities and differences in depression and schizophrenia. Curr Top Behav Neurosci. 2016;27:411–49
2016	Bischof M, et al.	The brief negative symptom scale: validation of the German translation and convergent validity with self-rated anhedonia and observer-rated apathy. BMC Psychiatry. 2016;16(1):415
2016	Bull H, et al.	Vocational functioning in schizophrenia spectrum disorders: does apathy matter? J Nerv Ment Dis. 2016;204(8):599–605
2016	Carpenter WT, et al.	Avolition, negative symptoms, and a clinical science journey and transition to the future. Nebr Symp Motiv. 2016;63:133–58
2016	Chang WC, et al.	Impact of avolition and cognitive impairment on functional outcome in first-episode schizophrenia-spectrum disorder: a prospective one-year follow-up study. Schizophr Res. 2016;170(2–3):318–21
2016	Kirschner M, et al.	Ventral striatal hypoactivation is associated with apathy but not diminished expression in patients with schizophrenia. J Psychiatry Neurosci. 2016;41(3):152–61
2016	Kos C, et al.	Neural correlates of apathy in patients with neurodegenerative disorders, acquired brain injury, and psychiatric disorders. Neurosci Biobehav Rev. 2016;69:381–401
2016	Nguyen A, et al.	Development of the Positive Emotions Program for Schizophrenia: an intervention to improve pleasure and motivation in schizophrenia. Front Psychiatry. 2016;7:13
2016	Pillny M, et al.	Predictors of improved functioning in patients with psychosis: the role of amotivation and defeatist performance beliefs. Psychiatry Res. 2016;244:117–22

Continued

Table 7.1 *Continued*

2016	Raffard S, et al.	Working memory deficit as a risk factor for severe apathy in schizophrenia: a 1-year longitudinal study. Schizophr Bull. 2016;42(3):642–51
2016	Reddy LF et al.	Predictors of employment in schizophrenia: the importance of intrinsic and extrinsic motivation. Schizophr Res. 2016;176(2–3):462–6
2016	Roth RM, et al.	Apathy is associated with ventral striatum volume in schizophrenia spectrum disorder. J Neuropsychiatry Clin Neurosci. 2016;28(3):191–4
2016	Tobe M, et al.	Characteristics of motivation and their impacts on the functional outcomes in patients with schizophrenia. Compr Psychiatry. 2016;65:103–9
2015	Cathomas F, et al.	The translational study of apathy—an ecological approach. Front Behav Neurosci. 2015;9:241
2015	Favrod J, et al.	Positive Emotions Program for Schizophrenia (PEPS): a pilot intervention to reduce anhedonia and apathy. BMC Psychiatry. 2015;15:231
2015	Fervaha G, et al.	Motivational deficits and cognitive test performance in schizophrenia. JAMA Psychiatry. 2014;71(9):1058–65
2015	Fervaha G, et al.	Motivational deficits in early schizophrenia: prevalent, persistent, and key determinants of functional outcome. Schizophr Res. 2015;166(1–3):9–16
2015	Fervaha G, et al.	Motivation and social cognition in patients with schizophrenia. J Int Neuropsychol Soc. 2015;21(6):436–43
2015	Fervaha G, et al.	Antipsychotics and amotivation. Neuropsychopharmacology. 2015;40(6):1539–48
2015	Fervaha G, et al.	Measuring motivation in people with schizophrenia. Schizophr Res. 2015;169(1–3):423–6
2015	Foussias G, et al.	Motivated to do well: an examination of the relationships between motivation, effort, and cognitive performance in schizophrenia. Schizophr Res.2015;166(1–3):276–82
2015	Hager OM, et al.	Reward-dependent modulation of working memory is associated with negative symptoms in schizophrenia. Schizophr Res. 2015;168(1–2):238–44
2015	Hanssen E, et al.	Neural correlates of reward processing in healthy siblings of patients with schizophrenia. Front Hum Neurosci. 2015;9:504
2015	Hartmann-Riemer MN, et al.	The association of neurocognitive impairment with diminished expression and apathy in schizophrenia. Schizophr Res. 2015;169(1–3):427–32
2015	Hartmann MN, et al.	Apathy in schizophrenia as a deficit in the generation of options for action. J Abnorm Psychol. 2015;124(2):309–18

Table 7.1 *Continued*

2015	Hartmann MN, et al.	Apathy but not diminished expression in schizophrenia is associated with discounting of monetary rewards by physical effort. Schizophr Bull. 2015;41(2):503–12
2015	Liemburg EJ, et al.	Neural correlates of planning performance in patients with schizophrenia—relationship with apathy. Schizophr Res. 2015;161(2–3):367–75
2015	Luther L, et al.	Intrinsic motivation and amotivation in first episode and prolonged psychosis. Schizophr Res. 2015;169(1–3):418–22
2015	Mørch-Johnsen L, et al.	Brain structure abnormalities in first-episode psychosis patients with persistent apathy. Schizophr Res. 2015;164(1–3):59–64
2015	Simon JJ, et al.	Reward system dysfunction as a neural substrate of symptom expression across the general population and patients with schizophrenia. Schizophr Bull. 2015;41(6):1370–8
2015	Tabak NT, et al.	Mindfulness in schizophrenia: associations with self-reported motivation, emotion regulation, dysfunctional attitudes, and negative symptoms. Schizophr Res. 2015;168(1–2):537–42
2015	Weiser M, et al.	Quantifying motivational deficits and apathy: a review of the literature. Eur Neuropsychopharmacol. 2015;25(8):1060–81
2014	Barch DM, et al.	Effort, anhedonia, and function in schizophrenia: reduced effort allocation predicts amotivation and functional impairment. J Abnorm Psychol. 2014;123(2):387–97
2014	Fervaha G, et al.	Motivational and neurocognitive deficits are central to the prediction of longitudinal functional outcome in schizophrenia. Acta Psychiatr Scand. 2014;130(4):290–9
2014	Fervaha G, et al.	Effect of intrinsic motivation on cognitive performance in schizophrenia: a pilot study. Schizophr Res. 2014;152(1):317–8
2014	Kirkpatrick B.	Recognizing primary vs secondary negative symptoms and apathy vs expression domains. J Clin Psychiatry. 2014;75(4):e09
2014	Kirkpatrick B.	Developing concepts in negative symptoms: primary vs secondary and apathy vs expression. J Clin Psychiatry. 2014;75(Suppl 1):3–7
2014	Schlosser DA et al.	Motivational deficits in individuals at-risk for psychosis and across the course of schizophrenia. Schizophr Res. 2014;158(1–3):52–7
2014	Wolf DH, et al.	Amotivation in schizophrenia: integrated assessment with behavioral, clinical, and imaging measures. Schizophr Bull. 2014;40(6):1328–37

Continued

Table 7.1 *Continued*

2014	Yazbek H, et al.	The Lille Apathy Rating Scale (LARS): exploring its psychometric properties in schizophrenia. Schizophr Res. 2014;157(1–3):278–84
2013	Choi KH, et al.	Beyond cognition: a longitudinal investigation of the role of motivation during a vocational rehabilitation program. J Nerv Ment Dis. 2013;201(3):173–8
2013	Faerden A, et al.	Apathy, poor verbal memory and male gender predict lower psychosocial functioning one year after the first treatment of psychosis. Psychiatry Res. 2013;210(1):55–61
2013	Fervaha G, et al.	Incentive motivation deficits in schizophrenia reflect effort computation impairments during cost-benefit decision-making. J Psychiatr Res. 2013;47(11):1590–6
2013	Fervaha G, et al.	Amotivation and functional outcomes in early schizophrenia. Psychiatry Res. 2013;210(2):665–8
2013	Liemburg EJ, et al.	Two subdomains of negative symptoms in psychotic disorders: established and confirmed in two large cohorts. J Psychiatr Res. 2013;47(6):718–25
2013	Strauss GP, et al.	Deconstructing negative symptoms of schizophrenia: avolition-apathy and diminished expression clusters predict clinical presentation and functional outcome. J Psychiatr Res. 2013;47(6):783–90
2013	Takayanagi Y, et al.	Hippocampal volume reduction correlates with apathy in traumatic brain injury, but not schizophrenia. J Neuropsychiatry Clin Neurosci. 2013;25(4):292–301
2012	Choi KH, et al.	The relationship of trait to state motivation: the role of self-competency beliefs. Schizophr Res. 2012;139(1–3):73–7
2012	Evensen J, et al.	Apathy in first episode psychosis patients: a ten year longitudinal follow-up study. Schizophr Res. 2012;136(1–3):19–24
2012	Green M, et al.	From perception to functional outcome in schizophrenia: modeling the role of ability and motivation. Arch Gen Psychiatry. 2012;69(12):1216–24
2011	Foussias G, et al.	Prediction of longitudinal functional outcomes in schizophrenia: the impact of baseline motivational deficits. Schizophr Res. 2011;132(1):24–7
2011	Konstantakopoulos G, et al.	Apathy, cognitive deficits and functional impairment in schizophrenia. Schizophr Res. 2011;133(1–3):193–8
2010	Cohen AS, et al.	A framework for understanding experiential deficits in schizophrenia. Psychiatry Res. 2010;178(1):10–6
2010	Faerden A, et al.	Apathy in first episode psychosis patients: one year follow up. Schizophr Res. 2010;116(1):20–6

Table 7.1 *Continued*

2010	Foussias G, et al.	Negative symptoms in schizophrenia: avolition and Occam's razor. Schizophr Bull. 2010;36(2):359–69
2010	Nakagami E, et al.	The prospective relationships among intrinsic motivation, neurocognition, and psychosocial functioning in schizophrenia. Schizophr Bull. 2010;36(5):935–48
2010	Silverstein SM, et al.	Bridging the gap between extrinsic and intrinsic motivation in the cognitive remediation of schizophrenia. Schizophr Bull. 2010;36(5):949–56
2010	Simon JJ, et al.	Neural correlates of reward processing in schizophrenia—relationship to apathy and depression. Schizophr Res. 2010;118(1–3):154–61
2009	Faerden A, et al.	Apathy is associated with executive functioning in first episode psychosis. BMC Psychiatry. 2009;9:1
2009	Gard DE	Motivation and its relationship to neurocognition, social cognition, and functional outcome in schizophrenia. Schizophr Res. 2009;115(1):74–81
2008	Faerden A et al.	Assessing apathy: the use of the Apathy Evaluation Scale in first episode psychosis. Eur Psychiatry. 2008;23(1):33–9
2008	Nakagami E, et al.	Intrinsic motivation, neurocognition and psychosocial functioning in schizophrenia: testing mediator and moderator effects. Schizophr Res. 2008;105(1–3):95–104
2008	Roth RM, et al.	Apathy and the processing of novelty in schizophrenia. Schizophr Res. 2008;98(1–3):232–8
2007	Padala PR, et al.	Treatment of apathy with methylphenidate. J Neuropsychiatry Clin Neurosci. 2007;19(1):81–3
2006	Velligan DI	Cognitive rehabilitation for schizophrenia and the putative role of motivation and expectancies. Schizophr Bull. 2006;32(3):474–85
2004	Arnold DS, et al.	Adjuvant therapeutic effects of galantamine on apathy in a schizophrenia patient. J Clin Psychiatry. 2004;65(12):1723–4
2004	Roth RM, et al.	Apathy in schizophrenia: reduced frontal lobe volume and neuropsychological deficits. Am J Psychiatry. 2004;161(1):157–9
2003	Kiang M, et al.	Apathy in schizophrenia: clinical correlates and association with functional outcome. Schizophr Res. 2003;63(1–2):79–88

Table 7.2 Assessment of apathy in different disorders (schizophrenia, dementia, traumatic brain injury, Parkinson's disease, Huntington's disease)

Item	Apathy Evaluation Scale (dementia, schizophrenia, Parkinson's disease, traumatic brain injury, Huntington's disease)
1	S/he is interested in things
2	S/he gets things done during the day
3	Getting things started on his/her own is important to him/her
4	S/he is interested in having new experiences
5	S/he is interested in learning new things
6	S/he puts little effort into anything
7	S/he approaches life with intensity
8	Seeing a job through to the end is important to her/him
9	S/he spends time doing things that interest her/him
10	Someone has to tell her/him what to do each day
11	S/he is less concerned about her/his problem
12	S/he has friends
13	Getting together with friends is important to her/him
14	When something good happens, s/he gets excited
15	S/he has an accurate understanding of her/his problem
16	Getting things done during the day is important to her/him
17	S/he has initiative
18	S/he has motivation

negative sub-symptoms (Table 7.3). The NIMH Consensus Statement on Negative Symptoms (1) addressed the shortcomings in these scales, highlighting that they did not reflect current knowledge. Therefore, development of new scales was encouraged. The Clinical Assessment Interview for Negative Symptoms (CAINS) and the Brief Negative Symptoms Scale (BNSS) were developed from this initiative. Both have subscales that assess motivation and avolition/apathy, in the CAINS named the motivation and pleasure subscale and in the BNSS, the avolition subscale (Table 7.3). As can be seen in Table 7.3, there are apparent differences in the way apathy is assessed across the different scales, such that in the CAINS the apathy subscale includes eight items, while the BNSS has two items (27, 28). Factor analysis of the negative scales also finds that negative symptoms cluster into two factors: the experiential domain

Table 7.3 Assessment of apathy in different negative symptom scales used in schizophrenia and other psychotic disorders

Name of scale	Name of subscale assessing apathy	Number of items assessing apathy
PANSS[a] (Positive and Negative Symptom Scale)	Seven items (N1–N7). No subscales. Factor analysis find two factors: the experiental and the expressive domain, where experiental domain represents apathy/amotivation	3
SANS[b] (Scale for Assessment of Negative Symptoms)	Avolition/apathy subscale	3 and a global rating
BNSS[c] (Brief Negative Symptom Scale)	Avolition subscale	2
CAINS[d] (Clinical Assessment Interview for Negative Symptoms)	Motivation and pleasure (MAP) scale	8

Sources: [a] British Journal of Psychiatry, 155 (suppl. 7), PANSS Rating Criteria: Negative Scale (N), pp. 66–67, Copyright (1989); [b] Arch Gen Psychiatry, 39(7), Andreasen NC, Negative symptoms in schizophrenia. Definition and reliability, pp. 784–8, Copyright (1982); [c] Schizophr Bull, 37(2), Kirkpatrick B, Strauss GP, Nguyen L, et al., The brief negative symptom scale: psychometric properties, pp. 300–305; [d] Am J Psychiatry, 170(2), Kring AM, Gur RE, Blanchard JJ, et al., The Clinical Assessment Interview for Negative Symptoms (CAINS): final development and validation, pp. 165–72, Copyright (2013).

(in some studies named PANSS amotivation) (29), including apathy/amotivation sub-symptom together with anhedonia and asociality, and the expressive domain, consisting primarily of alogia and affective flattening (30). This is another method to study apathy since the experiential domain is often used as the proxy for apathy or amotivation (29). These differences reflect the challenges in how we can best capture the symptom of apathy in the clinic.

The AES is a scale used extensively in patients with schizophrenia that only assesses apathy, and no other negative symptom (Table 7.2). It is widely used in neurology and increasingly also in psychiatry. It has been used in different studies of patients with schizophrenia (31–39) and was found to be reliable (40, 41). The AES has three forms—clinician, observer, and self-report—all with identical items (42). One study found a high association between clinician-rated apathy and self-report (33). Assessment of apathy and motivation in the SANS and PANSS are by observation by the clinician or report from others, but in the CAINS and BNSS also include patients' own reports.

Negative symptoms have been characterized as primary or secondary, where secondary symptoms are thought to be mainly due to antipsychotic medications, depression, or psychotic symptoms (43). It is acknowledged that it is clinically difficult to distinguish between the two and the terms are under debate (43). Another distinction that is also clinically difficult is that between deficit, enduring, persistent, and transient negative symptoms (44, 45). This differentiation of negative symptoms is also thought to reflect differences in underlying mechanisms, but this has not been confirmed sufficiently. The same distinctions have not been applied to the study of apathy, but apathy is present for some as enduring and for others it is transient (35, 46).

Despite the prominent position of apathy or avolition in the outcome of schizophrenia, it was not mentioned separately in the diagnostic criteria until recently. Indeed, negative symptoms were not introduced as a diagnostic criterion before the introduction of the International Classification of Diseases, tenth revision (ICD-10) and *Diagnostic and Statistical Manual of Mental Disorders*, fourth edition (DSM-IV) in the 1990s. In the DSM-IV, avolition is listed as one of five negative symptoms and in the ICD-10 as one of nine, but in neither are negative symptoms required for fulfilment of the diagnosis (47, 48). The current understanding of the negative symptoms as consisting of two dimensions is incorporated into the DSM-5 where negative symptoms are presented with the two subdomains and named avolition and affective flattening (49).

Cognitive Tests

Schizophrenia is characterized by cognitive impairment, affecting multiple domains such as attention, memory, and executive function (50). It could be hypothesized that a reduction in cognitive abilities may translate into apathy, for example, due to a diminished ability to set goals, plan, and execute the necessary actions. Alternatively, apathy itself, representing a reduction of motivation, could translate into poor performance on cognitive tests. With regard to schizophrenia, it is instructive to first evaluate the research regarding negative symptoms (of which apathy is a key component) and cognitive performance, as research has focused more often on negative symptoms taken together than on apathy separately. Nieuwenstein and colleagues reported a meta-analysis of two neuropsychological tests that have been shown to be robustly affected in patients with schizophrenia: the Wisconsin Card Sorting Test and the Continuous Performance Test (51). They found a mean weighted (for sample size) correlation of 0.27 between Wisconsin Card Sorting Test perseverations and negative symptoms, based on 15 studies (representing 699 patients). For accuracy on the Continuous Performance Test, they reported a mean weighted correlation of −0.31 with negative symptoms. The magnitude of these effect sizes is in the small to moderate range, according to the widely accepted nomenclature of Cohen. They are larger for negative symptoms than for positive symptoms. In a subsequent meta-analysis that pooled more neuropsychological tests together, de Gracia Dominguez and colleagues reported correlations varying from −0.12 to −0.29 with negative symptoms (52). The highest correlation for negative symptoms was observed with verbal fluency. This association has also been reported in elderly people with cognitive decline (53). Again, although significant, the association is in the small to moderate range, implying that cognitive impairment as measured with classical neuropsychological tests cannot fully explain the lack of initiative and goal-directed behaviour characteristic of apathy.

Studies investigating apathy proper find associations in the same range of magnitude. These have been reported for global cognitive functioning, for example, as assessed with the MATRICS test battery (54) and for executive functioning, including verbal fluency (31, 55). An interesting study that was recently published looked into longitudinal relationships between cognitive impairment and apathy in patients with schizophrenia (56). The authors followed 137 patients with apathy and tested them after 1 month and after 1 year (81 patients participated then). At baseline, only episodic verbal learning (as assessed with the California Verbal Learning Test) was associated with apathy. At the follow-up measurement after 1 year, working memory was associated with an increased risk of severe overall apathy (the investigators adjusted for baseline apathy). Executive functioning as assessed with the Trail Making Test, the Six Element Test, and the Stop Signal Paradigm was not associated with apathy.

In conclusion, although small to moderate correlations have been established between cognitive functioning and apathy, more specific cognitive functions than those measured in standardized neuropsychological tests might deserve investigation as putative underpinnings for apathy. For example, specific reward-related processes such as imagining positive events in the near future may be of relevance for apathy. Indeed, cognitive processes needed for motivated goal-directed behaviour can be broken down in several subprocesses, ranging from intention and goal selection to action planning and execution (57, 58). These subprocesses certainly deserve further study, as does their interrelationship.

Results of Studies on Apathy in Schizophrenia

The Assessment of Apathy, Amotivation, and Avolition

The different scales in use for assessment of apathy, amotivation, and avolition in schizophrenia differ in their definition, and for most scales, except the AES, this is not addressed. Table 7.2 and Table 7.3 show how the scales differ in number of items. The scales also differ in how changes are quantified, and whether anhedonia and consummatory or anticipatory anhedonia are assessed. Most scales do not have threshold values for a clinical state of apathy. This, together with other assessment issues, has been addressed in several recent studies (11, 59, 60). Also, the use of different words for apathy is confusing for at least readers outside the field and is in need of revision (11).

The Clinical Incidence of Apathy in Schizophrenia and Psychotic Disorders

The frequency of apathy at different stages of psychosis and schizophrenia has not been reported in many studies. Apathy has been reported to be present in first-episode psychosis at a level of 50%, reduced to 40% at 1-year follow-up and further reduction to 30% at 10-year follow-up (34, 36, 46). Motivational deficits are also found in at-risk individuals for psychosis (61), but most studies only report on negative symptoms. Negative symptoms are prevalent in early-onset schizophrenia, but no study so far has addressed the negative symptoms at the sub-symptom level (62).

The Association with Other Clinical Symptoms

Positive Symptoms
Very few studies report on the association between apathy and positive symptoms, and when they do, find a low correlation of either non-significance or in the range of 0.2–0.3 (34, 36, 63). This applies to first-episode samples as well as chronic patients.

Depression
Clinically, the symptoms of apathy and depression overlap with the reduced feeling of pleasure (anhedonia), loss of initiative, and affective flattening which makes the two challenging to differentiate and one may be taken for the other (64). Depression is a frequent symptom in schizophrenia, with high prevalence in the early stage, but with assumed different underlying mechanisms and pathways than negative symptoms (64). Studies show that depression and apathy can be present at the same time, or independent of each other (35). Depression has less influence on functioning, and in the presence of apathy the influence of depression on functioning is even less (35). In contrast to depression, apathy is not characterized by low self-esteem or feelings of hopelessness.

The correlation between apathy and depression varies from 0.2 to 0.5 across the different stages of illness (33, 65) and depends on assessment instruments as well as stage of illness (66). Apathy and depression differ in their association to outcome— whereas apathy more affects functional outcome, depression is more associated with poor quality of life and suicide (67).

Anhedonia and motivation are central to many mental disorders, cut across diagnoses, and are closely linked to each other, which is also the case in schizophrenia. Motivation is in part dependent on the feeling of pleasure in order to fulfil the goal (68). Delineating of anhedonia has given valuable insight into the understanding of the motivational process in schizophrenia. Studies have found that patients with depression have a reduced consummatory pleasure while patients with schizophrenia have reduced anticipatory pleasure (68, 69). For both groups, this can influence their motivation and degree of initiative and may explain the stable association when clinical assessment is used. This valuable knowledge is important for the next phase in treatment of apathy (70, 71).

Negative Symptoms

Factor analytic studies of the negative symptoms assessed with different scales find two factors in most studies using the older scales (30); an experiential and an expressive factor. A recent study of the factor structure of the BNSS in a large sample (>1500 patients) revealed a five-factor model with separate factors for blunted affect, alogia, anhedonia, avolition, and asociality (72).

The Association with Functioning

Apathy and functioning are closely associated in schizophrenia in such a way that high levels of apathy give rise to poor functioning both in the prodromal phase, first episode, 1-year follow-up, and 10-year follow-up, and high baseline apathy predicts poor functioning at follow-up (31, 34, 35, 46, 65, 73–81).

Apathy and Antipsychotic Medication

Antipsychotic medication can induce negative symptoms and also apathy, especially when dosed too high. It is important to note that negative symptoms are also found in patients who are unmedicated and in the prodrome. Longitudinal studies show reductions of negative symptoms and apathy even when patients remain on medication (30). Thus, medication is certainly not the main cause of negative symptoms and apathy in patients with schizophrenia.

Brain Structure

We will only briefly describe structural neural correlates of apathy in schizophrenia, as Chapter 10 in this book is devoted to structural imaging studies of apathy. In their review of neuroimaging correlates of apathy across disorders such as schizophrenia, depression, acquired brain injury, and dementias, Kos et al. (2016) concluded that abnormalities within frontal-striatal circuits are most consistently associated with apathy (82). The authors noted that abnormalities within the parietal cortex were also linked to apathy, a region previously not included in neuroanatomical models of apathy. Tumati and colleagues further discussed a possible role for the parietal lobe in the generation of goal-directed behaviour (57). Areas most consistently associated with apathy remain the medial prefrontal cortex, orbitofrontal cortex, basal ganglia, thalamus, and dorsolateral prefrontal cortex (55). A role for the cerebellum has also been suggested (83). The variance in brain regions implicated in apathy may suggest that different routes towards apathy are possible.

Two recent studies of grey matter density as measured with magnetic resonance imaging both reported frontal involvement of apathy in schizophrenia patients, albeit in different ways. Mørch-Johnsen and colleagues investigated magnetic resonance correlates of apathy in 70 first-episode patients who were divided into two groups based on the AES (84). The group (N = 18) with high apathy scores showed a significantly thinner left orbitofrontal cortex and left anterior cingulate cortex. This remained significant after controlling for depressive symptoms and antipsychotic medication. Caravaggio and colleagues investigated 20 stable patients with schizophrenia using the apathy/avolition subscale of the SANS (85). Apathy scores were negatively correlated with several grey matter clusters in frontal regions, including the frontal inferior operculum and the left dorsal anterior cingulate cortex. Such associations were not observed for affective flattening, a closely related negative symptom. Another study reported an association with ventral striatum volumes in 23 patients: higher apathy (self-report AES) was associated with reduced grey matter in the ventral striatum (38). Clearly, however, these studies may well be underpowered, as at least 30 participants per group (higher versus lower apathy scores, thus at least 60 in total) are necessary for establishing effects sizes of medium magnitude. More reliable results are to be expected from studies with larger samples.

Functional Neuroimaging Studies

Chapter 12 describes functional neuroimaging studies of apathy in more detail (in people with schizophrenia and for other conditions). Only a few studies have explicitly investigated the functional neuroimaging correlates of apathy in schizophrenia. Simon et al. (2010) investigated reward-related processing in relation to apathy (37). They compared brain activation of 15 patients with schizophrenia (who were all using antipsychotic medication) to that of 15 healthy control subjects using a probabilistic monetary incentive delay task. An interesting dissociation was observed: while ventral-striatal activation during reward anticipation was negatively correlated with apathy, activation during receipt of reward was negatively correlated with severity of depressive symptoms. Chapter 11 summarizes more recent studies into reward processing and apathy.

With regard to executive functioning, Liemburg and colleagues compared patients with schizophrenia or psychotic spectrum disorder (n = 47) and healthy controls (n = 20), while performing a planning task, the Tower of London task, during functional magnetic resonance imaging scanning (86). Apathy (or, more specifically, the social amotivation factor of the PANSS, comprising four items that correlate highly with the AES) was associated with less task-related activation within the inferior parietal lobule, precuneus, and thalamus.

A number of studies investigated resting-state connectivity in relationship to negative symptoms (and more specifically apathy) in schizophrenia. Brady and colleagues used a data-driven analysis and reported a reduced connectivity between the thalamus and dorsolateral prefrontal cortex with negative symptom severity in 44 patients with schizophrenia. In a subgroup of patients ($n = 11$) they were able to use brain stimulation with repetitive transcranial magnetic stimulation in an attempt to restore network connectivity (87). This was successful and corresponded to amelioration of negative symptoms. Regarding apathy proper, two studies reported a reduced connectivity from the ventral tegmental area (VTA) to frontal areas, among others. The VTA is a key region in the dopamine system, important for driving motivated behaviour (88). Giordano and colleagues reported findings from 28 patients with schizophrenia in whom significant negative correlations were found between avolition and resting-state functional connectivity of the VTA with the bilateral insula, right ventrolateral prefrontal cortex, and right lateral occipital complex (89). In 2019, Xu and colleagues correlated the social amotivation factor of the PANSS (the four items that correlate highly with the AES) to VTA connectivity in 84 patients with schizophrenia and reported associations with medial and lateral prefrontal cortex, the temporoparietal junction, and dorsal and ventral striatum (90). These associations were observed independently of depressive and positive symptoms.

Treatment

Psychosocial

The focus on apathy and motivation in schizophrenia has given rise to suggestions of different new psychosocial treatment options, some which first were found effectful for negative symptoms, such as cognitive training of defeatist beliefs. Defeatist beliefs are prominent in patients with negative symptoms (91, 92), and in recent studies linked also to amotivation (79, 93–97). The origin of defeatist beliefs could be from different sources, the experience of reduced motivation or neurocognitive dysfunction that give rise to the feeling of incompetence compared to one's peers. Currently no intervention study has been reported but it is known that several are underway. One study of extended early intervention over step-down treatment had an effect in alleviating motivation (98). For young individuals with schizophrenia, a mobile app to enhance and support motivation has been developed (99). However, few treatment studies have been published and we are only at the beginning in trying out new interventions.

Pharmacology

Antipsychotic drugs are thought to produce secondary negative symptoms, but little is known at the sub-symptom level and new approaches to the understanding of this 'secondarity' are needed (43). One recent study has reported on the impact on motivation from antipsychotics and found no reduction in motivation after 6 months of antipsychotic treatment (100). In schizophrenia, as in other fields of medicine, the pharmacological treatment of apathy or motivation is still at the beginning (101) with single-patient reports or single studies that have not been repeated (102, 103).

Transcranial Stimulation

There is evidence to suggest that repetitive transcranial magnetic stimulation may be effective in reducing negative symptoms in schizophrenia. No studies have focused exclusively on apathy; they are, in general, aimed at improving negative symptoms overall. A meta-analysis of 22 studies (encompassing 827 patients with schizophrenia) reported a mean weighted effect size of 0.64 as compared to sham stimulation. However, a considerable number of studies failed to find an improvement, thus raising the question of replicability and/or moderator variables that are relevant in determining response. Chapter 15 describes non-invasive neurostimulation approaches in more detail.

Future Directions

What do we know and what do we need to know to advance further?

Studies in the last 15 years have confirmed what Kraepelin observed 150 years ago, that apathy is closely linked to functional impairments. Focusing on the negative symptom of apathy has given valuable knowledge of the underlying mechanism of apathy in schizophrenia so that we are much closer to starting intervention studies. Studies are still exploring the underlying mechanisms, and comparing results with studies in the healthy populations and other disorders. The reduced prediction of reward as shown with reduced anticipation of pleasure, executive functioning, and studies showing that patients with schizophrenia are less able to weigh effort and reward valuation in reaching a goal are all results that give a base for future studies to build on and translate into a real-world setting. Indeed, studies are emerging in which psychosocial approaches are investigated to enhance anticipation of pleasure and increase motivation.

Apathy is a transdiagnostic symptom, not specific for schizophrenia but more specific to schizophrenia than other mental disorders, and often with the same frequency as other neuropsychiatric disorders such as Alzheimer's dementia and Parkinson's disease. The transdiagnostic feature of apathy is of great value for the understanding and development of new treatment interventions. We still are in need of further knowledge of apathy, such as understanding more of the underlying mechanisms, individual differences, and prognosis and treatment. Are defeatist beliefs more linked to those who also have depressive symptoms? Joining forces with researchers investigating apathy in other disorders, such as neurodegenerative conditions, holds promise for accelerating progress.

References

1. Kirkpatrick B, Fenton WS, Carpenter WT, Jr, Marder SR. The NIMH-MATRICS consensus statement on negative symptoms. Schizophr Bull. 2006;32(2):214–9.
2. Foussias G, Remington G. Negative symptoms in schizophrenia: avolition and Occam's razor. Schizophr Bull. 2010;36(2):359–69.
3. Strauss GP, Cohen AS. A transdiagnostic review of negative symptom phenomenology and etiology. Schizophr Bull. 2017;43(4):712–9.
4. Kreapelin E. Dementia Praecox and Paraphrenia. Huntington, NY: Robert E Krieger Publishing Co. Inc; 1971.
5. Bleuler E. Dementia Praecox or the Group of Schizophrenias. New York: International Universities Press; 1950.
6. Spitzer RL, Endicott J, Robins E. Research diagnostic criteria. Psychopharmacol Bull. 1975;11(3):22–5.
7. Carpenter WT. Shifting paradigms and the term schizophrenia. Schizophr Bull. 2016;42(4):863–4.
8. Carpenter WT, Frost KH, Whearty KM, Strauss GP. Avolition, negative symptoms, and a clinical science journey and transition to the future. Nebr Symp Motiv. 2016;63:133–58.
9. Marin RS. Differential diagnosis and classification of apathy. Am J Psychiatry. 1990;147(1):22–30.
10. Berrios GE, Gili M. Will and its disorders: a conceptual history. Hist Psychiatry. 1995;6(21):87–104.
11. Thant T, Yager J. Updating apathy: using research domain criteria to inform clinical assessment and diagnosis of disorders of motivation. J Nerv Ment Dis. 2019;207(9):707–14.
12. Andreasen NC, Olsen S. Negative v positive schizophrenia. Definition and validation. Arch Gen Psychiatry. 1982;39(7):789–94.
13. Reininghaus U, Priebe S, Bentall RP. Testing the psychopathology of psychosis: evidence for a general psychosis dimension. Schizophr Bull. 2013;39(4):884–95.
14. Tonna M, Ossola P, Marchesi C, Bettini E, Lasalvia A, Bonetto C, et al. Dimensional structure of first episode psychosis. Early Interv Psychiatry. 2019;13(6):1431–8.
15. Berrios GE. Positive and negative symptoms and Jackson. A conceptual history. Arch Gen Psychiatry. 1985;42(1):95–7.
16. Andreasen NC. Negative symptoms in schizophrenia. Definition and reliability. Arch Gen Psychiatry. 1982;39(7):784–8.
17. Erhart SM, Marder SR, Carpenter WT. Treatment of schizophrenia negative symptoms: future prospects. Schizophr Bull. 2006;32(2):234–7.
18. Insel T, Cuthbert B, Garvey M, Heinssen R, Pine DS, Quinn K, et al. Research domain criteria (RDoC): toward a new classification framework for research on mental disorders. Am J Psychiatry. 2010;167(7):748–51.
19. Marin RS. Apathy: a neuropsychiatric syndrome. J Neuropsychiatry Clin Neurosci. 1991;3(3):243–54.
20. Clarke DE, Ko JY, Kuhl EA, van RR, Salvador R, Marin RS. Are the available apathy measures reliable and valid? A review of the psychometric evidence. J Psychosom Res. 2011;70(1):73–97.
21. Santangelo G, Barone P, Cuoco S, Raimo S, Pezzella D, Picillo M, et al. Apathy in untreated, de novo patients with Parkinson's disease: validation study of Apathy Evaluation Scale. J Neurol. 2014;261(12):2319–28.
22. Raimo S, Trojano L, Spitaleri D, Petretta V, Grossi D, Santangelo G. Apathy in multiple sclerosis: a validation study of the apathy evaluation scale. J Neurol Sci. 2014;15;347(1–2):295–300.

23. Andersson S, Krogstad JM, Finset A. Apathy and depressed mood in acquired brain damage: relationship to lesion localization and psychophysiological reaction. Psychol Med. 1999;29(2):447–56.
24. Clarke DE, Reekum R, Simard M, Streiner DL, Freedman M, Conn D. Apathy in dementia: an examination of the psychometric properties of the apathy evaluation scale. J Neuropsychiatry Clin Neurosci. 2007;19(1):57–64.
25. Clarke DE, van RR, Patel J, Simard M, Gomez E, Streiner DL. An appraisal of the psychometric properties of the Clinician version of the Apathy Evaluation Scale (AES-C). Int J Methods Psychiatr Res. 2007;16(2):97–110.
26. Kay SR, Fiszbein A, Opler LA. The positive and negative syndrome scale (PANSS) for schizophrenia. Schizophr Bull. 1987;13(2):261–76.
27. Kring AM, Gur RE, Blanchard JJ, Horan WP, Reise SP. The Clinical Assessment Interview for Negative Symptoms (CAINS): final development and validation. Am J Psychiatry. 2013;170(2):165–72.
28. Kirkpatrick B, Strauss GP, Nguyen L, Fischer BA, Daniel DG, Cienfuegos A, et al. The brief negative symptom scale: psychometric properties. Schizophr Bull. 2011;37(2):300–5.
29. Luther L, Lysaker PH, Firmin RL, Breier A, Vohs JL. Intrinsic motivation and amotivation in first episode and prolonged psychosis. Schizophr Res. 2015;169(1–3):418–22.
30. Liemburg E, Castelein S, Stewart R, van der Gaag M, Aleman A, Knegtering H. Two subdomains of negative symptoms in psychotic disorders: established and confirmed in two large cohorts. J Psychiatr Res. 2013;47(6):718–25.
31. Konstantakopoulos G, Ploumpidis D, Oulis P, Patrikelis P, Soumani A, Papadimitriou GN, et al. Apathy, cognitive deficits and functional impairment in schizophrenia. Schizophr Res. 2011;133(1–3):193–8.
32. Fervaha G, Foussias G, Agid O, Remington G. Amotivation and functional outcomes in early schizophrenia. Psychiatry Res. 2013;210(2):665–8.
33. Faerden A, Lyngstad SH, Simonsen C, Ringen PA, Papsuev O, Dieset I, et al. Reliability and validity of the self-report version of the apathy evaluation scale in first-episode psychosis: concordance with the clinical version at baseline and 12 months follow-up. Psychiatry Res. 2018;267:140–7.
34. Evensen J, Rossberg JI, Barder H, Haahr U, Hegelstad W, Joa I, et al. Apathy in first episode psychosis patients: a ten year longitudinal follow-up study. Schizophr Res. 2012;136(1–3):19–24.
35. Lyngstad SH, Gardsjord ES, Simonsen C, Engen MJ, Romm KL, Melle I, et al. Consequences of persistent depression and apathy in first-episode psychosis—a one-year follow-up study. Compr Psychiatry. 2018;86:60–6.
36. Faerden A, Friis S, Agartz I, Barrett EA, Nesvag R, Finset A, et al. Apathy and functioning in first-episode psychosis. Psychiatr Serv. 2009; 60(11):1495–503.
37. Simon JJ, Biller A, Walther S, Roesch-Ely D, Stippich C, Weisbrod M, et al. Neural correlates of reward processing in schizophrenia—relationship to apathy and depression. Schizophr Res. 2010;118(1–3):154–61.
38. Roth RM, Garlinghouse MA, Flashman LA, Koven NS, Pendergrass JC, Ford JC, et al. Apathy is associated with ventral striatum volume in schizophrenia spectrum disorder. J Neuropsychiatry Clin Neurosci. 2016;28(3):191–4.
39. Ringen PA, Falk RS, Antonsen B, Faerden A, Mamen A, Rognli EB, et al. Using motivational techniques to reduce cardiometabolic risk factors in long term psychiatric inpatients: a naturalistic interventional study. BMC Psychiatry. 2018;18(1):255.
40. Faerden A, Nesvag R, Barrett EA, Agartz I, Finset A, Friis S, et al. Assessing apathy: the use of the Apathy Evaluation Scale in first episode psychosis. Eur Psychiatry. 2008;23(1):33–9.

41. Fervaha G, Foussias G, Takeuchi H, Agid O, Remington G. Measuring motivation in people with schizophrenia. Schizophr Res. 2015;169(1–3):423–6.

42. Marin RS, Biedrzycki RC, Firinciogullari S. Reliability and validity of the Apathy Evaluation Scale. Psychiatry Res. 1991;38(2):143–62.

43. Kirschner M, Aleman A, Kaiser S. Secondary negative symptoms—a review of mechanisms, assessment and treatment. Schizophr Res. 2017;186:29–38.

44. Mucci A, Merlotti E, Ucok A, Aleman A, Galderisi S. Primary and persistent negative symptoms: concepts, assessments and neurobiological bases. Schizophr Res. 2017;186:19–28.

45. Carpenter WT, Jr, Heinrichs DW, Wagman AM. Deficit and nondeficit forms of schizophrenia: the concept. Am J Psychiatry. 1988;145(5):578–83.

46. Faerden A, Finset A, Friis S, Agartz I, Barrett EA, Nesvag R, et al. Apathy in first episode psychosis patients: one year follow up. Schizophr Res. 2010;116(1):20–6.

47. World Health Organization. The ICD-10 Classification of Mental and Behavioural Disorders. Diagnostic Criteria for Research. Geneva: World Health Organization; 1993.

48. American Psychiatric Association. Diagnostic and Statistical Manual of Mental Disorders DSM IV. 4th ed. Washington DC: American Psychiatric Association; 1994.

49. American Psychiatric Association. Schizophrenia spectrum and other psychotic disorder. In: Diagnostic and Statistical Manual of Mental Disorders, fifth edition. Arlington, VA: American Psychiatric Association; 2013, pp. 87–122.

50. Heinrichs RW, Zakzanis KK. Neurocognitive deficit in schizophrenia: a quantitative review of the evidence. Neuropsychology. 1998;12(3):426–45.

51. Nieuwenstein MR, Aleman A, de Haan EH. Relationship between symptom dimensions and neurocognitive functioning in schizophrenia: a meta-analysis of WCST and CPT studies. J Psychiatr Res. 2001;35(2):119–25.

52. de Gracia Dominguez M, Viechtbauer W, Simons CJ, van OJ, Krabbendam L. Are psychotic psychopathology and neurocognition orthogonal? A systematic review of their associations. Psychol Bull. 2009;135(1):157–71.

53. van Reekum R, Stuss DT, Ostrander L. Apathy: why care? J Neuropsychiatry Clin Neurosci. 2005;17(1):7–19.

54. Nuechterlein KH, Green MF, Kern RS, Baade LE, Barch DM, Cohen JD, et al. The MATRICS Consensus Cognitive Battery, part 1: test selection, reliability, and validity. Am J Psychiatry. 2008;165(2):203–13.

55. Bortolon C, Macgregor A, Capdevielle D, Raffard S. Apathy in schizophrenia: a review of neuropsychological and neuroanatomical studies. Neuropsychologia. 2018;118(Pt B):22–33.

56. Raffard S, Gutierrez LA, Yazbek H, Larue A, Boulenger JP, Lancon C, et al. Working memory deficit as a risk factor for severe apathy in schizophrenia: a 1-year longitudinal study. Schizophr Bull. 2016;42(3):642–51.

57. Tumati S, Martens S, de Jong BM, Aleman A. Lateral parietal cortex in the generation of behavior: implications for apathy. Prog Neurobiol. 2019;175:20–34.

58. Levy R, Dubois B. Apathy and the functional anatomy of the prefrontal cortex-basal ganglia circuits. Cereb Cortex. 2006;16(7):916–28.

59. Luther L, Fischer MW, Firmin RL, Salyers MP. Clarifying the overlap between motivation and negative symptom measures in schizophrenia research: a meta-analysis. Schizophr Res. 2019;206:27–36.

60. Marder SR, Galderisi S. The current conceptualization of negative symptoms in schizophrenia. World Psychiatry. 2017;16(1):14–24.

61. Schlosser DA, Fisher M, Gard D, Fulford D, Loewy RL, Vinogradov S. Motivational deficits in individuals at-risk for psychosis and across the course of schizophrenia. Schizophr Res. 2014;158(1–3):52–7.

62. Petruzzelli MG, Margari L, Bosco A, Craig F, Palumbi R, Margari F. Early onset first episode psychosis: dimensional structure of symptoms, clinical subtypes and related neurodevelopmental markers. Eur Child Adolesc Psychiatry. 2018;27(2):171–9.

63. Fervaha G, Takeuchi H, Foussias G, Hahn MK, Agid O, Remington G. Achievement motivation in early schizophrenia: relationship with symptoms, cognition and functional outcome. Early Interv Psychiatry. 2018;12(6):1038–44.

64. Krynicki CR, Upthegrove R, Deakin JFW, Barnes TRE. The relationship between negative symptoms and depression in schizophrenia: a systematic review. Acta Psychiatr Scand. 2018;137(5):380–90.

65. Kiang M, Christensen BK, Remington G, Kapur S. Apathy in schizophrenia: clinical correlates and association with functional outcome. Schizophr Res. 2001;63(1–2):79–88.

66. Upthegrove R, Marwaha S, Birchwood M. Depression and schizophrenia: cause, consequence, or trans-diagnostic issue? Schizophr Bull. 2017;43(2):240–4.

67. Gardsjord ES, Romm KL, Rossberg JI, Friis S, Barder HE, Evensen J, et al. Depression and functioning are important to subjective quality of life after a first episode psychosis. Compr Psychiatry. 2018;86:107–14.

68. Gard DE, Kring AM, Gard MG, Horan WP, Green MF. Anhedonia in schizophrenia: distinctions between anticipatory and consummatory pleasure. Schizophr Res. 2007;93(1–3):253–60.

69. Barch DM, Pagliaccio D, Luking K. Mechanisms underlying motivational deficits in psychopathology: similarities and differences in depression and schizophrenia. Curr Top Behav Neurosci. 2016;27:411–49.

70. Nguyen A, Frobert L, McCluskey I, Golay P, Bonsack C, Favrod J. Development of the Positive Emotions Program for Schizophrenia: an intervention to improve pleasure and motivation in schizophrenia. Front Psychiatry. 2016;7:13.

71. Favrod J, Nguyen A, Chaix J, Pellet J, Frobert L, Fankhauser C, et al. Improving pleasure and motivation in schizophrenia: a randomized controlled clinical trial. Psychother Psychosom. 2019;88(2):84–95.

72. Ahmed AO, Kirkpatrick B, Galderisi S, Mucci A, Rossi A, Bertolino A, et al. Cross-cultural validation of the 5-factor structure of negative symptoms in schizophrenia. Schizophr Bull. 2019;45(2):305–14.

73. Fervaha G, Foussias G, Agid O, Remington G. Motivational and neurocognitive deficits are central to the prediction of longitudinal functional outcome in schizophrenia. Acta Psychiatr Scand. 2014;130(4):290–9.

74. Najas-Garcia A, Gomez-Benito J, Huedo-Medina TB. The relationship of motivation and neurocognition with functionality in schizophrenia: a meta-analytic review. Community Ment Health J. 2018;54(7):1019–49.

75. Chang WC, Hui CL, Chan SK, Lee EH, Chen EY. Impact of avolition and cognitive impairment on functional outcome in first-episode schizophrenia-spectrum disorder: a prospective one-year follow-up study. Schizophr Res. 2016;170(2–3):318–21.

76. Barch DM, Treadway MT, Schoen N. Effort, anhedonia, and function in schizophrenia: reduced effort allocation predicts amotivation and functional impairment. J Abnorm Psychol. 2014;123(2):387–97.

77. Bull H, Ueland T, Lystad JU, Evensen S, Martinsen EW, Falkum E. Vocational functioning in schizophrenia spectrum disorders: does apathy matter? J Nerv Ment Dis. 2016;204(8):599–605.

78. Faerden A, Barrett EA, Nesvag R, Friis S, Finset A, Marder SR, et al. Apathy, poor verbal memory and male gender predict lower psychosocial functioning one year after the first treatment of psychosis. Psychiatry Res. 2013;210(1):55–61.

79. Green MF, Hellemann G, Horan WP, Lee J, Wynn JK. From perception to functional outcome in schizophrenia: modeling the role of ability and motivation. Arch Gen Psychiatry. 2012;69(12):1216–24.

80. Foussias G, Mann S, Zakzanis KK, van RR, Agid O, Remington G. Prediction of longitudinal functional outcomes in schizophrenia: the impact of baseline motivational deficits. Schizophr Res. 2011;132(1):24–7.

81. Gard DE, Fisher M, Garrett C, Genevsky A, Vinograd S. Motivation and its relationship to neurocognition, social cognition, and functional outcome in schizophrenia. Schizophr Res. 2009;115(1):74–81.

82. Kos C, van Tol MJ, Marsman JB, Knegtering H, Aleman A. Neural correlates of apathy in patients with neurodegenerative disorders, acquired brain injury, and psychiatric disorders. Neurosci Biobehav Rev. 2016;69:381–401.

83. Schmahmann JD. Disorders of the cerebellum: ataxia, dysmetria of thought, and the cerebellar cognitive affective syndrome. J Neuropsychiatry Clin Neurosci. 2004;16(3):367–78.

84. Morch-Johnsen L, Nesvag R, Faerden A, Haukvik UK, Jorgensen KN, Lange EH, et al. Brain structure abnormalities in first-episode psychosis patients with persistent apathy. Schizophr Res. 2015;164(1–3):59–64.

85. Caravaggio F, Fervaha G, Menon M, Remington G, Graff-Guerrero A, Gerretsen P. The neural correlates of apathy in schizophrenia: an exploratory investigation. Neuropsychologia. 2018;118(Pt B):34–9.

86. Liemburg EJ, Dlabac-de Lange JJ, Bais L, Knegtering H, van Osch MJ, Renken RJ, et al. Neural correlates of planning performance in patients with schizophrenia—relationship with apathy. Schizophr Res. 2015;161(2–3):367–75.

87. Brady RO, Jr, Gonsalvez I, Lee I, Ongur D, Seidman LJ, Schmahmann JD, et al. Cerebellar-prefrontal network connectivity and negative symptoms in schizophrenia. Am J Psychiatry. 2019;176(7):512–20.

88. Lohani S, Poplawsky AJ, Kim SG, Moghaddam B. Unexpected global impact of VTA dopamine neuron activation as measured by opto-fMRI. Mol Psychiatry. 2017;22(4):585–94.

89. Giordano GM, Stanziano M, Papa M, Mucci A, Prinster A, Soricelli A, et al. Functional connectivity of the ventral tegmental area and avolition in subjects with schizophrenia: a resting state functional MRI study. Eur Neuropsychopharmacol. 2018;28(5):589–602.

90. Xu P, Klaasen NG, Opmeer EM, Pijnenborg GHM, van Tol MJ, Liemburg EJ, et al. Intrinsic mesocorticolimbic connectivity is negatively associated with social amotivation in people with schizophrenia. Schizophr Res. 2019;208:353–9.

91. Grant PM, Beck AT. Defeatist beliefs as a mediator of cognitive impairment, negative symptoms, and functioning in schizophrenia. Schizophr Bull. 2009;35(4):798–806.

92. Beck AT, Himelstein R, Grant PM. In and out of schizophrenia: activation and deactivation of the negative and positive schemas. Schizophr Res. 2019;203:55–61.

93. Couture SM, Blanchard JJ, Bennett ME. Negative expectancy appraisals and defeatist performance beliefs and negative symptoms of schizophrenia. Psychiatry Res. 2011;189(1):43–8.

94. Choi KH, Saperstein AM, Medalia A. The relationship of trait to state motivation: the role of self-competency beliefs. Schizophr Res. 2012;139(1–3):73–7.

95. Quinlan T, Roesch S, Granholm E. The role of dysfunctional attitudes in models of negative symptoms and functioning in schizophrenia. Schizophr Res. 2014;157(1–3):182–9.

96. Tabak NT, Horan WP, Green MF. Mindfulness in schizophrenia: associations with self-reported motivation, emotion regulation, dysfunctional attitudes, and negative symptoms. Schizophr Res. 2015;168(1–2):537–42.

97. Pillny M, Lincoln TM. Predictors of improved functioning in patients with psychosis: the role of amotivation and defeatist performance beliefs. Psychiatry Res. 2016;244:117–22.

98. Chang WC, Kwong VW, Chan GH, Jim OT, Lau ES, Hui CL, et al. Prediction of motivational impairment: 12-month follow-up of the randomized-controlled trial on extended early intervention for first-episode psychosis. Eur Psychiatry. 2017;41:37–41.
99. Schlosser DA, Campellone TR, Truong B, Etter K, Vergani S, Komaiko K, et al. Efficacy of PRIME, a mobile app intervention designed to improve motivation in young people with schizophrenia. Schizophr Bull. 2018;44(5):1010–20.
100. Fervaha G, Takeuchi H, Lee J, Foussias G, Fletcher PJ, Agid O, et al. Antipsychotics and amotivation. Neuropsychopharmacology. 2015;40(6):1539–48.
101. Chong TT, Husain M. The role of dopamine in the pathophysiology and treatment of apathy. Prog Brain Res. 2016;229:389–426.
102. Arnold DS, Rosse RB, Dickinson D, Benham R, Deutsch SI, Nelson MW. Adjuvant therapeutic effects of galantamine on apathy in a schizophrenia patient. J Clin Psychiatry. 2004;65(12):1723–4.
103. Padala PR, Burke WJ, Bhatia SC, Petty F. Treatment of apathy with methylphenidate. J Neuropsychiatry Clin Neurosci. 2007;19(1):81–3.

8

Apathy and Traumatic Brain Injury

Eliyas Jeffay, Kyrsten M. Grimes, and Konstantine K. Zakzanis

Traumatic Brain Injury

General Background

According to some estimates, a head injury occurs approximately once every 15–16 seconds (1). Globally, approximately 50 million traumatic brain injuries (TBIs) occur each year. The World Health Organization projected that neurological injury would be the most common cause of disability until 2030, a figure that is two to three times higher than contributions from Alzheimer's disease or cerebrovascular disorders combined (2). With an estimated total annual cost of US$400 billion (4), TBIs cost the international economy approximately 0.5% of the world's $73.7 trillion annual global output (4). These figures are theorized to be an underestimate, as not all persons sustaining milder TBIs may seek medical care.

Broadly speaking, a TBI can be defined as evidence of brain pathology or disruption in brain functioning due to an external force (3). In the United States, falls were the most common mechanism of TBI-related injury and accounted for 47.2% (413.2 per 100,000 population) of the combined total of TBI-related emergency department visits, hospitalizations, and deaths in 2013. Motor vehicle accident crashes were the second most common cause, accounting for 15.4% of total TBI-related injuries (142.1 per 100,000 population) in 2013. Lastly, TBIs that fell in the category of 'struck by/against' were the third most common mechanism of injury accounting for 13.7% of the total TBI-related injuries (121.7 per 100,000 population), which include sports-related and recreation-related injuries (5). Severity of TBI is important to articulate as it has important prognostic value and treatment implications.

Reliably, males have a higher risk of TBI-related injuries than do females. The Centers for Disease Control in the United States reported that males are 1.5 times more likely to sustain a TBI than are females (5). Canadian estimates are comparable with males having 60–80% higher rates of risk for TBI-related injuries than females over 8 years of data (2002–2009) (6, 7). Similarly, the World Health Organization reported that males have a two to three times greater likelihood of sustaining a TBI-related injury than females (2). This is postulated to be attributed to increased risk-taking behaviours and activities observed in men (8).

TBI severity can range from uncomplicated mild traumatic brain injury (mTBI), to complicated mTBI, to moderate TBI, and to severe TBI, and is determined by way of acute injury characteristics, such as the duration of post-traumatic amnesia (PTA), the Glasgow Coma Scale (GCS) score, duration of loss of consciousness, and absence/presence of neuroimaging findings (Table 8.1) (9–11). The GCS score is the most commonly employed scale for classifying TBI severity (11). This scale was first proposed by Teasdale and Jennett as an aid to the clinical assessment of post-traumatic (un)consciousness (12). It is typically employed by first responders and emergency triage personnel, as well as continuously during the acute periods of trauma in hospital. The scale has three components: eye opening, verbal response, and motor response. The eye-opening component score ranges from 1 (none) to 4 (spontaneous); verbal response score ranges from 1 (none) to 5 (oriented conversation); and the motor response score ranges from 1 (none) to 6 (obeys simple commands). The lowest possible score is 3 (deep coma or death) and the highest score is 15 (full wakefulness). It is generally agreed that following some sort of trauma to the head, a GCS score of 3–8 represents a severe TBI, 9–12 reflects a moderate TBI (9) and a score ranging from 13 to 15 would be indicative of a mTBI (10).

Several neurological organizations have published position statements on specific criteria to define TBI severity (11, 13–15) and specifically that of mTBI (10, 13, 16–18). The general consensus for the acute injury characteristics includes GCS score, PTA, loss of consciousness, and the presence or absence of neuroimaging findings after injury (Table 8.1). PTA is defined as the period from injury to the time when memory for day-to-day events continues. When PTA duration is less than 60 minutes, the severity falls in the mild category. A duration of 60 minutes to 24 hours is considered moderate TBI, and a duration greater than 24 hours is indicative of a severe injury (9). However, the reliability of using PTA data is poor, and data are inconsistent, and sometimes unavailable. PTA may also be a poor indicator of outcome in the absence of other information, such as injury characteristics, mechanism of injury, and neuroimaging findings (19). With respect to the latter, the role of neuroimaging in the clinical diagnosis of a TBI is limited to positive or negative findings. To this end, a positive finding on neuroimaging studies (i.e. contusion, haemorrhage) is commonly seen in moderate or severe TBI and less commonly observed in mTBI. As indicated in Table 8.1, when there is evidence of intracranial injury on a structural neuroimaging

Table 8.1 Classification of severity of traumatic brain injury

Variable	Uncomplicated mild	Complicated mild	Moderate	Severe
Glasgow Coma Scale	13–15	13–15	9–12	3–8
Loss of consciousness	<30 mins	<30 mins	30 mins–24 hours	>24 hours
Post-traumatic amnesia	<1 day	<1 day	1–7 days	>7 days
Positive neuroimaging	No	Yes	Yes or no	Yes

examination following a mTBI, it is termed a 'complicated' mTBI, to differentiate it from an uncomplicated (i.e. no evidence of intracranial injury on structural neuroimaging examination) mTBI.

Open/Closed

TBIs have been categorized into open and closed head injuries based on the pathophysiological processes that occur. Open head injuries are classified when something (e.g. bullets) penetrates the dura mater, resulting in an open wound and/or skull fracture. These injuries have higher fatality rates than do closed head injuries, especially if the object penetrates through the midline (20). Closed head injuries involve a blow to the head but do not necessarily penetrate the dura mater (21). In closed head injuries, the inertial forces cause the brain to move towards the direction of the locus of the blow (coup) and impact the bony protrusions of the interior of the cranial fossa. The brain then recoils to the opposite direction of the blow (contrecoup) and once again may collide with the bony protrusions of the interior cranial fossa (21, 22). During the coup and contrecoup, the brain may incur forces that cause it to accelerate and decelerate quickly, rotate, and twist. Events such as car accidents, athletic injuries, and falls are common causes of closed head injuries (21). Closed head injuries constitute the majority of head injuries (23, 24).

Primary/Secondary

The pathophysiology of TBI has been further classified into primary and secondary injuries in the literature. Primary injuries, also known as direct injury, result from the energy transfer of the impact to the brain (21, 25). For example, if a person is hit on the forehead with a baseball bat, the kinetic energy from the baseball bat will transfer to compress the head. The brain inside the skull will move towards the anterior cranial fossa due to inertial forces and possibly impact the surface of the bone. Bone, by definition, is hard, whereas the brain is soft and fragile. The results of the impact may cause stretching, twisting, and ultimately degeneration of axons. This may occur simultaneously, at a focal point, or across the entire brain (21, 25).

Clinically, the ensuing damage and symptomatology is generally presented in the form of secondary injury. Secondary injuries manifest following the initial impact and may be observed as multiple lesions in white matter tracts (e.g. diffuse axonal injury), cerebral contusions, and focal shear injury (21). A disruption to cortical vasculature can cause haemorrhages, which may lead to haematomas. Thus, secondary injuries include but are not limited to contusions, haemorrhage, increased intracranial pressure (e.g. hydrocephalus and cerebral oedema), hypoxia, and ischaemia. The onset of secondary injury can range from minutes to weeks after the date of injury, and the individual can experience symptoms that last from days to years (25). During trauma (e.g. a motor vehicle accident), the physical forces can act in a linear, transverse, or rotational direction. The head may undergo rapid acceleration and deceleration on multiple planes of axis, which may cause cellular disruption (e.g. altered conduction velocities, changes to mitochondrial energy output, oxidative stress, cytoskeleton degeneration, neuroinflammation, and ionic imbalance) that may be undetectable through current progresses in neuroimaging (4, 21, 25).

Typical Sequelae

The neuropathology following TBI can be described as both focal and diffuse. Penetrating objects clearly have focal disruption of the tissue they obliterate. They also cause diffuse effects throughout the brain as a result of disruption of interconnected neural networks, shock waves, and pressure effects. Similarly, closed head injuries cause diffuse effects and multifocal lesions as a result of contusions, ischaemia, and specific structures that are more prone to shearing effects. Moreover, the frontal and temporal lobes are more vulnerable due to the bony protrusions in the cranial fossa (26).

Due to the diffuse aspect of the injury, the typical sequelae of symptoms following a TBI may be all-encompassing and non-specific across physical, psychological, and cognitive domains. Somatic symptoms following a TBI can include headache, dizziness, sleep disturbance, fatigue, irritability, sensitivity to noise and light, and nausea (27–29). Emotional distress, such as depression, anxiety disorders (30), apathy (31), and other forms of psychopathology are also common (32). These symptoms may be a direct result of the injury or as a psychological reaction to the cognitive and physical changes (33). Regarding apathy specifically, neuroimaging studies have found associations between apathy and the anterior cingulate cortex, which is implicated in goal-directed behaviour, decision-making, and reward monitoring (34). Specifically, TBI with symptoms of apathy was associated with significant volume loss in the medial frontal and lateral areas such as the prefrontal cortex and insula (35). A myriad of neuropsychological impairments have been reported as well, including slowed information processing (36, 37), reduced visuomotor speed (38, 39), attentional deficits (40, 41), memory difficulties (39, 42), executive dysfunction (43–45), reduced expressive fluency (46, 47), and reduced awareness (48). Cognitive sequelae following a TBI shows a clear dose–response relationship between TBI severity and the breadth and severity of cognitive impairment (49). There is robust evidence of long-term (i.e. greater than 6 months) cognitive impairment associated with moderate to severe TBI (50, 51).

Disability

Although TBI was previously viewed as a single event that results in complete or incomplete recovery, it is now considered a chronic and often progressive disease with long-term consequences (8, 52, 53). It can impact a variety of activities of daily living, such as preparing meals, remembering appointments, managing finances, caregiving, home maintenance activities, self-care, mobility, shopping, and social and recreational activities (54). There is some evidence that PTA in conjunction with loss of consciousness is indirectly related to functional outcome (6, 55–59). As per the World Health Organization report on neurological disorders, approximately 50% of all trauma-related deaths are due to TBIs, and TBIs are the leading cause of death and disability in children and young adults (2).

Traumatic Brain Injury Lifespan

Regarding age ranges, many studies have indicated that the two age groups that are most at risk for TBIs are the very young (birth to 4 years old) and the elderly (5, 23, 60, 61). Race and socioeconomics appear to play a factor as well. The Healthy Aging in Neighborhoods of Diversity across the Life Span study reported that low-income, white males aged 30–36 years and low-income African Americans aged 56–64 years were found to be most at risk for TBI in an archival study on 2881 participants who self-reported lifetime history of TBI (62).

Prevalence of Apathy after Traumatic Brain Injury

Apathy, which is a 'lack of interest, enthusiasm, or concern' is of Greek origin (*apatheia*) and is derived from a- 'without' and pathos 'suffering' (63). It is not listed in the fifth edition of the *Diagnostic and Statistical Manual of Mental Disorders* (DSM-5) (64) as a distinct disorder or syndrome but rather a symptom that may be associated with a wide range of diagnostic categories (65). This symptom has gradually been referred to as a distinct syndrome and disorder. Although several specific definitions of apathy have been proposed (66–68), most agree that there are elements of reduced motivation, disinterest, lack of self-derived initiation, and emotional blunting.

Apathy is increasingly being recognized as a common symptom after a TBI, which affects behaviour, cognition, and emotion. Prevalence rates range from 11% to 71% (69–72). Accurately estimating the prevalence rate of apathy following a TBI is challenging, however, as there is a lack of agreement in the field regarding the operational definition of apathy.

Apathy is described in many ways: amotivation, anergia, avolition, indifference, insensitivity, lethargy, aloofness, coldness, coolness, detachment, disinterest, dispassion, disregard, dullness, emotionlessness, heedlessness, insensibility, insouciance, lazy, lassitude, listlessness, passiveness, passivity, stoicism, unconcern, unresponsiveness, half-heartedness, and so on. This heterogeneity of descriptors compounded with the heterogeneity of methodologies used across studies to measure apathy poses a challenge when determining the prevalence of apathy after TBI.

In addition to the many terms used to label apathy, depression is also common after TBI and overlaps with this construct, making it more difficult to estimate its true prevalence. Features of depression, such as significant weight loss, insomnia, psychomotor agitation or retardation, fatigue or loss of energy, and diminished ability to think or concentrate, are also observed in apathy. Combined with disinterest in activities, these five (out of nine) features of apathy would fulfil the diagnostic criteria for depression as per the DSM-5. Thus, there is potential for misdiagnosis of depression when apathy may be the primary concern.

While symptoms of depression and apathy may overlap to a degree, there is some evidence of dissociation, however. Kant and colleagues examined 83 patients who had sustained a TBI using the Apathy Evaluation Scale (AES (73)) and the Beck Depression Inventory (74) and found 71% of patients reported symptoms of apathy with or without depression but only 11% reported apathy without depression and another 11% reported symptoms of depression but not apathy (71). Similar dissociations of apathy and depression have been found in neurodegenerative disorders (75–77). More research is needed to elucidate the construct of apathy from depression to better understand the prevalence of apathy after TBI.

Finally, prevalence rates are also impacted by the way apathy is assessed. Self-reported apathy is questionable, as an individual's cognitive symptoms and potential lack of awareness may preclude reliable introspection and symptom reporting. Caregivers may misattribute apathetic behaviours as 'laziness', leading to inaccurate assessment of the prevalence of apathy. Symptoms of apathy increase caregiver burden, which decreases quality of life for both the patients and caregiver. In turn, this adds to the functional disability of the patient (78).

Assessment of Apathy

Measurement

Several measures have been developed to assess apathy in neurological disorders, including the Apathy Inventory (79), Neuropsychiatric Inventory (80), and Apathy Scale (81). While these measures are sometimes used in TBI research (82, 83) they are primarily utilized in studies examining neurodegenerative illnesses, such as Parkinson's disease.

Apathy Evaluation Scale
One of the most commonly used apathy measures in TBI research is the AES (73). It is an 18-item self-report questionnaire. Items are rated on a four-point Likert scale (not at all true to very true). An example of an item is, 'I get things done during the day'. There are three versions: informant, clinician, and self-rated. The initial validation

study was conducted on a sample of participants aged 55–85 years old who were diagnosed with stroke, probable Alzheimer's disease, or major depressive disorder. All three versions demonstrated adequate reliability and validity (73).

Even though this measure is widely used in TBI research, very few studies have examined the psychometric properties of the AES in this population. Lane-Brown and Tate found the measure to have adequate reliability and validity in a TBI sample (84). It was only moderately correlated with the apathy subscale of the Frontal Systems Behaviour Scale (FrSBe (85)), however. It was suggested that the AES taps into the emotional aspects of apathy, whereas the FrSBe taps into the behavioural aspects of apathy (84). This is in keeping with the multidimensional nature of apathy previously discussed.

Only two studies have attempted to establish a cut-off score for the diagnosis of apathy in TBI. Glenn and colleagues were unable to find a cut-off score that had adequate sensitivity and specificity (86). Lane-Brown and Tate proposed a cut-off score of 37 if using the measure to determine eligibility for interventions, resulting in 83% sensitivity and 67% specificity (84). They noted that within this context, it is better to be overinclusive than underinclusive, but 37 would not be an appropriate cut-off score in other contexts where specificity is also critical. Given these findings, it is recommended that the AES be utilized as a dimensional measure of apathy. This is in keeping with the overall trend in the field to move towards a dimensional model for understanding psychological symptoms.

Frontal Systems Behaviour Scale

The FrSBe, previously titled the Frontal Lobe Personality Scale, is another widely used measure to evaluate apathy in TBI (85). It was developed to assess behaviour changes associated with frontal lobe damage. It consists of three subscales—apathy, disinhibition, and executive functioning—and contains 46 items. The responder rates each item based on their behaviours or experiences prior to the brain injury or illness and after brain injury or illness. Items are rated on a five-point Likert-scale (almost never to almost always). An example of an item from the apathy subscale is 'Speaks only when spoken to'. There is both a self-rated and family-rated version.

The sample size in the initial validation study consisted of 87 participants between the ages of 19 and 78 years. The sample consisted of individuals with frontal lobe damage (i.e. diagnoses included closed head injury, stroke, tumour, and haemorrhage, among others), non-frontal lobe damage (i.e. stroke diagnosis), and healthy controls. The measure demonstrated adequate reliability and validity (85). It has similarly shown good psychometric properties in TBI samples (84, 87), although findings regarding its factor structure in this population are mixed (87–89).

Apathy Versus Depression

As previously discussed, the syndrome of apathy is not only thought to be distinct from depression but also hypothesized to have an organic basis. This is in comparison to the symptom of apathy observed in depression, which is thought to have a psychological cause (73). Given this, it is important to establish whether measures of apathy can discriminate between the syndrome and symptom of apathy.

In the initial validation study for the AES, only the clinician- and self-rated versions were able to discriminate between apathy and depression, but the authors suggested this was due to the use of an uncommon measure to evaluate depression (73). Other studies that attempted to discriminate between these two constructs using the AES in a TBI sample obtained mixed results (69, 71, 84). Comparably less research has examined the ability of the apathy subscale on the FrSBe to discriminate those with apathy versus those with depression.

Certainly, a low correlation between a scale measuring apathy and a scale measuring depression suggests that these are in fact two different constructs. This is perhaps unsurprising, however, as depression includes a host of other symptoms that are not part of apathy, such as low mood and fatigue. Thus, to correlate the AES or FrSBe apathy subscale with a measure of depression, one is correlating 18 items to a measure that perhaps has only two or three items explicitly tapping into the construct of apathy. The more critical question beyond the basic psychometric properties of the apathy measures is whether they can differentiate between the symptom and syndrome of apathy, which has yet to be examined. It is questionable whether the behavioural manifestations and subjective internal experiences of apathy in neurological and psychological disorders are qualitatively different. As such, the likelihood of a self-report measure being able to differentiate between these constructs is unlikely. Indeed, the AES was initially developed to measure apathy across neurological and psychological disorders (73). Further, individuals who experience TBI often experience significant psychological and environmental changes as a result. As such, identifying the cause of apathy is challenging.

Taken together, while there are various measures to assess apathy in neurological disorders, the AES and FrSBe are perhaps the most commonly used in TBI research. Further research is necessary to establish the psychometric properties of these measures in TBI populations, however. The research conducted thus far suggests that apathy can be differentiated from depression, although further research is needed to determine if there are qualitative differences between the syndrome and the symptom whether apathy measures are able to discriminate between these two constructs.

Neurobiology of Apathy after Traumatic Brain Injury

As previously stated, apathy is observed across a range of neurological disorders. Unfortunately, much of what we know regarding the neuroanatomical correlates of apathy in TBI is theoretical or based on isolated case studies. Numerous systematic reviews have been conducted on this topic with very few results. This often requires researchers to expand their search to studies of apathy in stroke to provide a more comprehensive explanation (90, 91). Of course, while stroke and TBI are both acquired brain injuries, the way in which the brain is impacted is distinctly different, which may also affect the way apathy develops and is expressed. To further complicate this, as previously stated, three subtypes of apathy have been proposed: emotional-affective (i.e. blunted affect, loss of interest in activities), cognitive (i.e. difficulty carrying out tasks and cognitive inflexibility), and auto-activation (i.e. lack of initiation of behaviours and thoughts), all of which are hypothesized to have different neuroanatomical correlates (92). Finally, given the significant life changes that often occur following a TBI, it would be difficult to disentangle whether apathy developed due to an organic or psychogenic cause or a combination of the two. This has implications for interpreting neuroimaging data. What follows is a review of the limited research conducted on the neuroanatomical correlates of apathy in TBI.

The frontal lobe is particularly susceptible to damage when a brain injury occurs (93). It is widely established that within this region the prefrontal cortex is responsible for executive functions and emotion regulation. Given that apathy is broadly defined as a reduction in goal-directed behaviours, which is largely an executive function, it has been hypothesized that damage to the prefrontal cortex is at least in part responsible for the development of apathy in TBI. It has further been proposed that damage to the amygdala may lead to apathy in TBI, given the role of the amygdala in the experience of emotions (90).

Andersson and colleagues examined apathy in acquired bran injury, including cerebrovascular, hypoxic, and TBI (70). Individuals with subcortical and right hemisphere damage exhibited significantly greater apathy than did those with left hemisphere or bilateral hemisphere damage. This finding was replicated in another sample of individuals with acquired brain injury (94). Unfortunately, because these were mixed samples, it is difficult to draw conclusions about the correlates of apathy in TBI specifically. Participants were categorized based on lesion location, but the groups were quite broad, providing little information about the specific brain structures involved. What can be gleaned from these studies is that the right hemisphere may play a greater role in the development of apathy in neurological disorders.

Paradiso and colleagues compared individuals with single lateral or single medial frontal lesions and found that individuals with lateral lesions exhibited greater apathy than did those with medial lesions (95). While this study looked at apathy exclusively in TBI, apathy was assessed by way of a mental status exam. As such, the reliability and validity of the assessment of apathy in this study is unknown.

These findings stand in contrast with the findings from Barrash and co-workers who found that individuals with bilateral ventromedial prefrontal lesions were significantly more apathetic, with a prevalence rate of 71%, than were those with prefrontal lesions with no bilateral ventromedial involvement or non-prefrontal lesions, with prevalence rates of 21% and 8% respectively (96). This is in contrast with previous findings that suggested apathy was less prevalent in those with bilateral lesions (70, 94).

The role of the ventromedial prefrontal cortex was further supported by the findings of Hogeveen et al. (97). Here, individuals with TBI were categorized based on lesion location: ventromedial prefrontal cortex, dorsolateral prefrontal cortex, other brain regions, and healthy controls (i.e. no brain lesion). Individuals with damage to the ventromedial prefrontal cortex exhibited significantly greater apathy than did the other groups. This study went one step further and attempted to understand the mechanisms involved in this relationship. Not only did this group exhibit greater apathy, but they also placed less value on a rewarding stimulus than did the other groups. This impaired valuation mediated the relationship between damage to the ventromedial prefrontal cortex and apathy scores. These findings suggest that damage to this region results in less perceived value of rewards, which leads to blunted affect and reduced goal-directed behaviour (97). This is one of the few empirical studies that evaluated the mechanism underlying apathy in TBI and warrants further exploration.

The findings support similar mechanisms proposed for apathy in neurodegenerative disorders. One model postulates that Alzheimer's-related apathy may result with damage to the circuit that connects the anterior cingulate cortex (attentional control/motivation) and insula (awareness) to the prefrontal cortex via the midbrain dopamine system (98, 99). Guild and Levine found that volume loss in these same midline and lateral regions were related to apathy in the chronic stages of TBI (34).

In contrast to Andersson and colleagues' findings that the right hemisphere plays a larger role in apathy after TBI (70), the left hemisphere may also be associated with apathy. The middle, superior, and inferior frontal regions (including the operculum and pars triangularis), supplementary motor area, anterior cingulate cortex, insula, corona radiata, and corpus callosum in the left hemisphere have all been implicated in apathy after penetrating TBI (34, 35). In support of this, Takayanagi and co-workers reported apathy scores were associated with reduced left hippocampal volume (100). They did not find a relationship between cortical thickness and apathy in individuals with severe TBI.

To summarize, much of what is known about the neuroanatomical correlates of apathy comes from isolated case studies. It is often necessary to draw on what is known about apathy in other neurological disorders, but it is unclear if these findings are generalizable to TBI. More research is needed before any strong conclusions can be drawn with respect to the neuroanatomical correlates of apathy in TBI.

Neuropsychology of Apathy after Traumatic Brain Injury

As noted previously, the neuropsychological profile after a TBI is non-specific and evidence for deficits across all domains have been reported (101). However, deficits in attention, executive functions, processing speed, memory acquisition, working memory, language, and visuospatial abilities are most commonly observed. Specifically, the domain of attention, difficulties with sustained, selective, and divided attention are characteristic following a TBI (102, 103). Reported symptoms such as difficulties with inhibitory control, being easily prone to distraction, and poor concentration are common following a TBI. Despite inconsistent test measures used to measure speed of processing, impairment in this domain has frequently been found following a TBI (104). Moreover, impairments in speed of processing may affect other cognitive domains, such as complex attention and executive functioning (102). Executive dysfunction, such as impaired working memory, planning, organization, problem-solving, and judgement, is also reported in this population and may manifest clinically as symptoms of poor self-control, insight, and self-awareness (104). Memory impairment is also prominent following a TBI, which some have argued may be due to impaired encoding. Encoding impairments might result from reduced speed of processing and poor working memory (104). To this end, difficulties with respect to encoding, storage, and retrieval have been reported (105). In more severe TBIs, deficits in language and visuoconstructional abilities have been documented. In the absence of a focal lesion to the language regions (left hemisphere in most individuals), classic aphasia is generally a rare occurrence following a TBI (106). More common are expressive difficulties such as word-finding problems with resultant circumlocutions, which may be due to impairments in working memory and reduced speed of processing (49). Similarly, visuoconstructional impairment is thought to be indirectly related to executive dysfunction such as impairments in working memory, planning, and organization and less so due to poor visual acuity (104).

Symptoms of depression, anxiety, disinhibition, and apathy may be a direct result of the brain injury or may manifest as a secondary reaction to the physical and cognitive changes following injury. At the risk of simplifying brain and behaviour relationships, the potential presence of neuroanatomical correlates of apathy implies that there may be associative, specific, and/or predictive cognitive dysfunction. Understanding the neuropsychological profile of apathy after TBI would be useful as efforts could be focused on the patient's strengths to aid in rehabilitating their weaknesses. Unfortunately, there is a dearth of studies examining the relationship between apathy and neuropsychological performance after TBI. Much is still unknown but patterns are emerging.

Andersson and Bergedalen sought to examine the cognitive profile of apathy in a sample ($N = 53$) of patients who had sustained a severe TBI (107). The AES along with a short neuropsychological battery were administered. Tests were grouped into seven cognitive domains: acquisition and memory, attention span, executive function, psychomotor speed, verbal skills, non-verbal skills, and motor speed. The authors found that endorsement of apathy as per the AES was not correlated with a global reduction in neuropsychological performance but rather with specific domains. Acquisition memory and executive functions were found to be significantly associated with higher scores on the AES. The authors noted that Pearson's product moment correlation of AES score and psychomotor speed was approaching significance ($r = -0.27$; $P = 0.06$). These three domains were included in a stepwise regression analysis to determine which cognitive variables predicted apathy. Acquisition memory was the only variable that was found to significantly predict apathy. A principal component analysis revealed that these three domains and the cognitive aspects of apathy from the AES loaded together. While this study did not explore any causal relationships between apathy and cognitive performance following a TBI, others have postulated a causal relationship between apathy and verbal memory impairment and phonemic fluency but small sample sizes ($N = 10$), heterogeneity of severity, and the lack of an appropriate control group (i.e. TBI without apathy) limit their findings (100). Andersson and Bergedalen's study did provide preliminary evidence to suggest specific deficits in the domains of acquisition memory along with executive functions (107). In other words, the presence of apathy after TBI may be associated with a patient's ability to learn, remember, and control behaviour in their daily life. Since these aspects of cognition are essential to activities of daily functioning (108, 109), patients with high apathy may appear to be slow to recover following a TBI. Thus, careful interpretation of the cognitive functions of patients with apathy in addition to highlighting behavioural observations during testing may be required as apathy may mask a patient's true cognitive ability, which in turn has implications for determining a patient's eligibility for treatment.

To examine if the findings from Andersson and Bergedalen (107) extended across all severities of TBI, a follow-up study was conducted (110). Patients who sustained a TBI were sequentially recruited from trauma units within 3 months of the date of injury. Sample sizes were not reported but the authors did report 57.3% had mild, 12.6% had moderate, and 16.5% had sustained a severe TBI. Patients were followed across four time points over the year (2 weeks, 3 months, 6 months, and 12 months post TBI) and evaluated on outcomes related to apathy and psychosocial functioning. Patients were also administered a cognitive battery but the specific tests were not reported. Results from a regression analysis indicated that higher AES scores less than 3 months post TBI were predictive of increased perseverative errors on the Wisconsin Card Sorting Test (111) at more than 3 months post TBI. A finding that was supported later by others (32). Rao and colleagues' study (110) provides additional support for the executive dysfunction associated with apathy following a TBI, but the lack of methodological elaboration and narrow neuropsychological battery limit the strength of these supportive findings. Furthermore, the results were not parsed by TBI severity groups. Thus, it is unclear what the impact of TBI severity and apathy may have on neuropsychological results.

Apathetic symptoms over the course of recovery were not explored in the study by Rao et al. (110). In an effort to elucidate the changes of apathy and cognition over 10 months after injury, a study with 32 patients with severe TBI and 36 community controls was conducted (31). Self-reported apathy and caregiver-reported apathy were assessed during inpatient rehabilitation stay and at 8–12-month follow-up. In addition to apathy questionnaires, patients were administered a cognitive battery with tests of working memory, verbal episodic memory, sensorimotor reaction time, cognitive flexibility, and executive functions. Across both time points, apathy was stable (i.e. no change in reported apathy) between the two time points for 27/32 patients (84.4%), increased for 4/32 patients (12.5%), and improved for 1/32 (3.1%) patients. Verbal memory and working memory performance during the inpatient rehabilitation stay was both associated and predictive of apathy at 8–12-month follow-up. To this end, verbal memory performance was related to caregiver apathy ratings rather than self-reported by the patient (31). Multitasking performance during the inpatient stay was also associated with apathy at follow-up but this relationship was not predictive as per regression analysis. The findings extend the work by Andersson and Bergedalen (107) in that memory difficulties are related to apathy and may be predictive of recovery after TBI. Moreover, the authors suggest that memory and working memory and predicted apathy may be related to return to productivity/work after TBI, as difficulties in updating and contents of working memory along with remembering information may be linked to poorer functional performance.

As noted in a previous section, disability following TBI may be long lasting and impacts instrumental activities of daily living, such as self-care, care-giving, mobility, home-maintenance activities, social and recreational activities, meal-preparation, and return to work (54). Indeed, typical referrals for a neuropsychological evaluation after a TBI pertain to a patient's cognitive strengths and weaknesses and how they may relate to their ability to engage in their instrumental activities of daily living. mTBIs are more common than moderate and severe TBIs combined. Assessment of mTBI contributes to the major proportion of private practice referrals with the most common question relating to capacity and prognosis of return to work (112). Neuropsychological impairment following a mTBI may be explained by factors such as pain disorders and headache (113), fatigue (36), stress at the time of injury (114, 115), post-traumatic stress (116–118), premorbid personality characteristic (119), involvement in litigation (27, 120–122), unremitting neuropathological alterations in mTBI that have yet to be fully understood (21, 93, 123), or depression and mood disorders (124–126). With respect to the latter, specific psychological symptomatology such as apathy may contribute greatly to the motivation to engage in activities of daily living, such as return to work.

Our group examined whether apathy could differentiate disability based on cognitive test performance (127). Patients were sourced from a large archival database of litigating patients who had incurred a mTBI and were referred for a neuropsychological evaluation. Diagnosis of mTBI was confirmed as per acute injury characteristics using the American Congress of Rehabilitation Medicine guidelines (Table 8.1) (10). Since patients were involved in litigation, a thorough and strict set of criteria for credible test performance was utilized, which included passing scores on symptom and performance validity tests, performance above known cut-off scores on embedded tests of effort, and lack of unusual symptom endorsement (i.e. painful hair, itchy finger nails). The final sample consisted of 104 participants who were on average 41.89 (standard deviation 13.45; range 19–78) years old. Sixty-six were in the disabled group whereas 38 were in the non-disabled group. Disability was assessed based on self-reported return to work in any capacity corroborated with their medical brief. Mean post-injury duration was approximately 2.87 years (Table 8.2). An analysis was conducted comparing neuropsychological test performance and reported apathy as per the AES between the two groups. We found significant differences between the

Table 8.2 Demographic information and injury characteristics of disabled and non-disabled mTBI patients

Variable	Disabled (N = 66)			Non-disabled (N = 38)		
	Mean	SD	%	Mean	SD	%
Age (years)	43.29	12.86		39.47	14.25	
Education (years)	13.62	2.74		13.78	2.67	
Gender ratio % (male/female)			56/44			42/58
Number of days since loss	987.11	837.41		1159.68	829.61	
Glasgow Coma Scale	14.66	0.59		14.53	0.61	

SD, standard deviation.

Reproduced from Applied Neuropsychology Adult, 24(6), Zakzanis KK, Grimes KM, Relationship among apathy, cognition, and real-world disability after mild traumatic brain injury, pp. 559–65, Copyright (2017), with permission from Taylor & Francis.

two groups on tests of verbal fluency, memory, and information processing. However, mean apathy scores did not significantly differ between the two groups. Further, an item analysis did not reveal significant difference across any items of the AES between disability groups (Table 8.3). These findings suggest that poorer cognitive performance was related to functional disability rather than apathy.

Of course, one cannot draw causal conclusions from our work, as there are several limitations hindering the generalization of the findings. The sample comprised a convenience sample of litigating patients with mTBI limiting the generalizability of the findings. The generalizability and reliability of the current findings need to be replicated in a non-litigating sample. Furthermore, all patients were in the post-acute period of recovery but time since injury was quite broad (102–5378 days). To this end, sequential recruitment of patients in a hospital setting with multiple follow-up assessments during the acute, subacute, and post-acute periods would control for potential recovery time effects. Including a matched control group would have improved the specificity of our findings and provided a clearer impact of the apathy after mTBI on return to work. Return to work was self-reported by each patient and was dichotomous as opposed to stratified, such as return to work with modified hours/duties as in other studies (128). Employment status confirmation by either the patient's employer or occupational therapist would have improved veracity of the patient's self-report. However, a follow-up with their employer may be considered intrusive and in breach of privacy. Despite these limitations, this study provided an important contribution to the ecological validity of apathy symptoms after mTBI.

The studies reviewed indicate that apathy after TBI is a common and elusive symptom with associated neuropsychological deficits. There is evidence that apathy

Table 8.3 Item analysis for the Apathy Evaluation Scale scores for disabled and non-disabled mTBI patients

AES	N	Disabled Mean (SD)	N	Non-disabled Mean (SD)	P
Total	66	38.29 (9.52)	38	36.08 (9.80)	n.s
AES 1		2.21 (0.79)		2.16 (0.86)	n.s.
AES 2		2.47 (0.77)		2.42 (0.72)	n.s.
AES 3		1.77 (0.84)		1.71 (0.90)	n.s.
AES 4		2.17 (0.92)		2.13 (1.11)	n.s.
AES 5		2.17 (1.00)		1.87 (0.99)	n.s.
AES 6		2.03 (1.08)		1.95 (0.90)	n.s.
AES 7		2.41 (0.99)		2.53 (1.03)	n.s.
AES 8		1.91 (1.76)		2.08 (1.14)	n.s.
AES 9		2.27 (0.89)		2.03 (0.97)	n.s.
AES 10		2.00 (1.02)		1.92 (1.14)	n.s.
AES 11		1.76 (1.03)		1.45 (0.86)	n.s.
AES 12		2.04 (0.90)		2.61 (5.13)	n.s.
AES 13		2.55 (2.61)		2.00 (1.07)	n.s.
AES 14		2.09 (0.87)		1.87 (0.88)	n.s.
AES 15		2.05 (0.75)		2.00 (0.81)	n.s.
AES 16		1.99 (0.95)		1.89 (0.92)	n.s.
AES 17		2.36 (0.87)		2.34 (0.91)	n.s.
AES 18		2.39 (0.89)		2.16 (0.97)	n.s.

M, mean; n.s., not significant; SD, standard deviation.

Reproduced from Applied Neuropsychology Adult, 24(6), Zakzanis KK, Grimes KM, Relationship among apathy, cognition, and real-world disability after mild traumatic brain injury, pp. 559–65, Copyright (2017), with permission from Taylor & Francis.

is not associated with global cognitive deficits but rather specific domains, such as executive functions and acquisition memory. At the moment, only associations between deficits in these domains and apathy after TBI can be made. Replication, strict methodology, and exploring the dissociation of apathy and other related symptoms and their effects on neurological functioning are necessary to elucidate robust patterns and the exploration of causal relationships. Future studies should also focus on the functional implications of apathy after TBI and attempt to delineate any associations with respect to TBI severity, acute injury characteristics, time since injury, demographics, comorbid psychiatric conditions, and self-reported versus observed apathy.

Treatment Considerations

The presence of apathy has significant implications for treatment and rehabilitation in TBI. Research indicates that individuals with high levels of apathy are at greater risk of dropping out of treatment (129). This is concerning, given that apathy is more prevalent in those with moderate to severe TBI where early intervention is critical. These individuals are not only at risk of not receiving treatment but also may receive less benefit. Andersson and colleagues had individuals with severe TBI engage in a therapeutic interaction in which they were asked to describe the event that resulted in the injury, the difficulties they are experiencing, and the long-term consequences of the injury (70). Not only did individuals in the apathetic group report less emotional discomfort during the interaction, they had a lesser physiological (i.e. blood pressure and heart rate) response than did the non-apathetic group. The authors suggested that this is indicative of a dampened emotional response, rather than a suppressed emotional reaction, where there may be low self-reported distress but high physiological activity. While emotional involvement may be less critical for neurocognitive rehabilitation, the authors highlight that it is essential for psychotherapy. As such, apathy may reduce patients' responsivity to treatment.

Apathy is not only potentially therapy-interfering but also may have detrimental effects on long-term outcomes. A longitudinal study conducted by Arnould and colleagues found that apathy levels remained the same over a 10-month period for individuals with severe TBI, and for a small percentage of these individuals, apathy symptoms increased (31). Patients with worsening apathetic symptoms exhibited greater memory impairments at 10 months than did those whose symptoms remained the same. In contrast, DeBoussard and co-workers assessed individuals with severe TBI at 3 weeks, 3 months, and 1 year post injury and found that apathy was significantly less common at 3 months than at 3 weeks (130). For those patients who did exhibit apathy at 3 months, however, it was associated with poor outcomes at 1 year post injury. Apathy has also been associated with poor interpersonal functioning (131), reduced self-efficacy (31), and fewer coping strategies (94).

Despite these consequences, very few studies have explicitly looked at the treatment of apathy in TBI. No high-quality studies have examined the use of pharmacological interventions, although some initial support has been established for the use of dopamine agonists (72) and acetylcholinesterase inhibitors (132, 133) in this population.

With respect to non-pharmacological interventions, only a small number of preliminary investigations have been undertaken. Lane-Brown and Tate conducted a single-patient case study to examine the effectiveness of motivational interviewing and external rewards to treat apathy in a patient with a severe TBI (134). Apathy decreased as a result of the intervention, which was maintained at 1-month follow-up. Tate and colleagues employed a single-case experimental design utilizing a novel intervention titled the Programme for Engagement, Participation, and Activities (135). The intervention included three stages: (i) assessment and goal planning, (ii) weekly individual sessions to assist patients in implementing target behaviours at home, and (iii) maintenance of therapeutic gains. Target behaviours were developed collaboratively with the patient and focused on increasing meaningful activities. The study included seven participants with severe TBI. Six of the seven participants showed improvements in being able to carry out the target behaviours independently with large effect sizes. These results are promising but need to be tested in a randomized controlled trial with a larger sample.

Wiart and colleagues employed a neuro-systemic psychotherapy with 47 participants to address the emotional and behavioural symptoms observed in TBI, including apathy (136). While the nature of the intervention was not clearly described, it appeared to focus on improving the participants' functioning within their interpersonal relationships. Improvements were observed for anxiety, depressed mood, and hostility but not for apathy.

Given the lack of research, it may prove useful to consider how apathy is treated in other neurological disorders. Holmes and co-workers found that exposing patients with moderate to severe dementia to live music resulted in greater positive engagement relative to pre-recorded music or no music (137). Positive engagement was assessed qualitatively based on video recordings. As such, it is possible that this intervention resulted in improvements in mood, rather than apathy per se. While the results are positive, it is likely that this intervention is less applicable to a TBI population. In individuals with severe dementia, activities of daily living and the ability to function independently are already severely impaired. Thus, the goal of treatment may be different than in patients with TBI, where the aim is to improve engagement in rehabilitation and increase goal-directed behaviour, rather than simply increasing engagement with the environment.

Given the impact apathy has on treatment responsivity, as well as the psychological and social outcomes associated with apathy in TBI, treatment for this condition is critical. Very few studies have examined the use of pharmacological and psychosocial interventions for apathy in this population. Of the non-pharmacological treatments, interventions are primarily behavioural (e.g. rewards) and closely resemble intervention strategies employed in depression (e.g. motivational interviewing, behavioural activation). This leads one to question the utility or meaningfulness of distinguishing the syndrome of apathy from the symptom if they are treated similarly. It may be beneficial to consider how apathy is treated in psychiatric disorders and whether this can be applied to a neurological population. Given the organic basis of apathy in TBI, it might also be important to incorporate the treatment of apathy into neurocognitive rehabilitation programmes, which has yet to be examined.

Conclusion

In sum, despite the lack of studies and heterogeneity in methodologies, one certainty that can be gleaned is that apathy after TBI is common and may be associated with cognitive and affective symptoms post injury. There are still many aspects that are poorly understood such as the neuroanatomical, neurocognitive, psychological, and even environmental factors that may impact apathy after TBI. Initial hypotheses regarding the neuroanatomical basis of apathy in TBI were derived from studies on apathy in neurodegenerative disorders (65). Neuroanatomically, the prefrontal cortex and the anterior cingulate cortex, in conjunction with the insula and motor areas, appear to be involved in motivation, attentional control, and self-awareness, which are all aspects of apathy and regions of the brain that are commonly disrupted following brain injury. There is preliminary evidence that apathy may be associated with cognitive deficits in memory and executive functioning, rather than a global reduction of neurocognitive functioning (107). Moreover, there may be an interaction between TBI severity and functional impact of apathy (127). Replication is necessary to validate and generalize these initial findings, however. A major gap in apathy research is defining apathy and how it differentiates from depression (65). The assessment of apathy is largely completed through self-reported questionnaires and may involve caregivers. Ideally, self-reported questionnaires would be used in combination with psychological, neuropsychological, and neuroimaging data in an effort to determine one's risk for developing apathy, types of apathy, and stability of apathy over the course of recovery. Greater understanding of the factors involved in apathy following brain injury would improve research and development of targeted treatments, such as cognitive, behavioural, and pharmacological interventions.

References

1. Signoretti S, Vagnozzi R, Tavazzi B, Lazzarino G. Biochemical and neurochemical sequelae following mild traumatic brain injury: summary of experimental data and clinical implications. Neurosurg Focus. 2010;29(5):E1.
2. World Health Organization. Neurological Disorders: Public Health Challenges. Geneva: World Health Organization; 2006.
3. The World Bank. World Development Indicators database. 2017. https://databank.worldbank.org/data/download/GDP.pdf
4. Maas AIR, Menon DK, Adelson PD, Andelic N, Bell MJ, Belli A, et al. Traumatic brain injury: integrated approaches to improve prevention, clinical care, and research. Lancet Neurol. 2017;16(12):987–1048.
5. Taylor CA, Bell JM, Breiding MJ, Xu L. Traumatic brain injury-related emergency department visits, hospitalizations, and deaths—United States, 2007 and 2013. MMWR Surveill Summ. 2017;66(9):1–16.
6. Colantonio A, Mroczek D, Patel J, Lewko J, Fergenbaum J, Brison R. Examining occupational traumatic brain injury in Ontario. Can J Public Health. 2010;101(Suppl 1):S58–62.

7. Fu TS, Jing R, Fu WW, Cusimano MD. Epidemiological trends of traumatic brain injury identified in the emergency department in a publicly-insured population, 2002–2010. PLoS One. 2016;11(1):e0145469.
8. Corrigan JD, Hammond FM. Traumatic brain injury as a chronic health condition. Arch Phys Rehabil Med. 2013;94(6):1199–201.
9. Bryant RA, O'Donnell ML, Creamer M, McFarlane AC, Clark CR, Silove D. The psychiatric sequelae of traumatic injury. Am J psychiatry. 2010;167(3):312–20.
10. Kay T, Harrington D, Adams R, Anderson T, Berrol S, Cicerone K, et al. Definition of mild traumatic brain injury. J Head Trauma Rehabil. 1993;8(3):86–7.
11. Menon DK, Schwab K, Wright DW, Maas AI. Position statement: definition of traumatic brain injury. Arch Phys Rehabil Med. 2010;91(11):1637–40.
12. Teasdale G, Jennett B. Assessment of coma and impaired consciousness. A practical scale. Lancet. 1974;2(7872):81–4.
13. Management of Concussion/mTBI Working Group. VA/DoD clinical practice guideline for management of concussion/mild traumatic brain injury. J Rehabil Res Dev. 2009;46(6):Cp1–68.
14. Malec JF, Brown AW, Leibson CL, Flaada JT, Mandrekar JN, Diehl NN, et al. The mayo classification system for traumatic brain injury severity. J Neurotrauma. 2007;24(9):1417–24.
15. McCrory P, Meeuwisse W, Dvořák J, Aubry M, Bailes J, Broglio S, et al. Consensus statement on concussion in sport—the 5(th) international conference on concussion in sport held in Berlin, October 2016. Br J Sports Med. 2017;51(11):838–47.
16. Practice parameter: the management of concussion in sports (summary statement). Report of the Quality Standards Subcommittee. Neurology. 1997;48(3):581–5.
17. Holm L, Cassidy JD, Carroll LJ, Borg J. Summary of the WHO Collaborating Centre for Neurotrauma Task Force on mild traumatic brain injury. J Rehabil Med. 2005;37(3):137–41.
18. Ruff RM, Iverson GL, Barth JT, Bush SS, Broshek DK. Recommendations for diagnosing a mild traumatic brain injury: a National Academy of Neuropsychology education paper. Arch Clin Neuropsychol. 2009;24(1):3–10.
19. Shames J, Treger I, Ring H, Giaquinto S. Return to work following traumatic brain injury: trends and challenges. Disabil Rehabil. 2007;29(17):1387–95.
20. Ball CG. Penetrating nontorso trauma: the head and the neck. Can J Surg. 2015;58(4):284–5.
21. Bigler ED. Distinguished Neuropsychologist Award Lecture 1999. The lesion(s) in traumatic brain injury: implications for clinical neuropsychology. Arch Clin Neuropsychol. 2001;16(2):95–131.
22. Gennarelli TA, Thibault LE, Graham DI. Diffuse axonal injury: an important form of traumatic brain damage. Neuroscientist. 1998;4:202–15.
23. Faul MXL, Wald MM, Coronado VG. Traumatic Brain Injury in the United States. Atlanta, GA: Centers for Disease Control and Prevention, National Center for Injury Prevention and Control; 2010.
24. León-Carrión J, Domínguez-Morales M. del R, Barroso y Martín JM, Murillo-Cabezas F. Epidemiology of traumatic brain injury and subarachnoid hemorrhage. Pituitary. 2005;8(3–4):197–202.
25. Bigler ED. Neuropsychology and clinical neuroscience of persistent post-concussive syndrome. J Int Neuropsychol Soc. 2008;14(1):1–22.
26. Katz DI. Neuropathology and neurobehavioral recovery from closed head injury. J Head Trauma Rehabil. 1992;7(2):1–15.
27. Binder LM. A review of mild head trauma. Part II: clinical implications. J Clin Exp Neuropsychol. 1997;19(3):432–57.
28. Christensen BK, Colella B, Inness E, Hebert D, Monette G, Bayley M, et al. Recovery of cognitive function after traumatic brain injury: a multilevel modeling analysis of Canadian outcomes. Arch Phys Rehabil Med. 2008;89(12 Suppl):S3–15.

29. Gasquoine PG. Postconcussion symptoms. Neuropsychol Rev. 1997;7(2):77–85.
30. Hibbard MR, Uysal S, Kepler K, Bogdany J, Silver J. Axis I psychopathology in individuals with traumatic brain injury. J Head Trauma Rehabil. 1998;13(4):24–39.
31. Arnould A, Rochat L, Azouvi P, Van der Linden M. Longitudinal course and predictors of apathetic symptoms after severe traumatic brain injury. Arch Clin Neuropsychol. 2018;33(7):808–20.
32. Bivona U, Costa A, Contrada M, Silvestro D, Azicnuda E, Aloisi M, et al. Depression, apathy and impaired self-awareness following severe traumatic brain injury: a preliminary investigation. Brain Inj. 2019;33(9):1245–56.
33. Prigatano GP. Neuropsychological rehabilitation after brain injury: scientific and professional issues. J Clin Psychol Med Settings. 1996;3(1):1–10.
34. Guild EB, Levine B. Functional correlates of midline brain volume loss in chronic traumatic brain injury. J Int Neuropsychol Soc. 2015;21(8):650–5.
35. Knutson KM, Dal Monte O, Raymont V, Wassermann EM, Krueger F, Grafman J. Neural correlates of apathy revealed by lesion mapping in participants with traumatic brain injuries. Human Brain Mapp. 2014;35(3):943–53.
36. Johansson B, Berglund P, Rönnbäck L. Mental fatigue and impaired information processing after mild and moderate traumatic brain injury. Brain Inj. 2009;23(13–14):1027–40.
37. Mathias JL, Beall JA, Bigler ED. Neuropsychological and information processing deficits following mild traumatic brain injury. J Int Neuropsychol Soc. 2004;10(2):286–97.
38. Cremona-Meteyard SL, Geffen GM. Event-related potential indices of visual attention following moderate to severe closed head injury. Brain Inj. 1994;8(6):541–58.
39. Levin HS, Mattis S, Ruff RM, Eisenberg HM, Marshall LF, Tabaddor K, et al. Neurobehavioral outcome following minor head injury: a three-center study. J Neurosurg. 1987;66(2):234–43.
40. Chan RC. Sustained attention in patients with mild traumatic brain injury. Clin Rehabil. 2005;19(2):188–93.
41. Ziino C, Ponsford J. Selective attention deficits and subjective fatigue following traumatic brain injury. Neuropsychology. 2006;20(3):383–90.
42. McAllister TW, Saykin AJ, Flashman LA, Sparling MB, Johnson SC, Guerin SJ, et al. Brain activation during working memory 1 month after mild traumatic brain injury: a functional MRI study. Neurology. 1999;53(6):1300–8.
43. Nolin P. Executive memory dysfunctions following mild traumatic brain injury. J Head Trauma Rehabil. 2006;21(1):68–75.
44. Ord JS, Greve KW, Bianchini KJ, Aguerrevere LE. Executive dysfunction in traumatic brain injury: the effects of injury severity and effort on the Wisconsin Card Sorting Test. J Clin Exp Neuropsychol. 2010;32(2):132–40.
45. Vasquez BP, Tomaszczyk JC, Sharma B, Colella B, Green REA. Longitudinal recovery of executive control functions after moderate-severe traumatic brain injury: examining trajectories of variability and ex-gaussian parameters. Neurorehabil Neural Repair. 2018;32(3):191–9.
46. Henry JD, Crawford JR. A meta-analytic review of verbal fluency performance in patients with traumatic brain injury. Neuropsychology. 2004;18(4):621–8.
47. Zakzanis KK, McDonald K, Troyer AK. Component analysis of verbal fluency scores in severe traumatic brain injury. Brain Inj. 2013;27(7–8):903–8.
48. Sherer M, Bergloff P, Levin E, High WM, Jr, Oden KE, Nick TG. Impaired awareness and employment outcome after traumatic brain injury. J Head Trauma Rehabil. 1998;13(5):52–61.
49. Dikmen SS, Corrigan JD, Levin HS, Machamer J, Stiers W, Weisskopf MG. Cognitive outcome following traumatic brain injury. J Head Trauma Rehabil. 2009;24(6):430–8.

50. Colantonio A, Ratcliff G, Chase S, Kelsey S, Escobar M, Vernich L. Long-term outcomes after moderate to severe traumatic brain injury. Disabil Rehabil. 2004;26(5):253–61.

51. Green RE, Colella B, Hebert DA, Bayley M, Kang HS, Till C, et al. Prediction of return to productivity after severe traumatic brain injury: investigations of optimal neuropsychological tests and timing of assessment. Arch Phys Rehabil Med. 2008;89(12 Suppl):S51–60.

52. Green RE, Colella B, Maller JJ, Bayley M, Glazer J, Mikulis DJ. Scale and pattern of atrophy in the chronic stages of moderate-severe TBI. Front Hum Neurosci. 2014;8:67.

53. Masel BE, DeWitt DS. Traumatic brain injury: a disease process, not an event. J Neurotrauma. 2010;27(8):1529–40.

54. Marcotte TD, Grant I (Eds). Neuropsychology of Everyday Functioning. New York: Guilford Press; 2010.

55. Cattelani R, Tanzi F, Lombardi F, Mazzucchi A. Competitive re-employment after severe traumatic brain injury: clinical, cognitive and behavioural predictive variables. Brain Inj. 2002;16(1):51–64.

56. Dawson DR, Levine B, Schwartz ML, Stuss DT. Acute predictors of real-world outcomes following traumatic brain injury: a prospective study. Brain Inj. 2004;18(3):221–38.

57. Fleming J, Tooth L, Hassell M, Chan W. Prediction of community integration and vocational outcome 2–5 years after traumatic brain injury rehabilitation in Australia. Brain Inj. 1999;13(6):417–31.

58. van der Naalt J, van Zomeren AH, Sluiter WJ, Minderhoud JM. One year outcome in mild to moderate head injury: the predictive value of acute injury characteristics related to complaints and return to work. J Neurol Neurosurg Psychiatry. 1999;66(2):207–13.

59. Ruff RM, Marshall LF, Crouch J, Klauber MR, Levin HS, Barth J, et al. Predictors of outcome following severe head trauma: follow-up data from the Traumatic Coma Data Bank. Brain Inj. 1993;7(2):101–11.

60. Langlois JA, Rutland-Brown W, Wald MM. The epidemiology and impact of traumatic brain injury: a brief overview. J Head Trauma Rehabil. 2006;21(5):375–8.

61. Rutland-Brown W, Langlois JA, Thomas KE, Xi YL. Incidence of traumatic brain injury in the United States, 2003. J Head Trauma Rehabil. 2006;21(6):544–8.

62. Evans MK, Lepkowski JM, Powe NR, LaVeist T, Kuczmarski MF, Zonderman AB. Healthy aging in neighborhoods of diversity across the life span (HANDLS): overcoming barriers to implementing a longitudinal, epidemiologic, urban study of health, race, and socioeconomic status. Ethn Dis. 2010;20(3):267–75.

63. Definition of apathy. Oxford University Press. 2021. Available at: https://www.lexico.com/definition/apathy.

64. American Psychiatric Association. Diagnostic and Statistical Manual of Mental Disorders, fifth edition. Arlington, VA: American Psychiatric Association; 2013.

65. Thant T, Yager J. Updating apathy: using research domain criteria to inform clinical assessment and diagnosis of disorders of motivation. J Nerv Ment Dis. 2019;207(9):707–14.

66. Levy R, Czernecki V. Apathy and the basal ganglia. J Neurol. 2006;253(Suppl 7):Vii54–61.

67. Marin RS. Apathy: concept, syndrome, neural mechanisms, and treatment. Semin Clin Neuropsychiatry. 1996;1(4):304–14.

68. Stuss DT. Disturbance of self-awareness after frontal system damage. In: Prigatano GP, Schacter DL (Eds), Awareness of Deficit after Brain Injury: Clinical and Theoretical Issues. Oxford: Oxford University Press; 1991, pp. 63–83.

69. Al-Adawi S, Dorvlo AS, Burke DT, Huynh CC, Jacob L, Knight R, et al. Apathy and depression in cross-cultural survivors of traumatic brain injury. J Neuropsychiatry Clin Neurosci. 2004;16(4):435–42.

70. Andersson S, Krogstad JM, Finset A. Apathy and depressed mood in acquired brain damage: relationship to lesion localization and psychophysiological reactivity. Psychol Med. 1999;29(2):447–56.

71. Kant R, Duffy JD, Pivovarnik A. Prevalence of apathy following head injury. Brain Inj. 1998;12(1):87–92.
72. Newburn G, Newburn D. Selegiline in the management of apathy following traumatic brain injury. Brain Inj. 2005;19(2):149–54.
73. Marin RS, Biedrzycki RC, Firinciogullari S. Reliability and validity of the Apathy Evaluation Scale. Psychiatry Res. 1991;38(2):143–62.
74. Beck AT, Ward CH, Mendelson M, Mock J, Erbaugh J. An inventory for measuring depression. Arch Gen Psychiatry. 1961;4:561–71.
75. Kirsch-Darrow L, Fernandez HH, Marsiske M, Okun MS, Bowers D. Dissociating apathy and depression in Parkinson disease. Neurology. 2006;67(1):33–8.
76. Marin RS, Fogel BS, Hawkins J, Duffy J, Krupp B. Apathy: a treatable syndrome. J Neuropsychiatry Clin Neurosci. 1995;7(1):23–30.
77. Thompson JC, Snowden JS, Craufurd D, Neary D. Behavior in Huntington's disease: dissociating cognition-based and mood-based changes. J Neuropsychiatry Clin Neurosci. 2002;14(1):37–43.
78. Stanton BR, Carson A. Apathy: a practical guide for neurologists. Pract Neurol. 2016;16(1):42–7.
79. Robert PH, Clairet S, Benoit M, Koutaich J, Bertogliati C, Tible O, et al. The apathy inventory: assessment of apathy and awareness in Alzheimer's disease, Parkinson's disease and mild cognitive impairment. Int J Geriatr Psychiatry. 2002;17(12):1099–105.
80. Cummings JL, Mega M, Gray K, Rosenberg-Thompson S, Carusi DA, Gornbein J. The Neuropsychiatric Inventory: comprehensive assessment of psychopathology in dementia. Neurology. 1994;44(12):2308–14.
81. Starkstein SE, Mayberg HS, Preziosi TJ, Andrezejewski P, Leiguarda R, Robinson RG. Reliability, validity, and clinical correlates of apathy in Parkinson's disease. J Neuropsychiatry Clin Neurosci. 1992;4(2):134–9.
82. Arnould A, Rochat L, Azouvi P, Van der Linden M. Apathetic symptom presentations in patients with severe traumatic brain injury: assessment, heterogeneity and relationships with psychosocial functioning and caregivers' burden. Brain Inj. 2015;29(13–14):1597–603.
83. Castaño Monsalve B, Bernabeu Guitart M, López R, Bulbena Vilasar A, Ignacio Quemada J. [Psychopathological evaluation of traumatic brain injury patients with the Neuropsychiatric Inventory]. Revista Psiquiatr Salud Ment. 2012;5(3):160–6.
84. Lane-Brown A, Tate R. Interventions for apathy after traumatic brain injury. Cochrane Database Syst Rev. 2009;2:CD006341.
85. Grace J, Stout JC, Malloy PF. Assessing frontal lobe behavioral syndromes with the frontal lobe personality scale. Assessment. 1999;6(3):269–84.
86. Glenn MB, Burke DT, O'Neil-Pirozzi T, Goldstein R, Jacob L, Kettell J. Cutoff score on the apathy evaluation scale in subjects with traumatic brain injury. Brain Inj. 2002;16(6):509–16.
87. Niemeier JP, Perrin PB, Holcomb MG, Nersessova KS, Rolston CD. Factor structure, reliability, and validity of the Frontal Systems Behavior Scale (FrSBe) in an acute traumatic brain injury population. Rehabil Psychol. 2013;58(1):51–63.
88. Carvalho JO, Ready RE, Malloy P, Grace J. Confirmatory factor analysis of the Frontal Systems Behavior Scale (FrSBe). Assessment. 2013;20(5):632–41.
89. Stout JC, Ready RE, Grace J, Malloy PF, Paulsen JS. Factor analysis of the frontal systems behavior scale (FrSBe). Assessment. 2003;10(1):79–85.
90. Arnould A, Rochat L, Azouvi P, Van der Linden M. A multidimensional approach to apathy after traumatic brain injury. Neuropsychol Rev. 2013;23(3):210–33.
91. Le Heron C, Apps MAJ, Husain M. The anatomy of apathy: a neurocognitive framework for amotivated behaviour. Neuropsychologia. 2018;118(Pt B):54–67.

92. Levy R, Dubois B. Apathy and the functional anatomy of the prefrontal cortex-basal ganglia circuits. Cereb Cortex. 2006;16(7):916–28.
93. Bigler ED. Neurobiology and neuropathology underlie the neuropsychological deficits associated with traumatic brain injury. Arch Clin Neuropsychol. 2003;18(6):595–621.
94. Finset A, Andersson S. Coping strategies in patients with acquired brain injury: relationships between coping, apathy, depression and lesion location. Brain Inj. 2000;14(10):887–905.
95. Paradiso S, Chemerinski E, Yazici KM, Tartaro A, Robinson RG. Frontal lobe syndrome reassessed: comparison of patients with lateral or medial frontal brain damage. J Neurol Neurosurg Psychiatry. 1999;67(5):664–7.
96. Barrash J, Tranel D, Anderson SW. Acquired personality disturbances associated with bilateral damage to the ventromedial prefrontal region. Dev Neuropsychol. 2000;18(3):355–81.
97. Hogeveen J, Hauner KK, Chau A, Krueger F, Grafman J. Impaired valuation leads to increased apathy following ventromedial prefrontal cortex damage. Cereb Cortex. 2017;27(2):1401–8.
98. Guimarães HC, Levy R, Teixeira AL, Gomes Beato R, Caramelli P. Neurobiology of apathy in Alzheimer's disease. Arq Neuro Psiquiatr 2008;66(2B):436–43.
99. Tunnard C, Whitehead D, Hurt C, Wahlund LO, Mecocci P, Tsolaki M, et al. Apathy and cortical atrophy in Alzheimer's disease. Int J Geriatr Psychiatry. 2011;26(7):741–8.
100. Takayanagi Y, Gerner G, Takayanagi M, Rao V, Vannorsdall TD, Sawa A, et al. Hippocampal volume reduction correlates with apathy in traumatic brain injury, but not schizophrenia. J Neuropsychiatry Clin Neurosci. 2013;25(4):292–301.
101. Sherer M, Sander AM. Handbook on the Neuropsychology of Traumatic Brain Injury. New York: Springer; 2014.
102. Kinsella GJ. Traumatic brain injury and processing speed. In: DeLuca J, Kalmar JH (Eds) Information Processing Speed in Clinical Populations (Studies on Neuropsychology, Neurology and Cognition). New York: Psychology Press; 2008, pp. 173–94.
103. Stuss DT, Stethem LL, Hugenholtz H, Picton T, Pivik J, Richard MT. Reaction time after head injury: fatigue, divided and focused attention, and consistency of performance. J Neurol Neurosurg Psychiatry. 1989;52(6):742–8.
104. Deluca J, Kalmar JH (Eds). Information Processing Speed in Clinical Populations (Studies on Neuropsychology, Neurology and Cognition). New York: Psychology Press; 2008.
105. Ponsford J, Kinsella G. Attentional deficits following closed-head injury. J Clin Exp Neuropsychol. 1992;14(5):822–38.
106. Sohlberg MM, Mateer CA. Cognitive Rehabilitation: An Integrative Neuropsychological Approach. New York: Guilford Press; 2001.
107. Andersson S, Bergedalen AM. Cognitive correlates of apathy in traumatic brain injury. Neuropsychiatry Neuropsychol Behav Neurol. 2002;15(3):184–91.
108. Lillie RA, Kowalski K, Patry BN, Sira C, Tuokko H, Mateer CA. Everyday impact of traumatic brain injury. In: Marcotte TD, Grant I (Eds), Neuropsychology of Everyday Functioning. New York: Guilford Press; 2010, pp. 302–30.
109. Rapoport MJ, Herrmann N, Shammi P, Kiss A, Phillips A, Feinstein A. Outcome after traumatic brain injury sustained in older adulthood: a one-year longitudinal study. Am J Geriatr Psychiatry. 2006;14(5):456–65.
110. Rao V, McCann U, Bergey A, Han D, Brandt J, Schretlen DJ. Correlates of apathy during the first year after traumatic brain injury. Psychosomatics. 2013;54(4):403–4.
111. Kongs SK, Thompson LL, Iverson GL, Heaton RK. Wisconsin Card Sorting Test—64 Card Version Professional Manual. Odessa, FL: Psychological Assessment Resources; 2000.

112. Rabin LA, Paolillo E, Barr WB. Stability in test-usage practices of clinical neuropsychologists in the United States and Canada over a 10-year period: a follow-up survey of INS and NAN members. Arch Clin Neuropsychol. 2016;31(3):206–30.

113. Iverson GL, McCracken LM. 'Postconcussive' symptoms in persons with chronic pain. Brain Inj. 1997;11(11):783–90.

114. Alexander MP. Mild traumatic brain injury: pathophysiology, natural history, and clinical management. Neurology. 1995;45(7):1253–60.

115. Bryant RA. Disentangling mild traumatic brain injury and stress reactions. N Engl J Med. 2008;358(5):525–7.

116. Hoge CW, McGurk D, Thomas JL, Cox AL, Engel CC, Castro CA. Mild traumatic brain injury in U.S. soldiers returning from Iraq. N Engl J Med. 2008;358(5):453–63.

117. Kennedy JE, Leal FO, Lewis JD, Cullen MA, Amador RR. Posttraumatic stress symptoms in OIF/OEF service members with blast-related and non-blast-related mild TBI. NeuroRehabilitation. 2010;26(3):223–31.

118. Nelson LA, Yoash-Gantz RE, Pickett TC, Campbell TA. Relationship between processing speed and executive functioning performance among OEF/OIF veterans: implications for postdeployment rehabilitation. J Head Trauma Rehabil. 2009;24(1):32–40.

119. Mittenberg W, Strauman S. Diagnosis of mild head injury and the postconcussion syndrome. J Head Trauma Rehabil. 2000;15(2):783–91.

120. Belanger HG, Vanderploeg RD. The neuropsychological impact of sports-related concussion: a meta-analysis. J Int Neuropsychol Soc. 2005;11(4):345–57.

121. Greiffenstein MF, Baker WJ, Gola T. Validation of malingered amnesia measures with a large clinical sample. Psychol Assess. 1994;6(3):218–24.

122. Lees-Haley PR, Brown RS. Neuropsychological complaint base rates of 170 personal injury claimants. Arch Clin Neuropsychol. 1993;8(3):203–9.

123. Bigler ED. Neuropsychological results and neuropathological findings at autopsy in a case of mild traumatic brain injury. J Int Neuropsychol Soc. 2004;10(5):794–806.

124. Garden N, Sullivan KA. An examination of the base rates of post-concussion symptoms: the influence of demographics and depression. Appl Neuropsychol. 2010;17(1):1–7.

125. Iverson GL. Sensitivity of computerized neuropsychological screening in depressed university students. Clin Neuropsychol. 2006;20(4):695–701.

126. Suhr JA, Gunstad J. Postconcussive symptom report: the relative influence of head injury and depression. J Clin Exp Neuropsychol. 2002;24(8):981–93.

127. Zakzanis KK, Grimes KM. Relationship among apathy, cognition, and real-world disability after mild traumatic brain injury. Appl Neuropsychol Adult. 2017;24(6):559–65.

128. Wäljas M, Iverson GL, Lange RT, Liimatainen S, Hartikainen KM, Dastidar P, et al. Return to work following mild traumatic brain injury. J Head Trauma Rehabil. 2014;29(5):443–50.

129. Gray JM, Shepherd M, McKinlay WW, Robertson I, Pentland B. Negative symptoms in the traumatically brain-injured during the first year postdischarge, and their effect on rehabilitation status, work status and family burden. Clin Rehabil. 1994;8(3):188–97.

130. Nygren DeBoussard C, Lannsjö M, Stenberg M, Stålnacke BM, Godbolt AK. Behavioural problems in the first year after severe traumatic brain injury: a prospective multicentre study. Clin Rehabil. 2017;31(4):555–66.

131. Rosenberg H, McDonald S, Rosenberg J, Frederick Westbrook R. Amused, flirting or simply baffled? Is recognition of all emotions affected by traumatic brain injury? J Neuropsychol. 2018;12(2):145–64.

132. Masanic CA, Bayley MT, VanReekum R, Simard M. Open-label study of donepezil in traumatic brain injury. Arch Phys Rehabil Med. 2001;82(7):896–901.

133. Tenovuo O. Central acetylcholinesterase inhibitors in the treatment of chronic traumatic brain injury-clinical experience in 111 patients. Prog Neuropsychopharmacol Biol Psychiatry. 2005;29(1):61–7.

134. Lane-Brown A, Tate R. Evaluation of an intervention for apathy after traumatic brain injury: a multiple-baseline, single-case experimental design. J Head Trauma Rehabil. 2010;25(6):459–69.

135. Tate RL, Wakim D, Sigmundsdottir L, Longley W. Evaluating an intervention to increase meaningful activity after severe traumatic brain injury: a single-case experimental design with direct inter-subject and systematic replications. Neuropsychol Rehabil. 2020;30(4):641–72.

136. Wiart L, Richer E, Destaillats JM, Joseph PA, Dehail P, Mazaux JM. Psychotherapeutic follow up of out patients with traumatic brain injury: preliminary results of an individual neurosystemic approach. Ann Phys Rehabil Med. 2012;55(6):375–87.

137. Holmes C, Knights A, Dean C, Hodkinson S, Hopkins V. Keep music live: music and the alleviation of apathy in dementia subjects. Int Psychogeriatr. 2006;18(4):623–30.

9
Apathy

A Pathology of Goal-Directed Behaviour and Prefrontal Cortex–Basal Ganglia Circuits

Richard Levy

Introduction

Let's imagine that someone who was previously active and busy is now spending their time lying on a bed, or seated on a chair watching TV. Relatives do not recognize them anymore. What is happening? Does this person occupy their mind by building a novel philosophical theory? Do they ruminate dark thoughts? Or, is their mind empty? The last proposal seems odd; however, when questioned, it is very likely that such a person declares that their 'mind is empty'. This sentence could be conceived as a way of expressing the idea that brain signals corresponding to thoughts are not consciously perceived by this person at a given time/period. In other words, unconscious messages, such as adaptive neurovegetative signals or those triggering automatic actions, are present and lead to normal brain/behaviour responses, but thoughts and therefore actions that require higher level of consciousness are not fully activated in one's mind/brain. Such a fascinating situation does exist in neurology. It is called 'auto-activation' deficit (AAD) or 'psychic self-activation' deficit or 'athymhormia' (1–4). AAD can be considered as the most severe existing form of apathy. Therefore, it can be used as a model of description of apathy to depict the clinical syndrome that usually corresponds to apathy but also to discuss the underlying psychological/cognitive mechanisms and the neuroanatomy of apathy.

Auto-Activation Deficit

AAD, the most severe form of apathy, is associated with stereotypic and pseudo-compulsive behaviours or thoughts (such as arithmomania, the compulsion of mentally counting). In other words, there is a sharp contrast between the drastic quantitative reduction of self-generated actions and the relatively normally executed externally driven behaviours and automatic thoughts and actions. Such a syndrome raises the central issues of how voluntary and self-initiated behaviour is generated in terms of mental/psychological/cognitive mechanisms and how these mechanisms relate to human biology (i.e. the macro- and microscopic brain structure).

From Auto-Activation Deficit to Apathy

According to a recent conceptual shift in definition (5, 6), AAD could be considered as a prototypical case description of apathy. Indeed, apathy is here defined from a behaviourist point of view (the clinical observation of one's behaviour) rather than from the underlying presumed psychological mechanism, in accordance with the recent international consensus group (6). Following this perspective, apathy can be seen as a quantitative reduction of adaptive behaviour despite the patient's environmental or physical constraints remaining unchanged (5). In the particular case of AAD, patients' ability to execute externally driven behaviour is preserved and unwanted automatic behaviour (such as stereotypies or compulsions) is associated with the quantitative reduction of behaviour. In consequence, in order to accurately describe apathetic situations, we propose to narrow the definition of apathy to voluntary (or 'purposeful' or 'internally generated' or 'goal-directed') actions. In other words, apathy can be defined as 'the quantitative reduction of self-generated voluntary and purposeful behaviours' (5, 7). As such, a given patient may, at the same time, be inert when he has to self-initiate actions, but capable of adequate adaptive behaviour to strong external solicitations and may present with spontaneous automatic behaviour such as stereotypies/compulsions, such as in AAD.

The Presumed Underlying Psychological/ Cognitive Mechanisms of Apathy

It is important to note that, at the present time, the precise pathophysiology of apathy, including from the psychological/cognitive perspective and the underlying biological mechanisms, is only partially understood. Many future studies relying on clinical observation, cognitive neuroscience, functional neuroanatomy, modelling, and strong theoretical models (to be confirmed or refuted) are required.

As a theoretical framework, we propose that apathy is the observable clinical output resulting from several different underlying mechanisms, all arising from pathological changes in the brain system that allows us to generate, execute, and control voluntary actions or goal-directed behaviours (GDBs (8)). As several steps are necessary to achieve GDB (processing of external and internal determinants that influence the intention to act, elaboration of the plan of actions, initiation, execution, feedback control, etc.), apathy may arise from dysfunctions occurring at any of the steps required to achieve a GDB. It is thus likely that the pathophysiology of apathy is not a single entity but multiple, depending on which specific process is disrupted during the completion of GDB (Fig. 9.1). Grossly, we propose that apathy may results from:

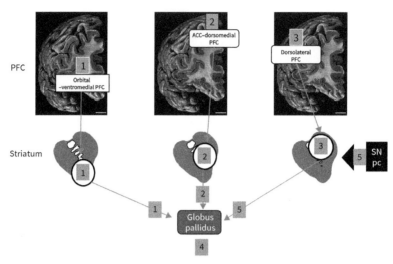

Fig. 9.1 Neural bases of apathy. 1. A lesion in the ventral circuit (at the prefrontal cortex (PFC) level, striatum, globus pallidus, or the thalamic output system and white fibre tracts connecting these areas) is associated with an affective valuation disorder: 'amotivation'; 2. A lesion in the dorsal circuit (at the PFC level, striatum, globus pallidus, or the thalamic output system and white fibre tracts connecting these areas) is associated with impairment in elaborating strategies and plan of actions: 'cognitive inertia'; 3. A lesion in the dorsal mesial intermediate circuit (at the PFC level, striatum, globus pallidus, or the thalamic output system and white fibre tracts connecting these areas) is associated with a default in transferring affective values to the executive system that generates voluntary actions: 'invigoration deficit'; 4. Summation of lesions of the three circuits leads to the absence of amplification of the signal reaching the PFC: 'empty mind'; 5. A lesion in the dopaminergic nigrostriatal pathway leads to a loss of spatial and temporal focalization of signals within the basal ganglia. Decision-making is difficult because signals are not correctly disambiguated: 'loss of focalization'. ACC, anterior cingulate cortex. SN pc, substantia nigra pars compacta.

A. *A dysfunction in the valuation system* (Fig. 9.1, point 1). Apathy may result from an inability to accurately translate determinants of actions (signals form the 'internal milieu' or from the environment) into one's corresponding implemented values. Values relate to our innate elementary valuation system and to values and beliefs acquired during personal experiences. Values may be absolute in an invariant situation but also relative depending on specific contexts (9, 10). For instance, if someone dislikes spinach, they would not eat it when they are given the choice of chocolate, which they like more. However, if the same person is following diet, then although they prefer chocolate, they would choose spinach. Therefore, as GDB requires to use values in a way adapted to the context, one may hypothesize that apathy results from an inability to contextualize, that is, to attribute a relative weight to a given value in order to generate a behaviour, that is, to translate a given contextual value into reward (the object that we would like to obtain) and the punishment (the object that we would like to avoid). Reward and punishment are crucial to trigger an operating response (the 'incentive behaviour') such as producing enough energy to generate an action, disambiguating decision-making by selecting and increasing the signal-to-noise ratio corresponding to a specific decision, learning new things through reinforcement ('the carrot or the stick'), and evaluate in real-life situations the consequences of future actions. Altogether, the first presumed psychological/ cognitive mechanism could be summarized as a motivation ('what pushes us to act') problem and we may name this pathological mechanism 'amotivation'. Such a mechanism would be at play when dysfunctions or lesions are observed in areas/networks involved in valuation processing.

B. *A dysfunction in the elaboration of the plan of actions* (Fig. 9.1, point 2). Let's imagine that someone's motivational processing is intact, could it nevertheless be possible for them to be apathetic? Theoretically, yes: what would happen if the cognitive system that allows us to generate strategies, to retrieve relevant information from our memory systems, to organize them in multiple forthcoming steps to perform future actions (planning), to shift from one idea to another, and to allocate attention resources to several parallel tasks is altered? Among the possible consequences, difficulties in completing cognitive programmes required to achieve complex voluntary actions would likely lead to the abortion of many potential actions and therefore lead to a decrease in the number of GDBs (i.e. apathy). This mechanism is part of the cognitive dysexecutive syndrome. In this case, apathy would be the consequence of a psychological/cognitive mechanism that we may name 'cognitive inertia'. Such a mechanism would be at play when dysfunctions or lesions are observed in brain areas/networks involved in the generation and control of cognitive executive functions.

C. *A disconnection between motivation and action or a summation all mechanisms* (Fig. 9.1, points 3 and 4). We hypothesize that the most severe form of apathy such as that seen in AAD may be secondary either to:

- A disconnection between motivation and actions (cognitive executive functions), both being potentially intact but uncoupled one from the other. Therefore, incentives would not influence the generation of actions. Such a mechanism has been strongly suggested in AAD patients in work by Schmidt et al. (4). We, therefore, could name this mechanism 'invigoration deficit'.
- The summation of the above-described mechanisms due to lesions that affect all the brain system involved in generating and controlling GDB, leading to a global decrease of the signals that should trigger action. This situation may lead to the impression of 'empty mind' described by some patients. We shall name this mechanism 'empty mind'.

D. *Could we conceptualize other mechanism(s) for apathy?* Is it possible to observe apathy without structural damage affecting the networks serving the generation and control of GDB? Yes indeed. Changes in the striatal phasic dopaminergic flow in these networks such as seen in Parkinson's disease may also produce a quantitative reduction in GDB, through a loss of temporal and/or spatial discrimination of relevant signals leading to difficulties in decision-making secondary to the inability to disambiguate relevant signals for others that are now blended together (11). We may call this mechanism 'loss of focalization' (Fig. 9.1, point 5).

These mechanisms relate apathy to problems (structural damage or demodulation) in the brain systems that process voluntary/willed/intentional/conscious actions. However, GDBs also depend on other brain functions not directly involved in their generation but necessary to activate the brain system that generates and controls GDB. To translate this idea into a real-life situation, let's imagine a patient presenting with significant episodic memory impairment. Entering into his living room with the intention of reading a book, once arrived in the room, he does not remember the reason why he came in. Then, he sat on the sofa. A GDB was aborted and replaced by a non-activity that corresponds to the definition of apathy. Stated differently, we may hypothesize that the causes of apathy may be more numerous that the main presumed mechanisms depicted previously.

Do these proposed cognitive mechanisms correspond to what we see in clinical practice? Does each mechanism evoked have its own pathophysiology and does it rely on relatively separate brain network dysfunctions/lesions?

Neuroanatomy of Apathy

A First Lesson from Auto-Activation Deficit

This apathetic syndrome is in general due to restricted and specific lesions within the basal ganglia, in most cases affecting bilaterally the internal portion of the pallidum (1, 2) or bilateral striato-pallidal lesions, uni- or bilateral lesions of the head of the caudate nucleus, and lesions of the medial-dorsal and anterior nuclei of the thalamus and the deep frontal white matter (1, 12–19). The topography of lesions associated with AAD indicates that this syndrome is the clinical consequence of damage to limbic and cognitive territories of the basal ganglia (and to the tracts that are connected to them), which probably explains the absence of extrapyramidal motor signs in this syndrome. It is likely that it results from the disruption of the prefrontal cortex (PFC)–basal ganglia system, the functional systems involved in the generation and control of GDB (5, 20, 21, 22). And indeed, the very small bi-pallidal lesions observed in AAD are associated with a major hypometabolism in the PFC (2), supporting a PFC deafferentation syndrome. The strong connectivity between the PFC and the basal ganglia has been demonstrated in monkeys (23) and more recently *in vivo* in humans using magnetic resonance diffusion tensor fibre tracking (24). As a consequence, a prefrontal-like syndrome (including apathy as one of its clinical manifestations) can be encountered following diseases that mainly involve the basal ganglia, such as AAD, as well as in neurodegenerative diseases associated with direct lesions of the striatum, globus pallidus, and the subthalamic nucleus, such as in progressive supranuclear palsy and Huntington's disease (25, 26). Similarly, physiological and lesion studies in monkeys found a similarity in neuronal activation or deficits in behavioural tasks whether the target was within the PFC or in the basal ganglia (27–30). Obviously, direct focal lesions of the PFC are associated with severe apathy (21, 31–33). For instance, apathy is almost constantly present in the behavioural variant of frontotemporal lobar degeneration (34–37). Altogether, this indicates that, above all, apathy results from damage or dysfunction affecting the cognitive and/or limbic territories of the frontal lobes, the basal ganglia, or the frontal–basal ganglia circuits that could be gathered under the general framework of the 'prefrontal–basal ganglia system', a system particularly dedicated to the generation and control of GDB.

The Functional and Anatomical Heterogeneity of the Prefrontal–Basal Ganglia System

The PFC represents almost one-third of the human brain volume and can therefore be divided anatomically and functionally into several subregions (20, 21, 31, 38–40). Similarly, prefrontal–basal ganglia anatomical and functional networks are multiple, according to the relative segregation of PFC–basal ganglia–PFC circuits (23, 41, 42). Three relatively segregated circuits, of importance in the context of apathy, have been identified in primates: (i) the orbital–ventromedial circuit grossly linking the orbital and ventromedial PFC to the ventral regions of the basal ganglia; (ii) the dorsal circuit linking the dorsolateral PFC to the dorsal regions of the basal ganglia, and, (iii) the anterior cingulate–dorsomedial circuit linking the medial wall of the PFC to basal ganglia portions located between the dorsal and the ventral regions.

Given the heterogeneity of the anatomical and functional organization of the 'prefrontal–basal ganglia system', several questions can be raised regarding apathy: do the PFC and the basal ganglia contribute equally to apathy? Does one prefrontal–basal ganglia circuit contribute more than others to apathy? Do all the prefrontal–basal ganglia circuits contribute to apathy but through different mechanisms?

Here, we support the idea that each of the three above-mentioned circuits, when damaged, may lead to apathy, but each in a different manner (Fig. 9.1): the orbital–ventromedial circuit for 'amotivation', the dorsolateral circuit for 'cognitive inertia', and the anterior cingulate–dorsomedial circuit for 'invigoration deficit'. In addition, as lesions in general do not strictly follow this functional neuroanatomy, a mix of these three different mechanisms often occurs and when lesions are massive in the frontal lobes (such as in frontotemporal lobar degeneration) or small but affecting all territories in the basal ganglia, apathy could result from alterations of all of these mechanisms ('empty mind'). In the following sections we will discuss the evidence leading to the proposal of this idea.

The Neuroanatomy of 'Amotivation'

We propose that alteration in the contextual behavioural valuation processing of GDB leads to apathy via a general mechanism that we named 'amotivation'. This valuation brain system belongs to a 'prefrontal–basal ganglia system', itself integrated in the so-called limbic system. Within this system, it corresponds to the orbital and ventro-medial prefrontal–basal ganglia circuit. Orbital and ventromedial PFC projects to the medial and ventral portion of the head, body, and tail of the caudate nuclei (43, 44) as well as to the ventral striatum (43, 45). Output from these striatal regions termin-ates in the medial and ventral pallidum and in the medial portion of the substantia nigra pars reticulata (42, 45). The pallido-thalamic projections terminate in the magnocellular part of the medial-dorsal thalami, which in turn project to the orbital and ventromedial PFC (42).

Direct focal or degenerative lesions of the orbital and ventromedial PFC in hu-mans are almost constantly accompanied by apathy (32, 36). In behavioural variant frontotemporal dementia, where apathy is a major criterion for the clinical diagnosis and almost universal, the neurodegeneration mostly affects the orbital and the ven-tral parts of the PFC (34, 46, 47). A default of the valuation system has been clearly demonstrated in behavioural variant frontotemporal dementia patients as well as in human and non-human primates with ventromedial focal lesions (48–53). Single-cell recordings in monkeys as well as recent neuroimaging studies in humans indicate that the orbital and ventromedial PFC is essential to provide the contextual (or relative) value of reward and to transfer this rewarding value into behaviour (9, 10, 54–62). In particular, the influence of the orbital and ventromedial PFC is essential when the context requires the subject to adapt his/her behaviour to maintain a positive out-come and anticipate the rewarding value of a forthcoming behaviour. Taken together, these data indicate that lesions or dysfunctions of the orbital and ventromedial PFC can lead to an insensitivity to reward, which may in turn lead to a decreased number of voluntary actions.

With regard to the basal ganglia territories of this circuit, several physiological studies (cell recordings) in monkeys have confirmed the involvement of the ventral portion of the striatum in a functional axis with the orbital–ventromedial PFC: in-deed, the ventral striatal neurons seem to play a major role in integrating the affective value of a given stimulus into the ongoing behaviour (63, 64). The main patterns of neural discharge are an anticipatory response to a forthcoming reward and double coding (reward and motor preparation). Accordingly, the few reports or lesion studies published that focused on the ventral striatum in humans and monkeys showed that lesions to the ventral striatum have consequences for affective, emotional, and motivational evaluation of a given environmental context (15, 65, 66).

The Neuroanatomy of 'Cognitive Inertia'

Apathy related to 'cognitive inertia' refers to the reduction in GDB due to impairments in the executive cognitive functions needed to elaborate the plan of actions, especially difficulties in generating new rules or strategies or difficulty in shifting from one mental and behavioural set to another. These cognitive functions are supported by the dorsolateral prefrontal–basal ganglia circuit. In the PFC, this circuit is represented by the dorsolateral (Brodmann area 9/46), ventrolateral (12, 44, 45, 47), and frontopolar (lateral 10) regions (for reviews see (20, 21, 67)). The lateral portion of the PFC is tightly connected with the dorsal and anterior portion of the striatum, particularly to the head of the caudate nucleus (43, 44, 68). This striatal territory projects itself to the dorsal and lateral portion of the globus pallidus and to the rostral and lateral part of the substantia nigra pars reticulata (42, 45). The pallido-thalamic projections terminate in the parvocellular part of the medial-dorsal and ventral-anterior thalami, which in turn project to lateral part of the PFC (42).

Cognitive inertia is frequently observed in patients with lateral PFC lesions. It consists of difficulties in maintaining and manipulating mental representations such as goals and subgoals in short-term memory (working memory), activating mental strategies, generating rules, planning, shifting from one strategy to another, and retrieving words or information from declarative memory. It is easily understandable that impairments in these processes may lead to problems in the elaboration of GDB, thereby quantitatively (and qualitatively) reducing GDB. And indeed, all the experimental approaches including neuropsychology and functional imaging studies in humans and single-cell recording and lesion studies in monkeys converge towards the idea that the dorsolateral PFC is an essential node in the neural network subserving executive functions such as planning, rule-finding, set-shifting, working memory, and the self-activation of strategies for retrieval in declarative memory (20–22, 31, 39, 69–74).

Lesions of the dorsal portion of the dorsal caudate nucleus induce impairments in tasks that are also altered after dorsolateral PFC lesions, such as spatial delayed and delayed alternation tasks (27, 28). Moreover, electrophysiological studies focusing on the head of the caudate nuclei have demonstrated patterns of neural activation similar to those observed in the dorsolateral PFC during working memory or sequencing tasks (30, 75, 76). In functional imaging, activation in the dorsal portion of the head of the caudate nuclei was found during working memory tasks and, more importantly, during planning tasks (29, 73, 77). Taken together, these data suggest that the dorsal portion of the caudate nuclei (in particular the head) is a key structure in an anatomical–functional network in combination with the dorsolateral PFC that mostly contributes to executive functions required to elaborate strategies and planned actions.

Therefore, it is not surprising that, in humans, unilateral or bilateral lesions of the dorsal portion of the head of the caudate nucleus are associated with a massive apathetic syndrome (15, 16, 19). In patients with dorsal caudate lesions, cognitive inertia is very likely the mechanism that explains apathy through difficulty in generating new rules or strategies or difficulty in shifting from one mental and behavioural set to another. Indeed, in patients with caudate lesions, impairment of executive functions includes planning, working memory, set shifting, ability to activate or generate cognitive strategies (for instance, those used to retrieve semantic or episodic information from memory), and temporal ordering.

The Neuroanatomy of 'Invigoration Deficit', 'Empty Mind', and Other Lessons from Auto-Activation Deficit

In both the PFC and the basal ganglia, cognitive and limbic territories are represented in the (dorso)lateral and the ventral portions of these brain regions, respectively. In order for motivation to influence action (or to invigorate it), both aspects of mental processing of GDB should interact. A third circuit links the medial wall of the PFC (mostly the dorsal anterior cingulate cortex) to the basal ganglia (the 'anterior cingulate–dorsomedial circuit'). Interestingly, within the basal ganglia and especially in the striatum, this circuit is anatomically positioned between the cognitive (also called the 'associative') and the affective/motivational (also called the 'limbic') territories (42–45). Firstly, in this intermediary territory, there are interdigitated connections arising from the two other territories according to a dorsal–ventral gradient (the fibres originated from the orbital–ventromedial PFC are mostly located in the ventral part of this area while those originated from the dorsolateral PFC are mostly located in the dorsal part). This may have a functional significance as this territory may allow communication between the system of valuation and the one that generates the plan of actions. This hypothesis is supported by a study performed in AAD patients (4), where the lesions were bilaterally located in discrete portions of the striatum or the globus pallidus. Participants squeezed a handgrip in order to produce different levels of force in association with a strong external solicitation or with different monetary incentives. First, AAD patients could generate a high level of force (even higher than normal controls at the lowest level of incentive). Second, in both AAD patients and controls, skin conductance varied according to the level of monetary incentives, suggesting that in both groups, participants took into account the incentive at stake. Third, in normal controls, the more the reward at stake, the more force was developed. Fourth and importantly, although the perception of values and motor force were normal, AAD patients were not able to modulate (invigorate) their performance according to the monetary incentive at stake while being able to emotionally perceive the odds at stake. It suggests that strategic lesions in the brain may disconnect the executive output (that generates the level of force) from the affective valuation of the potential rewards.

Secondly, in AAD, the sharp contrast between the absence of self-initiated actions and the relative sparing of externally driven ones (at least after strong external solicitations), indicates that the brain system that is mostly affected is the one central to the generation, initiation, or execution of self-generated behaviour. In line with this idea, AAD bears similarities with the impact of direct lesions of the dorsomedial PFC (in general including the anterior cingulate cortex): indeed, extensive bilateral lesions of the medial PFC result in an 'akinetic mutism', a clinical state in which patients do not spontaneously speak or move (78–80). Further, lesions affecting the anterior portion of the medial PFC of the dominant hemisphere may produce a motor transcortical aphasia, in which one can observe a sharp decrease in spontaneous speech contrasting with normal language abilities in repetition tasks, again indicating that the impairment mostly concerns the ability to self-generate verbal output (81). In addition, more caudal lesions of the medial PFC (affecting mostly the supplementary motor area and the contiguous anterior cingulate region) are responsible for a reduction of self-initiated movement, called 'motor neglect', characterized by an underutilization of the contralateral arm in spontaneous conditions (17, 82). In monkeys, a syndrome of this type is induced by experimental lesions of the medial PFC (including the dorsal portion of the anterior cingulate cortex): the monkeys exhibit a sharp decrease in self-initiation of voluntary movements, contrasting with the total sparing of externally triggered actions (83). Several studies using positron emission tomography scanning in humans have shown that the regional cerebral blood flow in the medial frontal cortex (and, in particular, in the rostral supplementary motor area) was associated with the self-generation of motor actions but not with externally cued ones (84, 85). This set of clinical, behavioural, and imaging data suggest that lesions of the dorsomedial PFC are associated with an apathetic syndrome largely explained by the subject's inability to self-activate (or generate) actions, whereas these very actions can be elaborated and performed under strong and sustained external stimulation. As the dorsomedial PFC (including dorsal anterior cingulate cortex) is the cortical node of the circuit linking anterior cingulate cortex to basal ganglia (the anterior cingulate cortex/medial 'dorsal circuit') and that the striatal, pallidal, or thalamic subregions lesions responsible for ADD are likely located in this circuit, we may propose that damage to this circuit may affect the self-generation of GDB by 'switching off' the medial PFC and lead to deep apathy (86).

Thirdly, the severity of the apathetic syndrome in AAD, affecting both the cognitive and the affective dimensions of behaviour could indicate that this syndrome reflects the summation (or even the synergy) of the disruption of three circuits linking the PFC to the basal ganglia. It may lead to a failure for the signal that represents self-generated thoughts and actions channelled by the frontal–basal ganglia circuits to reach the threshold of initiation/activation. According to the latter hypothesis, AAD may represent one of the pathological mirrors of central functions of the basal ganglia, that is, the selection and amplification of the most relevant actions and thoughts for adaptive behaviour (11, 30, 87). We propose that, in normal conditions, the PFC represents the mental space that allows voluntary and conscious decisions about potential actions to be elaborated and performed (20). Neural signals corresponding to the thoughts or actions generated by PFC are then processed by the basal ganglia in order to validate the most relevant signal. Validation processing may be translated into the extraction of the relevant signal from noise to be re-addressed to the output target, namely the PFC. The very specific general architecture of the basal ganglia combining the relative spatial segregation into parallel anatomical circuits and the relative progressive concentration of fibres throughout the basal ganglia may favour the extraction of the relevant signal from the background noise by selecting (through the parallel loops) and amplifying (by concentrating) it. These 'extracted' signals are ultimately transferred to the PFC where a clear-cut signal can be detected and contributes to disambiguating decision-making and maintaining or modifying the ongoing behaviour. In pathological situations, if there is a focal destruction within the basal ganglia subregions involved in affective–cognitive processing, the signal emerging from the basal ganglia is diminished, the ongoing behaviour is not validated (i.e. not amplified) at the level of the PFC and could be difficult to maintain, and the forthcoming one (if it is not reflexive) is not activated. Above all, if the destruction is massive in these areas, no signal is ultimately transferred to the PFC. In other words, the 'empty mind' described by AAD patients may reflect the sharp decrease of relevant signals above threshold in the prefrontal representational space.

What about Monoaminergic Neurotransmission in Apathy?

In PD patients, we demonstrated a significant difference in the severity of apathy between the 'off' and 'on' states in fluctuating PD patients, indicating that apathy in PD is at least partly a dopamine-dependent syndrome (88, 89). Apathy is also inversely correlated to a marker of dopamine transporter in the ventral striatum (90). Therefore, this dopamine-dependent apathy is likely to occur via the impact of striatal dopamine dysfunction and the cascade of dysfunctions within the frontal–basal ganglia circuits.

Classically, dopamine is associated with reward processing as demonstrated by studies in rodents and monkeys using the techniques of electrical self-stimulation of the brain under dopamine-receptor blockade (91), self-administration of dopaminergic substances (92), behavioural observation following dopamine release (93), and single-cell recordings in dopamine neurons coupled with behaviour (94). Learning through positive reinforcement is thought to be an important mechanism of striatal dopamine phasic release within the striatum (94). Learning made by trials/errors triggers dopamine phasic release, reinforces positive choices, and therefore contributes to stabilize the newly established behaviour. Specifically, dopamine neurons may signal discrepancies between the predicted reward as the result of a given behaviour and the reward that the subject eventually receives (94, 95). In addition, dopamine may also code uncertainty of reward delivery (96). Both mechanisms may suggest a possible role for dopamine signals in attention-based learning and evaluating the odds in decision-making based on potentially unpredicted rewarding events. In this line of ideas, Frank and colleagues showed, in a probabilistic selection task in which subjects should learn by trials/errors to choose the stimulus which is the most frequently associated with a reward, that PD patients 'on' dopa-therapy are better at reward learning while being 'off' dopa-therapy, they are better at punishment avoidance (97). The presumed underlying learning rule is that phasic release of striatal dopamine activates the so-called direct output striatal pathway, via D_1-dopamine receptors onto the surface of the striatal output medium spiny neurons, mediating a facilitating signal ('go-signal') to thalamocortical pathways favouring the release of actions. Inversely, dopamine depletion releases the inhibition of the 'indirect' pathway ('no-go' pathway). This circuit inhibits the thalamocortical pathway, which may in turn lead to a 'no-go' cortical signal. As a whole, the consequence of excess dopamine release is likely to trigger impulsive behaviour towards positively reinforced stimuli while dopamine depletion may lead to excessively avoiding punishment with a possible risk of decreasing voluntary GDB.

Striatal dopamine depletion also diminishes spatial focalization of signals in the striatum, leading to the transmission of this modified signal to its output structures (11). A loss of spatial focalization by decreasing the ratio of the relevant signals to noise may lead to a failure to extract the relevant signal in the output structures (the frontal cortex). The decreased signal/noise ratio may lead to apathy because the output structures can no longer disambiguate the relevant signal and this may cause problems in decision-making, inducing aborted or delayed responses.

However, in PD, apathy cannot be fully related to the dopamine denervation (88, 89, 98). In Parkinson's disease, structural direct lesions in the three circuits of GDB are sparse. In contrast, in Parkinson's disease, noradrenergic, serotoninergic, and cholinergic neurotransmission systems are affected to various degrees and may impact cognition and behaviour. Recently, Barber et al. (99) showed a relation between lesions in the raphe serotoninergic system and apathy in Parkinson's disease. Further, several studies in Lewy body and Alzheimer's diseases showed that anticholinesterase medications have a positive (but moderate) effect on treating apathy, indicating a relationship between the loss of cholinergic brain innervation and apathy (100–102).

Conclusion

We would like to assert the three following ideas: (i) apathy is only an output syndrome of several different underlying cognitive and neural mechanisms; (ii) all or most of these mechanisms are related to damage or dysfunction of three PFC–basal ganglia circuits directly involved in the willed/intentional/conscious generation and control of thoughts and actions; and (iii) each of these circuits has its functional and anatomical specificities in contributing to GDB.

These ideas open the way for a clinical diagnosis of apathetic syndromes based on their different dimensions (amotivation, cognitive inertia, invigoration deficit, empty mind, loss of focalization), leading to the development of dimensional tools to assess apathy (this research is ongoing by several different teams). It should also lead to the therapeutic approach to apathy being viewed not in a single unitary way but, on the contrary, in multiple ways, targeted towards the specific underlying mechanism(s) identified for each patient.

References

1. Ali-Cherif A, Royere ML, Gosset A, Poncet M, Salamon G, Khalil R. Behavior and mental activity disorders after carbon monoxide poisoning. Bilateral pallidal lesions. Rev Neurol (Paris). 1984;140(6–7):401–5.
2. Laplane D, Levasseur M, Pillon B, Dubois B, Baulac M, Mazoyer B, et al. Obsessive-compulsive and other behavioural changes with bilateral basal ganglia lesions. A neuro-psychological, magnetic resonance imaging and positron tomography study. Brain. 1989;112(3):699–725.
3. Starkstein SE, Berthier ML, Leiguarda R. Psychic akinesia following bilateral pallidal lesions. Int J Psychiatry Med. 1989;19(2):155–64.
4. Schmidt L, Forgeot d'Arc B, Galanaud D, Czernecki V, Grabli D, Schüpbach M, et al. Disconnecting force from money: effects of basal ganglia damage on incentive motivation. Brain. 2008;131(Pt 5):1303–10.
5. Levy R, Dubois B. Apathy and the prefrontal cortex-basal ganglia circuits. Cereb Cortex. 2006;16(7):916–28.
6. Robert P, Lanctôt KL, Agüera-Ortiz L, Aalten P, Bremond F, Defrancesco F, et al. Is it time to revise the diagnostic criteria for apathy in brain disorders? The 2018 international consensus group. Eur Psychiatry. 2018;54:71–6.
8. Brown RG, Pluck G. Negative symptoms: the 'pathology' of motivation and goal-directed behaviour. Trends Neurosci. 2000;23(9):412–7.
7. Levy R, Czernecki V. Apathy and the basal ganglia. J Neurol. 2006;253(Suppl 7):54–61.
9. Tremblay L, Schultz W. Relative reward preference in primate orbitofrontal cortex. Nature. 1999;398(6729):704–8.
10. Padoa-Schioppa C. Range-adapting representation of economic value in the orbitofrontal cortex. J Neurosci. 2009;29(44):14004–14.
11. Tremblay L, Filion M, Bedard PJ. Responses of pallidal neurons to striatal stimulation in monkeys with MPTP-induced parkinsonism. Brain Res. 1989;498(1):17–33.
12. Pardal MM, Micheli F, Asconape J, Paradiso G. Neurobehavioral symptoms in caudate hemorrhage: two cases. Neurology. 1985;35(12):1806–7.
13. Richfield EK, Twyman R, Berent S. Neurological syndrome following bilateral damage to the head of the caudate nuclei. Ann Neurol. 1987;22(6):768–71.
14. Laplane D, Dubois B, Pillon, Baulac M. Perte d'auto-acitvation psychique et activité mentale stéréotypée par lésion frontale. Rev Neurol (Paris). 1988;144(10):564–70.
15. Mendez MF, Adams NL, Lewandowski KS. Neurobehavioral changes associated with caudate lesions. Neurology. 1989;39(3):349–54.
16. Bhatia KP, Marsden CD. The behavioural and motor consequences of focal lesions of the basal ganglia in man. Brain. 1994;117(4):859–76.

17. von Giesen HJ, Schlaug G, Steinmetz H, Benecke R, Freund HJ, Seitz RJ. Cerebral network underlying unilateral motor neglect: evidence from positron emission tomography. J Neurol Sci. 1994;125(1):29–38.

18. van Domburg PH, Donkelaar HJ, Notermans SL. Akinetic mutism with bithalamic infarction. Neurophysiological correlates. J Neurol Sci. 1996;139(1):58–65.

19. Cognat E, Lagarde J, Decaix C, Hainque E, Azizi L, Gaura-Schmidt V, et al. "Habit" gambling behaviour caused by ischemic lesions affecting the cognitive territories of the basal ganglia. J Neurol. 2010;257(10):1628–32.

20. Goldman-Rakic PS. Circuitry of primate prefrontal cortex and regulation of behaviour by representational memory. In: Plum F, Mouncastle U (Eds), Handbook of Physiology (Vol. 5). Washington, DC: The American Physiological Society; 1987, pp. 373–417.

21. Fuster JM. The Prefrontal Cortex. New York: Raven Press; 1997.

22. Miller EK, Cohen JD. An integrative theory of prefrontal cortex function. Annu Rev Neurosci. 2001;24:167–202.

23. Middleton FA, Strick PL. Basal-ganglia 'projections' to the prefrontal cortex of the primate. Cereb Cortex. 2002;12(9):926–35.

24. Lehéricy S, Ducros M, Van de Moortele PF, Francois C, Thivard L, Poupon C, et al. Diffusion tensor fiber tracking shows distinct corticostriatal circuits in humans. Ann Neurol. 2004;55(4):522–9.

25. Aarsland D, Litvan I, Larsen JP. Neuropsychiatric symptoms of patients with progressive supranuclear palsy and Parkinson's disease. J Neuropsychiatry Clin Neurosci. 2001;13(1):42–9.

26. Craufurd D, Thompson JC, Snowden JS. Behavioral changes in Huntington disease. Neuropsychiatry Neuropsychol Behav Neurol. 2001;14(4):219–26.

27. Battig K, Rosvold HE, Mishkin M. Comparison of the effect of frontal and caudate lesions on delayed response and alternation in monkeys. J Comp Physiol Psychol. 1960;53:400–4.

28. Divac I, Rosvold HE, Scwarcbart MK. Behavioural effects of selective ablation of the caudate nucleus. J Comp Physiol Psych. 1967;63(2):184–90.

29. Levy R, Friedman HR, Davachi L, Goldman-Rakic PS. Differential activation of the caudate nucleus in primates performing spatial and nonspatial working memory tasks. J Neurosci. 1997;17(10):3870–82.

30. Kimura M, Matsumoto N, Okahashi K, Ueda Y, Satoh T, Minamimoto T, et al. Goal-directed, serial and synchronous activation of neurons in the primate striatum. Neuroreport. 2003;14(6):799–802.

31. Luria AR. Higher Cortical Functions in Man. New York: Basic Books; 1980.

32. Eslinger PJ, Damasio AR. Severe disturbance of higher cognition after bilateral frontal lobe ablation: patient EVR. Neurology. 1985;35(12):1731–41.

33. Alexander MP, Stuss DT. Disorders of frontal lobe functioning. Semin Neurol. 2000;20(4):427–37.

34. Rosen HJ, Hartikainen KM, Jagust W, Kramer JH, Reed BR, Cummings JL, et al. Utility of clinical criteria in differentiating frontotemporal lobar degeneration (FTLD) from AD. Neurology. 2002;58(11):1608–15.

35. Chow TW, Binns MA, Cummings JL, Lam I, Black SE, Miller BL, et al. Apathy symptom profile and behavioral associations in frontotemporal dementia vs dementia of Alzheimer type. Arch Neurol. 2009;66(7):888–93.

36. Rascovsky K, Hodges JR, Knopman D, Mendez MF, Kramer JH, Neuhaus J, et al. Sensitivity of revised diagnostic criteria for the behavioural variant of frontotemporal dementia. Brain. 2011;134(9):2456–77.

37. Batrancourt B, Lecouturier K, Ferrand-Verdejo J, Guillemot V, Azuar C, Bendetowicz D, et al. Exploration deficits under ecological conditions as a marker of apathy in frontotemporal dementia. Front Neurol. 2019;10:941.

38. Levy R, Goldman-Rakic PS. Segregation of working memory functions within the dorso-lateral prefrontal cortex. Exp Brain Res. 2000;133(1):23–32.

39. Volle E, Kinkinghehun S, Pochon JB, Mondon K, Thiebaut de Schotten M, et al. The functional architecture of the posterior and lateral prefrontal cortex. Cereb Cortex. 2008;18(10):2460–9.

40. Thiebaut de Schotten M, Urbanski M, Batrancourt B, Levy R, Dubois B, Cerliani L, Volle E. Rostro-caudal architecture of the frontal lobes in humans. Cereb Cortex. 2017;27(8):4033–47.

41. Alexander GE, Delong MR, Strick PL. Parallel organization of functionally segregated circuits linking basal ganglia and cortex. Ann Rev Neurosci. 1986;9:357–81.

42. Haber SN. The primate basal ganglia: parallel and integrative networks. J Chem Neuroanat. 2003;26(4):317–30.

43. Selemon LD, Goldman-Rakic PS. Longitudinal topography and interdigitation of corticostriatal projections in the rhesus monkeys. J Neurosci. 1985;5(3):776–94.

44. Yeterian EH, Pandya DN. Prefrontostriatal connections in relation to cortical architectonic organization in rhesus monkeys. J Comp Neurol. 1991;312(1):43–67.

45. Haber SN, Kunishio K, Mizobuchi M, Lynd-Balta E. The orbital and medial prefrontal circuit through the primate basal ganglia. J Neurosci. 1995;15(7 Pt 1):4851–67.

46. Rahman S, Sahakian BJ, Hodges JR, Rogers RD, Robbins TW. Specific cognitive deficits in mild frontal variant frontotemporal dementia. Brain. 1999;122(8):1469–93.

47. Lough S, Gregory C, Hodges JR. Dissociation of social cognition and executive function in frontal variant frontotemporal dementia. Neurocase. 2001;7(2):123–30.

48. Grossman M, Eslinger PJ, Troiani V, Anderson C, Avants B, Gee JC, et al. The role of ventral medial prefrontal cortex in social decisions: converging evidence from fMRI and frontotemporal lobar degeneration. Neuropsychologia. 2010;48(12):3505–12.

49. Camille N, Griffiths CA, Vo K, Fellows LK, Kable JW. Ventromedial frontal lobe damage disrupts value maximization in humans. J Neurosci. 2011;31(20):7527–32.

50. Massimo L, Powers JP, Evans LK, McMillan CT, Rascovsky K, Eslinger P, et al. Apathy in frontotemporal degeneration: neuroanatomical evidence of impaired goal-directed behavior. Front Hum Neurosci. 2015;109:611.

51. Delgado M, Beer J, Fellows L, Huettel S, Platt M, Quirk G, et al. Viewpoints: dialogues on the functional role of the ventromedial prefrontal cortex. Nat Neurosci. 2016;19(12):1545–52.

52. Manohar SG, Husain M. Human ventromedial prefrontal lesions alter incentivisation by reward. Cortex. 2016;76:104–20.

53. Schneider B, Koenigs M. Human lesion studies of ventromedial prefrontal cortex. Neuropsychologia. 2017;107:84–93.

54. Hollerman JR, Tremblay L, Schultz W. Involvement of basal ganglia and orbitofrontal cortex in goal-directed behavior. Prog Brain Res. 2000;126:193–215.

55. Rolls ET. The orbitofrontal cortex and reward. Cereb Cortex. 2000;10(3):284–94.

56. Schultz W, Tremblay L, Hollerman JR. Reward processing in primate orbitofrontal cortex and basal ganglia. Cereb Cortex. 2000;10(3):272–84.

57. O'Doherty J, Kringelbach ML, Rolls ET, Hornak J, Andrews C. Abstract reward and punishment representations in the human orbitofrontal cortex. Nat Neurosci. 2001;4(1):95–102.

58. Knutson B, Fong GW, Bennett SM, Adams CM, Hommer D. A region of mesial prefrontal cortex tracks monetarily rewarding outcomes: characterization with rapid event-related fMRI. Neuroimage. 2003;18(1):263–72.

59. Elliott R, Newman JL, Longe OA, Deakin JF. Differential response patterns in the striatum and orbitofrontal cortex to financial reward in humans: a parametric functional magnetic resonance imaging study. J Neurosci. 2003;23(1):303–7.
60. Wallis, JD. Cross-species studies of orbitofrontal cortex and value-based decision-making. Nat Neurosci. 2011;15(1):13–9.
61. Clithero JA, Rangel A. Informatic parcellation of the network involved in the computation of subjective value. Soc Cog Affect Neurosci. 2014;9(9):1289–302.
62. Ruff CC, Fehr E. The neurobiology of rewards and values in social decision making. Nat Rev Neurosci. 2104;15(8):549–62.
63. Schultz W, Apicella P, Scarnati E, Ljungberg T. Neuronal activity in monkey ventral striatum related to the expectation of reward. J Neurosci. 1992;12(12):4595–610.
64. Hollerman JR, Tremblay L, Schultz W. Influence of reward expectation on behavior-related neuronal activity in primate striatum. J Neurophysiol. 1998;80(2):947–63.
65. Stern CE, Passingham RE. The nucleus accumbens in monkeys (Macaca fascicularis): II. Emotion and motivation. Behav Brain Res. 1995;75(1–2):179–93.
66. Calder AJ, Keane J, Lawrence AD, Manes F. Impaired recognition of anger following damage to the ventral striatum. Brain. 2004;127(9):1958–69.
67. Petrides M, Pandya DN. Dorsolateral prefrontal cortex: comparative cytoarchitectonic analysis in the human and the macaque brain and corticocortical connection patterns. Eur J Neurosci. 1999;11(3):1011–36.
68. Arikuni T, Kubota K. The organization of prefronto-caudate projections and their laminar origin in the macaque monkey: a retrograde study using HRP-gel. J Comp Neurol. 1986;244(4):492–510.
69. Milner B. Some cognitive effects of frontal-lobe lesions in man. Philos Trans R Soc Lond B. 1982;298(1089):211–26.
70. Petrides M, Milner B. Deficits on subject-ordered tasks after frontal- and temporal-lobe lesions in man. Neuropsychologia. 1982;20(3):249–62. doi:10.1016/0028-3932(82)90100-2. PMID: 7121793.
71. Shallice T. Specific impairments of planning. Philos Trans R Soc Lond B. 1982;298(1089):199–209.
72. Stuss DT, Benson DF. Neuropsychological studies of the frontal lobes. Psychol Bull. 1984 Jan;95(1):3–28. PMID: 6544432.
73. Owen AM, Doyon J, Petrides M, Evans AC. Planning and spatial working memory: a positron emission tomography study in humans. Eur J Neurosci. 1996;158(2):353–64.
74. Stuss DT, Knight RT. Principles of Frontal Lobe Function. Oxford: Oxford University Press; 2002.
75. Rolls ET, Thorpe SJ, Maddison SP. Responses of striatal neurons in the behaving monkey. 1. Head of the caudate nucleus. Behav Brain Res. 1983 Feb;7(2):179–210. doi:10.1016/0166-4328(83)90191-2. PMID: 6830651.
76. Hikosaka O, Sakamoto M, Usui S. Functional properties of monkey caudate neurons. III. Activities related to expectation of target and reward. J Neurophysiol. 1989;61(4):814–32.
77. Baker SC, Rogers RD, Owen AM, Frith CD, Dolan RJ, Frackowiak RS, et al. Neural systems engaged by planning: a PET study of the Tower of London task. Neuropsychologia. 1996;34(6):515–26.
78. Mega MS, Cohenour. Akinetic mutism: disconnection of frontal-subcortical circuits. Neuropsychiatry Neuropsychol Behav Neurol. 1997;10(4):254–9.
79. Anderson CA, Arciniegas DB, Huddle DC, Leehey MA. Akinetic mutism following unilateral anterior cerebral artery occlusion. J Neuropsychiatry Clin Neurosci. 2003;15(3):385–6.

80. Nagaratnam N, Nagaratnam K, Ng K, Diu P. Akinetic mutism following stroke. J Clin Neurosci. 2004;1(1):25–30.

81. Ardila A, Lopez MV. Transcortical motor aphasia: one or two aphasias? Brain Lang. 1984;2(2):350–3.

82. Laplane D, Degos JD. Motor neglect. J Neurol Neurosurg Psychiatry. 1983;46(2):152–8.

83. Thaler DE, Rolls ET, Passingham RE. Neuronal activity of the supplementary motor area (SMA) during internally and externally triggered wrist movements. Neurosci Lett. 1988;93(2–3):264–9.

84. Deiber MP, Passingham RE, Colebatch JG, Friston KJ, Nixon PD, Frackowiak RS. Cortical areas and the selection of movement: a study with positron emission tomography. Exp Brain Res. 1991;84(2):393–402.

85. Jenkins IH, Jahanshahi M, Jueptner M, Passingham RE, Brooks DJ. Self-initiated versus externally triggered movements. II. The effect of movement predictability on regional cerebral blood flow. Brain. 2000;123(6):1216–28.

86. Le Heron C, Apps MAJ, Husain M. The anatomy of apathy: a neurocognitive framework for amotivated behaviour. Neuropsychologia. 2018;118(B):54–67.

87. Brotchie P, Iansek R, Horne MK. Motor function of the monkey globus pallidus. 1. Neuronal discharge and parameters of movement. Brain. 1991 Aug;114 (Pt 4):1667–83. doi:10.1093/brain/114.4.1667. PMID: 1884172.

88. Czernecki V, Pillon B, Houeto JL, Pochon JB, Levy R, Dubois B. Motivation, reward and Parkinson's disease: influence of dopatherapy. Neuropsychologia. 2002;40(13):2257–67.

89. Czernecki V, Schüpbach M, Yaici S, Levy R, Bardinet E, Yelnik J, et al. Ropinerole improves apathy in patients with Parkinson disease and subthalamic nucleus stimulation. Mov Disord. 2008;23(7):964–9.

90. Remy P, Doder M, Lees A, Turjanski N, Brooks D. Depression in Parkinson's disease: loss of dopamine and noradrenaline innervation in the limbic system. Brain. 2005;128(6):1314–22.

91. Rolls ET. The neurophysiological basis of brain-stimulation reward. In: Wauquier A, Rolls ET (Eds), Brain Stimulation Reward. Amsterdam: NorthHolland; 1976, pp. 65–87.

92. Koob GF. Neural mechanisms of drug reinforcement. Ann N Y Acad Sci. 1992;654:171–91.

93. Robbins TW, Everitt BJ. Neurobehavioural mechanisms of reward and motivation. Curr Opin Neurobiol. 1996;6(2):228–36.

94. Schultz W, Dayan P, Montague PR. A neural substrate of prediction and reward. Science. 1997;275(5306):1593–9.

95. Tobler PN, Dickinson A, Schultz W. Coding of predicted reward omission by dopamine neurons in a conditioned inhibition paradigm. J Neurosci. 2003;23(32):10402–10.

96. Fiorillo CD, Tobler PN, Schultz W. Discrete coding of reward probability and uncertainty by dopamine neurons. Science. 2003;299(5614):1898–902.

97. Frank MJ, Seeberger LC, O'Reilly RC. By carrot or by stick: cognitive reinforcement learning in parkinsonism. Science. 2004;306(5703):1940–3.

98. Le Heron C, Plant O, Manohar S, Ang YS, Jackson M, Lennox G, et al. Distinct effects of apathy and dopamine on effort-based decision-making in Parkinson's disease. Brain. 2018;141(5):1455–69.

99. Barber TR, Griffanti L, Muhammed K, Drew DS, Bradley KM, McGowan DR, et al. Apathy in rapid eye movement sleep behaviour disorder is associated with serotonin depletion in the dorsal raphe nucleus. Brain. 2018;141(10):2848–54.

100. McKeith IG, Grace JB, Walker Z, Byrne EJ, Wilkinson D, Stevens T, et al. Rivastigmine in the treatment of dementia with Lewy bodies: preliminary findings from an open trial. Int J Geriatr Psychiatry. 2000;15(5):387–92.

101. Gauthier S, Feldman H, Hecker J, Vellas B, Ames D, Subbiah P, et al. Efficacy of donepezil on behavioral symptoms in patients with moderate to severe Alzheimer's disease. Int Psychogeriatr. 2002;14(4):389–404.
102. Edwards KR, Hershey L, Wray L, Bednarczyk EM, Lichter D, Farlow M, et al. Efficacy and safety of galantamine in patients with dementia with Lewy bodies: a 12-week interim analysis. Dement Geriatr Cogn Disord. 2004;17(Suppl 1):40–8.

10
Neural Basis of Apathy

Structural Imaging Studies

Ingrid Agartz and Lynn Mørch-Johnsen

Structural Brain Imaging

Neuroimaging of brain anatomy and tissue composition in neurodevelopmental and neurodegenerative diseases is an important field of research. The development of *in vivo* neuroimaging methods such as computed tomography (CT) and magnetic resonance imaging (MRI) has had an immense impact on obtaining new knowledge about the central nervous system (CNS). CT was introduced in the 1970s. In more recent decades, MRI has dominated the neuroimaging field of both research and clinical imaging. CT and/or magnetic resonance (MR) scanners are now available at most radiology units in the world.

Paul Lauterbur and Peter Mansfield were awarded the Nobel Prize in Physiology or Medicine in 2003 for their work leading to MRI. Using different MR techniques, it is possible to characterize brain structures based on tissue biochemistry sensitive to the MR phenomenon and reconstructed into a three-dimensional image. At a structural level, MRI allows for excellent estimation of tissue contrast and spatial image resolution along with quantitative tissue measurements in discrete anatomical areas. Grey and white matter cortical or subcortical structure volumes as well as estimation of cortical surface area, cortical thickness, and cortical folding at submillimetre levels can be obtained. The anatomical positions can be determined or mapped in three-dimensional brain image reconstructions using brain atlases. Measures of white matter integrity and white matter tracts using diffusion methods (diffusion-weighted (tensor) imaging (DWI or MR-DWI)) can also be obtained. Although direct methods of quantifying white matter microstructure *in vivo* are not applicable, DWI represents a tool for non-invasive observation of structural organization in the human brain. DWI maps the Brownian movement of water molecules and as axonal membranes and myelin provide natural barriers for water diffusion it is used to infer local tissue properties. Diffusion tensor imaging (DTI) measures indirectly reflect white matter microstructure, fibre orientation and degree of co-linearity often indicated by the fractional anisotropy (FA) measure, and aspects of myelination (1). Free-water DWI is a new application to separate extracellular water from the diffusion of water molecules inside the fibre tracts, leading to a higher specificity in detecting structural changes (2). Methods for mapping white matter myelin allow for an even closer characterization and are of great potential value since many CNS disorders affect the white matter early in the disease process.

The methods previously mentioned, together called structural MRI (sMRI) methods, have become standard for delineating and measuring anatomical brain structure characteristics—their volume, shape, thickness, surface area expansion, texture, fibre direction, and other morphology among available applications. With MR spectroscopy, it is possible to measure spectra of metabolic compounds such as, for example, N-acetyl aspartate, or glutamate/glutamine in discrete volume elements (voxels) in the image. In other words, it is possible to take a 'biopsy' of the image for investigating a number of biochemical parameters. Functional MRI is described elsewhere in this book (see Chapter 12). Structural and functional brain networks or connectivity are of great interest to study in CNS disorders, as many of the CNS disorders are considered to be systemic diseases. Schizophrenia is suggested to be a disorder of connectivity (dysconnectivity) across brain regions. DWI and functional MRI are often used to describe structural and functional connectivity, respectively, at a network level. Structural covariance attempts to define regions that co-vary in brain space and complementary measures of time and functionality need to be integrated with the structural covariance. Combining different MRI modalities (multimodal imaging) increases specificity. This is advantageous since there is typically a large overlap between structural MR measures across different CNS diseases as well as with the healthy population. Many neurological and neuropsychiatric disorders also show systemic pathology which is less characterized than the neurological symptoms, and whole-body imaging may be a valuable future tool.

The concept of apathy has been described in previous chapters. In this chapter, we will discuss structural brain findings, mainly from sMRI in the clinical apathy syndrome occurring in severe illnesses such as schizophrenia and neurodegenerative disorders, including Alzheimer's disease (AD), mild cognitive impairment (MCI), Parkinson's disease (PD), Huntington's disease (HD), and cerebrovascular brain disease or stroke. We will also discuss if the results point to a common structural apathy network or not, and discuss the limitations of structural neuroimaging in characterizing the neuropathology of apathy.

Alzheimer's Disease

AD occurs in about 50–70% of dementia cases (3). Dysfunction in frontal brain systems, co-occurring with deficits in executive function, is thought to be an important neurobiological basis for the onset of apathy. Structural brain imaging shows variability when examining grey matter changes and apathy in AD. Two well-conducted studies using different analysis methods identified atrophy within the anterior cingulate cortex (ACC), dorsolateral prefrontal cortex, putamen, and caudate nuclei in

AD apathy (4, 5), while two other investigations of over 50 patients did not find an association between apathy and grey matter volume (6, 7). As reviewed by Theleritis et al. in 2014 (8), neuroimaging findings have substantiated the involvement of the frontal–subcortical networks in apathy in AD. Based on a systematic review, Stella et al. (9) in 2014 reported that prefrontal regions and the ACC were the leading brain areas associated with apathy in AD and MCI. Other cortical regions and subcortical structures were also implicated. They concluded that abnormalities in frontal regions (associated with impairment in planning and decision-making) and in the ACC (related to emotional blunting and loss of motivation) were the crucial structures associated with apathy in AD and MCI.

Abnormalities of white matter tracts can occur directly from local pathology or indirectly from pathology in the grey matter regions the tracts connect. Kim et al. (6) found that apathy was associated with reduced FA, a DWI measure, in the left ACC (a tract that connects limbic structures including ACC but no other regions). The frontal cortex (mostly ACC and orbitofrontal cortex (OFC)) and ventral striatum (VS), medial thalamus, and ventral tegmental area (VTA) show the strongest association with apathy in AD. This appears similar to reports of apathy correlates in PD.

In summary, abnormalities in frontal regions (associated with impairments in planning and decision-making), including ACC (related to emotional blunting and loss of motivation), appear to be the crucial structures associated with apathy in AD and MCI (10).

Mild Cognitive Impairment

MCI refers to cognitive decline that does not meet the clinical criteria for dementia. MCI arises in many populations, including the aged. It is unclear whether the mechanisms are similar across different diseases and if MCI is a disease precursor or represents a risk state. MCI assessment accuracy based on cognitive batteries is relatively poor. As such, neuroimaging techniques have been used to better identify its neural signature. MCI is a heterogeneous entity and thereby often divided into two different subtypes. The amnestic MCI subtype (aMCI) is considered a precursor to AD development and shows memory loss as predominant feature (11) while the non-amnestic MCI subtype (naMCI) has its main impairments in attention, language, visuospatial, and executive functions and is more related to vascular or Lewy body dementia (12). Structural differences between aMCI and naMCI in the right hippocampus, bilateral amygdala, left precuneus, and left transverse temporal gyrus have been related to specific neuropsychological features of the MCI subtypes (13). In an aMCI population of 756 individuals followed over a 9-year period, cognitive scores and MRI biomarkers combined to predict the onset of dementia due to AD (14). Notably, both neurocognitive scores and MRI biomarkers were required to obtain high predictive sensitivity and specificity, especially for longer follow-ups. The MRI features appeared more sensitive, while cognitive features increased the specificity of the prediction.

MCI is a comorbid factor in PD. The search for PD-MCI biomarkers has employed an array of neuroimaging techniques, but still yields divergent findings. This may in part be due to the broad definition of MCI, including heterogeneous cognitive domains, only some of which show subtle deficits in PD. Structural changes in PD-MCI have been associated with overall cognitive function. Frontal deficit areas have been more associated with executive dysfunction and limbic system areas more associated with executive dysfunction (15).

Using DTI, FA differences between PD-aMCI and cognitively normal individuals with PD found in the white matter were memory related but also influenced by motor function. The commonality between memory and motor function in FA differences suggests that there is a common dopaminergic mechanism underlying both motor and memory impairment in PD-aMCI (16). A characteristic MRI pattern of grey matter atrophy is found in early stages of AD but atrophy patterns at different stages of PD have been inconclusive. Kunst et al. (17) reported a direct comparison of 144 individuals investigated at different stages of both PD and AD and age-matched healthy controls using different image analysis techniques: voxel-based morphometry and source-based morphometry, and cortical thickness. None of the methods could differentiate between PD-MCI and AD-MCI. Both MCI groups showed distinct limbic and frontotemporoparietal neocortical atrophy compared to healthy controls with no specific between-group differences. AD individuals, however, showed the typical pattern of major temporal lobe atrophy, which was associated with broad cognitive deficits.

Parkinson's Disease

The pathological hallmark of PD is a loss of nigrostriatal dopamine cells and an accumulation of intracellular inclusions of alpha-synuclein aggregates (Lewy bodies). Brainstem degeneration associated with the initial progression of Lewy body deposits may be the first identifiable stage in PD, as originally proposed by Braak et al. (18). Several other neurotransmitter systems also degenerate, and in later stages Lewy body pathology spreads to the cortex. This makes PD a systems disorder, understood at the level of brain networks of molecular, structural, and functional abnormalities (19). Monosynaptic dopaminergic projections from the VTA spread to the frontal regions (20). Structural and functional networks disruption of subcortical structures that link the prefrontal cortex with the limbic system underlie the clinical manifestations of apathy in PD (21). Since in PD the dopaminergic systems are primarily affected, apathy is likely to be a prevalent symptom.

The typical onset of PD is over 60 years of age. Individuals with PD have two to six times the risk of developing dementia compared to the general population and up to 80% of individuals with PD have dementia. Apathy affects about 40% of PD patients (22). The level of cognitive function predicts apathy severity in PD, and cognitive performance and dementia need to be corrected for when investigating apathy specifically. An attempt to isolate apathy from cognitive impairments and depression was made by Martínez-Horta et al. (23) who compared non-apathetic PD patients to non-demented and non-depressed PD patients with apathy. Apathetic patients showed grey matter volume loss in cortical and subcortical brain structures with clusters of cortical grey matter decrease in the parietal, lateral prefrontal cortex, and OFC. The second largest cluster of grey matter volume loss was located in the left nucleus accumbens (NAc), a key node of the human reward circuit. Apathy in PD correlated with atrophy in the left dorsal NAc and the dorsolateral head of the caudate (24) but showed no association with cortical thickness. The lack of association between grey matter volumes and apathy status has been corroborated by Bagiio et al. (25), although other studies have reported associations with several cortical regions (26).

A multimodal imaging approach at the systems level was used by Lucas-Jiménez et al. (27) to study PD patients divided into low-subclinical symptoms of apathy and high-subclinical symptoms of apathy and healthy controls with T1-weighted MRI, diffusion-weighted MRI, and resting-state functional MRI using a region-of-interest (ROI) approach. There were no significant grey matter differences across groups. Frontostriatal functional connectivity decreased and white matter axial and mean diffusivity increased in high-subclinical symptom apathy PD compared to lower-apathy PD or controls. The frontostriatal connectivity increased in lower-apathy PD compared with controls and decreased compared with high-subclinical symptom apathy PD. Increased axial diffusivity can be interpreted as axon and myelin loss expanding the extracellular space. However, white matter axial diffusivity results should be interpreted with caution and the study sample was small.

DWI is promising as a marker of both cognitive function and motor symptoms in PD. Free-water diffusion imaging shows promise as a biomarker of progression in early-stage PD and in substantia nigra imaging. Neuromelanin-sensitive and iron-sensitive imaging also have potential to track progression of PD (28). High-field imaging at 7 Tesla makes it possible to segment the substantia nigra, subthalamic nucleus, and the red nucleus. Tracers (radioligands) that specifically bind to alpha-synuclein in the body (e.g. the gut) or in smaller cerebral nuclei using positron emission tomography (PET) will be part of future developments. These imaging advancements have not yet made their way to routine patient studies but have the potential to elucidate different pathways in PD apathy development.

To summarize, neuroimaging studies of apathy in PD have implicated the VS and dorsal ACC together with interconnected regions: medial and lateral prefrontal cortex and the midbrain that contains the key dopaminergic VTA, and NAc (20). Some of the structural findings have been substantiated by functional findings.

Huntington's Disease

HD is an inherited, progressive, and fatal neurodegenerative disease caused by an expanded trinucleotide CAG sequence in the huntingtin gene (*HTT*) on chromosome

4. HD pathology is characterized by the formation of intranuclear inclusions of mu-tated huntingtin protein in the brain. These aggregates impair the function of a number of transcription factors leading to the loss of GABAergic medium spiny neurons in the striatum but also in cortical areas as reviewed by Niccolini and Politis, in 2014 (29). Neuropathological studies in HD have demonstrated neuronal loss in the striatum, as well as in other brain regions including the cortex. Numerous sMRI studies have dem-onstrated widespread striatal and cortical atrophy and microstructural white matter loss in premanifest and manifest HD gene carriers (30).

The most consistent structural change in the brain in patients with HD is a sig-nificant progressive volumetric loss of the striatum. A reduction of 50–54% in mean putamen volume and 28–29% in mean caudate volume has been reported in patients with mild to moderate HD (31). Striatal atrophy has been documented in early HD and even in premanifest HD gene carriers who were 15–20 years before predicted disease onset (29). The amount of volume loss in the striatum correlates with the age of onset, the disease duration, and the CAG repeat length. While motor impairment correlates with increased putamen atrophy, cognitive assessments correlate inversely with caudate volume loss.

Cortical volume loss has also been reported in HD patients. Cortical thinning occurs early in the disease course and seems to proceed from posterior to anterior cortical regions as the disease progresses. Individual variability in regional cortical thinning may also have a role in explaining phenotypic variability. For example, HD patients with more prominent bradykinesia showed significant cortical volume loss in frontal regions including the premotor and supplementary motor areas compared to HD patients with chorea. Widespread white matter atrophy has been identified in HD patients and has been associated with longer CAG length and decline in cognitive and motor performance. Changes in white matter volume are detectable up to 12–15 years before the predicted onset and correlate with cognitive functions, which underlines the role of structural connectivity degeneration in HD pathogenesis. DWI studies have reported white matter tract abnormalities in premanifest HD gene carriers and alterations in diffusion indices correlate with cognitive performance. Abnormal white matter connections of the sensory-motor cortex correlated with a 5-year probability for symptomatic conversion. Using specific DWI metrics, Zhang et al., in 2018 (32), reported reduced axonal density as one of the major factors underlying white matter pathology in pre-HD, coupled with altered local organization in areas surrounding the basal ganglia.

Apathy has a high incidence in HD and follows the disease progression. A DWI study of 80 early-stage HD patients failed to find a relationship between apathy and FA throughout the whole brain (33). In contrast, a single, smaller investigation re-ported FA in the bilateral rectus gyrus white matter of HD patients to be negatively correlated with apathy score (34). This area contains fibres connecting the OFC and subcortical structures, including the VS. In a 2-year follow-up study by Baake et al. (35), apathy at baseline was associated with thalamic atrophy but there was no asso-ciation with an increase in severity of apathy over a 2-year time period for any of the subcortical structures. As reported by McColgan et al. (36), increased functional connections between the default-mode functional brain network were associated with depressive and apathy symptoms in presymptomatic HD, while reduced structural connections between the basal ganglia and the default-mode network were associated with depressive symptoms but not apathy.

In summary, the number of imaging studies of apathy in HD is comparatively low. The results are generally in concordance with results reported for AD and PD, with disruption of mainly the medial prefrontal cortex and the VS being associated with apathy. An integrative multimodal imaging approach, which combines different MRI and PET techniques in HD at different stages of apathy, would be valuable.

Stroke

The pathophysiology of a stroke involves an acute reduction in blood flow to brain tissue. The most common type is ischaemic, due to a thrombosis or an embolus. Around 15% of strokes results from intracranial haemorrhage. In any event, local ischaemia leads to a cascade of events resulting in localized neuronal cell death. Eventually, more widespread neuropathology may evolve, such as descending fibre tract damage and remote alterations of tissue volume (37).

Apathy is present in about 20–30% of patients after stroke (38) and has been associated with older age, decreased global cognition, and worse daily functioning (38). Although apathy can be associated with depression, it has also been shown to occur separately from affective symptom correlates (38–40).

It could be hypothesized that strokes affecting certain regions, for instance, regions involved in reward processing, would be associated with an increased risk of apathy. Results from CT or MRI studies investigating the association between the location of a stroke and post-stroke apathy have not been consistent as concluded by different reviews (10, 39, 40). An association between apathy and basal ganglia lesions appears to be reported most consistently (40), but associations with the medial frontal cortex and medial thalamic nuclei have also been reported (20). Douven et al. (39) performed a meta-analysis on studies investigating brain structural correlates of post-stroke apathy and post-stroke depression. Post-stroke depression in the acute phase was reported more frequently in patients with frontal or basal ganglia lesions. Regarding apathy, no significant association was found between post-stroke apathy and lesions in frontal, subcortical, or basal ganglia regions. It should be cautioned that the results on apathy were based on a small number of studies, such as for the analysis on subcortical regions where only two studies were included. Left hemisphere strokes were numerically associated with an increased odds of post-stroke apathy, but this association was not statistically significant.

Neuropsychiatric symptoms after stroke can be associated with the lesion itself, or with secondary effects of the lesion, such as degeneration of white matter tracts and associated postsynaptic regions (37, 41). In a relatively small yet interesting study,

Matsuoka et al. (41) investigated delayed cortical grey matter volume changes in patients with subcortical infarcts. MRI was performed first at 10–28 days after stroke onset, and again 6 months later. Compared to healthy controls, patients had significant volume reductions in anterior parts of the posterior cingulate cortex over this period of time. The reduction in posterior cingulate cortex volume was significantly associated with increased severity of the apathy score over the same time. This association was significant after controlling for effects of age, sex, laterality of the infarction, and acute stroke size. The authors suggest that the delayed volume change in the posterior cingulate cortex post stroke, remote to the original location of the stroke, may reflect degeneration secondary to neuronal loss.

Evidence associating white matter alterations with apathy has been indicated from a few studies. Brodaty et al. (38) studied clinical neuroradiological ratings of severity of periventricular and deep white matter hyperintensities, and cortical and subcortical atrophy in stroke patients assessed 3–6 months post stroke. No significant associations were found between apathy scores and stroke volume, number of prior strokes, or ratings of atrophy. An association was seen between apathy and right-sided and right frontal–subcortical circuit hyperintensity scores; however, this association was not significant after correcting for multiple statistical comparisons. In a DTI study, Yang et al. (42) investigated the association of apathy and brain white matter networks in patients within 7 days after stroke onset. Both tissue damage related to the brain lesion and topological properties of white matter networks were explored. Apathy was not found to be associated with regional tissue damage, but with global and local efficiencies of an apathy-related subnetwork. Subnetwork nodes were located across the brain in the limbic system, frontal lobe, basal ganglia, temporal lobe, parietal lobe, insula, and occipital lobe.

Cerebral small vessel disease affects the small vessels of the brain, such as the small arteries that supply deep white matter and grey matter structures (43). The disease is associated with lacunar infarcts which constitute about 20% of strokes. A high prevalence of apathy as well as cognitive impairment and depression has been reported in cerebral small vessel disease. It has been proposed that the neuropsychiatric symptoms may arise due to disruption of white matter tracts involved in subcortical–cortical circuits. In support of this, Hollocks et al. (44), using DTI, found that apathy was associated with widespread white matter microstructural changes in patients with small vessel disease and lacunar strokes. Changes were found particularly in anterior brain regions such as the anterior cingulum but also within the parietal and temporal lobes. Apathy and depression were both highly prevalent in this patient group, with apathy being present in 52% of the patients, and depression in 56% of the patients. Despite a large overlap of symptoms, approximately 18% of the patients showed high levels of apathy and low levels of depression. No significant association was seen between white matter integrity and depression. In another DTI study, Lisiecka-Ford et al. (45) used DTI and graph theory to investigate structural brain network efficiency in relation to apathy in patients with cerebral small vessel disease. They found that apathy was significantly correlated with reduced connectivity in network clusters involving medial frontal lobes, basal ganglia, parietal lobes, and temporal lobes. The authors also investigated the correlation between apathy and network efficiency in three predefined networks: a reward network, a motor network, and a visual network. Efficiency in the reward network was significantly correlated with severity of apathy after controlling for the efficiency of the motor and visual networks. Nodes in the reward network included bilateral ACC, putamen, inferior OFC, medial OFC, superior medial cortex, amygdala, superior temporal pole, and middle temporal pole.

In summary, no clear association between location of stroke lesion and severity of apathy has been observed; however, the number of studies is quite small. Some evidence suggests that instead, post-stroke apathy is related to damage in white matter tracts and alterations in brain network connectivity. Such findings have also been reported in patients with small vessel disease and lacunar infarcts. However, in general, there are very few studies and various methods have been employed, limiting the conclusion.

Schizophrenia and Psychotic Disorders

The pathophysiology underlying severe psychotic disorders such as schizophrenia is not fully known. Underlying causes most likely involve a complex interaction between genetic and environmental factors involved in neurodevelopment. Suggested pathophysiological mechanisms include genetic vulnerability, neurodevelopmental abnormalities, dopamine and glutamate dysregulation, and immune system activation (46). Brain imaging has limited clinical utility as no diagnostic marker has been identified. However, structural neuroimaging studies report subtle, yet consistent brain structure alterations when schizophrenia patients are compared to healthy controls on a group level. These alterations include reductions in cortical grey matter, increased ventricle size, and decreased volumes of several deeper grey matter structures, as well as widespread abnormalities in the structural integrity of white matter tracts (47–49).

Apathy is present in around 50% of schizophrenia patients (50) and is part of the negative symptom construct, which also includes expressive deficits such as blunted affect and alogia. Negative symptoms have been associated with cognitive deficits and social and functional decline in schizophrenia. For many patients, the negative symptoms are enduring and respond poorly to pharmacological treatment.

Severity of apathy has been linked to reductions in bilateral frontal lobe volume in schizophrenia patients (51), and a thinner cortex in frontal cortex regions of the ACC and OFC in first-episode psychosis (52). Two independent studies have also reported associations between apathy and reduced grey matter volume of the VS (53, 54) VS dysfunction during reward anticipation has been reported from functional MRI studies (see Chapter 12).

Most studies to date have been so-called ROI studies, limiting the specificity of findings. A recently published study by Caravaggio and colleagues (54) explored the correlation between grey matter volumes and subdomains of negative symptoms. They found that the Avolition–Apathy score, as measured by the Scale for the Assessment of Negative Symptoms, was negatively correlated with grey matter volume in grey matter clusters in bilateral frontal inferior operculum, bilateral post-central gyrus, bilateral hypothalamus, and left caudal anterior cingulate; however, results were not statistically significant after correction for multiple comparisons.

Chuang et al. (55) studied the neural correlates of negative symptoms in patients with major depressive disorder and schizophrenia. The results suggested differential pathophysiological mechanisms of negative symptoms in depression and schizophrenia. In schizophrenia patients, white matter volume *decrease* in the left anterior limb of the internal capsule and *increase* in the left superior longitudinal fasciculus was correlated with a pleasure/motivation domain derived from principal component analysis of ten different negative symptom rating scales. In contrast to the aforementioned studies, no association was seen with grey matter volume.

In DWI studies, the severity of apathy has been associated with reductions in white matter structural integrity (as measured by FA) between the left medial OFC and the rostral ACC (56), and in the anterior part of the corpus callosum (57). Amodio et al. (58) used probabilistic tractography to investigate connectivity strength and structural integrity of pathways between important regions within the motivational reward system. ROIs included the amygdala, VTA, striatum, insula, and OFC, as well as the dorsolateral prefrontal cortex. Reduced FA was found in connections between the left amygdala and the insular cortex in schizophrenia patients compared to healthy controls, and was negatively correlated with avolition/apathy scores, but not with expressive deficits negative symptoms. The authors argued that these pathways are 'involved in updating and retrieving the value information to support motivated behaviour'.

In summary, apathy in schizophrenia has been associated with regional volumetric reductions in the frontal lobes, including the ACC, the OFC, and the striatum, although some studies have also failed to find such an association. Most studies to date have been ROI studies, which may bias the specificity of the regional findings. Studies have also reported white matter volumetric alterations as well as alterations in white matter structural integrity associated with apathy.

Is There a Common Apathy Circuitry Network Across Disorders with a Clinical Apathy Syndrome?

Apathy manifests in many brain or neurological disorders including several of the common neurodegenerative disorders such as PD, HD, and AD as well as in schizophrenia and other brain syndromes. This raises the question of whether the brain structure findings associated with the clinical apathy syndrome (see earlier; e.g. frontal brain regions including OFC and ACC, and the VS, VTA, and NAc) point to a common brain circuitry or network. The structural neuroimaging studies that have investigated apathy so far appear to point to commonalities across brain regions and across patient populations, implicating abnormalities within frontostriatal circuits as the most consistently associated with apathy across the different pathological conditions. In 2018, Le Heron and colleagues performed a similar review of structural imaging correlates of apathy, attempting to define a neurocognitive framework common to all brain disorders (20). They concluded that apathy across diagnostic categories was consistently associated with disruption in an interconnected group of brain regions with the dorsal ACC and the VS including the NAc. These interconnected regions correspond to observations from experimental studies on the motivational system in humans, primates, and rodents, and from studies on addiction behaviour in mice and men, that also engages reward circuits (59, 60). It could be hypothesized that different pathological processes, such as regional neuronal cell death in stroke, basal ganglia pathology in PD, and microstructural alterations in white matter tracts as seen across disorders all contribute to dysfunctions of these motivational networks, resulting in the clinical syndrome of apathy.

Although the dysfunction of the motivational reward system appears closely associated with apathy, differential processes may underlie the complex clinical syndrome of apathy such as pointed out by Kos et al. (61) in a systematic review of apathy in patients with neurodegenerative disorders, acquired brain injury, and psychiatric disorders. Kos et al. (61) concluded that abnormalities within frontostriatal circuits (frontal, striatal, anterior cingulate, and parietal regions) were most consistently associated with apathy across different pathological conditions. However, the authors also pointed to the variance in the implicated brain regions, which suggested different routes towards apathy that can vary across patient populations. The authors identified a 'need to study possible differential processes underlying different aspects of goal-directed behaviour, from intention and goal selection to action planning and execution'.

Different 'routes to apathy' have been theorized. Levy and Dubois (62) who defined apathy as a 'quantitative reduction of voluntary, goal-directed behaviours', suggested three subtypes of mechanisms that could lead to apathy: 'emotional-affective', 'cognitive', and 'auto-activation'. Those authors further suggested that dysfunction in emotional-affective processing includes problems with linking the affective-emotional signal to ongoing and forthcoming behaviour, and could correspond to lesions in orbital medial prefrontal cortex or regions in the basal ganglia such as VS and ventral pallidum. Several of the above-mentioned studies point to alterations in these circuits, but these regions may also be the most frequently investigated in ROI-based studies. Dysfunction of cognitive functioning may lead to difficulties in the planning of necessary actions for goal-directed behaviour, and may result from alterations in the dorsolateral prefrontal cortex and associated regions in the basal ganglia such as the dorsal caudate. Associations between cognitive dysfunction and apathy have been reported in studies of patients with stroke and AD, and associations between apathy and executive functioning have been shown in schizophrenia, supporting the involvement of this mechanism in apathy. Levy and Dubois also suggested a third mechanism, disruption of 'auto-activation' of thoughts or self-initiated action associated with lesions of pallidum affecting basal ganglia output. Combining clinical, cognitive, and neuroimaging methods to disentangle putative differential mechanisms may be a target for future studies.

Strengths and Limitations of Structural Imaging Studies of the Clinical Apathy Syndrome

Discrepant results across MR studies can be explained by using different inclusion criteria for diseases, comorbidity that is not accounted for, unwarranted age effects, and a low statistical power. Diverging definitions of apathy and lack of a consensual (still evolving) validation of the multidimensional concept of apathy across disorders may hamper progress of research. Effects of apathy can be difficult to disentangle from effects such as depression or fatigue. Apathy may not only be related to specific brain dysfunctions but to other underlying more disease-specific phenomena. There are also no quantitative measures from neurophysiological studies or reliable biomarkers for more precise disease stage definitions, which touch not only on limitations in the apathy construct as such, but also on limitations in conducting well-designed imaging studies. Investigating the neural correlates of apathy across different clinical diseases through direct comparisons, and in comparisons with healthy control groups, could also be helpful. Discoveries from addiction disorders that have mapped the dopaminergic system in reward and compulsive behaviours circuits in animal as well as in human studies could be valuable as hypothesis generators since apathy appears to represent an antithesis to motivational behaviour.

MR studies of CNS disorders also harbour limitations. First, particularly in psychiatric disorders, studies have been conducted at the group level with, so far, little, if any, clinical use in the individual case. Second, although group differences can show robust and significant differences at group level, the distributional overlap can be considerably greater. A large within-syndrome heterogeneity and overlap with healthy controls has been shown, for example, in schizophrenia (63, 64). Often, as in schizophrenia, the most severe cases do not show up for examination. Third, longitudinal studies need to overcome methodological changes over time and follow-up studies using the same equipment are difficult to do. Fourth, the specificity of regional findings calls for caution in that many of the studies have used a restricted ROI-based approach, rather than exploring the whole brain.

Non-standardized MRI methods and underpowered studies are also problematic. Despite these shortcomings, MRI has a potential important role for improving our understanding of different clinical syndromes such as apathy.

Future Directions

The neuroimaging field is developing rapidly, thanks to advances in both neuro-imaging techniques and computer technology. Higher MRI resolution (7-Telsa scanners) can demonstrate the details of smaller brain structures. Imaging animal models and patients for translational research questions is advantageous. Use of artificial intelligence in multimodal imaging which sets to develop algorithms for disease prediction and outcome, stratification, and treatment selection and to address the heterogeneity across diseases as well as within disease may also provide novel contributions. Development of new biomarkers, whole-body imaging, and physiological assessments in integrated models is also a way forward. Cross-site collaboration with larger structural and functional MR data sets can help address the clinical heterogeneity since many of the studies presented here have been small and thus likely to be underpowered. Using different neuroimaging modalities simultaneously may aid our understanding of the complex mechanisms underlying the CNS disorders and contributing to transdiagnostic clinical syndromes, such as apathy. The new possibilities of combining PET and MRI in PET-MR machines, which allow for near-simultaneous functional and structural imaging, will undoubtedly increase information extraction. Often, functional MRI activation pattern studies temporarily forego the structural findings in brain disorders but functional MRI normally has lower spatial resolution than sMRI. A better understanding of the biological underpinnings of the respective CNS disorders and a better understanding of the apathy phenotypic components will lead to more precise imaging study designs. Finally, today's large-scale collaborative ventures and novel imaging approaches hold promise for new discoveries.

Conclusion

Across the different neurological disorders and neuropsychiatric disorders reviewed in this chapter, structural regional alterations in frontal, striatal, anterior cingulate, and parietal brain regions, as well as alterations in white matter microstructure and connectivity appear to be involved in the apathy syndrome. Several of the structural brain findings map to regions and circuits in the human motivational reward system, but regions outside of these circuits have been observed, implicating different routes to the clinical syndrome of apathy. So far, no clear disorder-specific mechanisms have been demonstrated and it is possible that the neural correlates of apathy can differ across clinical populations and that apathy subtypes can be identified. More in-depth studies of different processes within the apathy syndrome are called for. Integrative multimodal imaging, which combines different high-resolution MRI, MR diffusion, and PET techniques, could be helpful in resolving these. Transdiagnostic approaches and large-scale collaborations enabling better statistically powered studies are future prospects.

References

1. Alexander AL, Lee JE, Lazar M, Field AS. Diffusion tensor imaging of the brain. Neurotherapeutics. 2007;4(3):316–29.
2. Pasternak O, Sochen N, Gur Y, Intrator N, Assaf Y. Free water elimination and mapping from diffusion MRI. Magn Reson Med. 2009;62(3):717–30.
3. Mega MS, Cummings JL, Fiorello T, Gornbein J. The spectrum of behavioral changes in Alzheimer's disease. Neurology. 1996;46(1):130–5.
4. Bruen PD, McGeown WJ, Shanks MF, Venneri A. Neuroanatomical correlates of neuropsychiatric symptoms in Alzheimer's disease. Brain. 2008;131(Pt 9):2455–63.
5. Tunnard C, Whitehead D, Hurt C, Wahlund LO, Mecocci P, Tsolaki M, et al. Apathy and cortical atrophy in Alzheimer's disease. Int J Geriatr Psychiatry. 2011;26(7):741–8.
6. Kim JW, Lee DY, Choo IH, Seo EH, Kim SG, Park SY, et al. Microstructural alteration of the anterior cingulum is associated with apathy in Alzheimer disease. Am J Geriatr Psychiatry. 2011;19(7):644–53.
7. Starkstein SE, Mizrahi R, Capizzano AA, Acion L, Brockman S, Power BD. Neuroimaging correlates of apathy and depression in Alzheimer's disease. J Neuropsychiatry Clin Neurosci. 2009;21(3):259–65.
8. Theleritis C, Politis A, Siarkos K, Lyketsos CG. A review of neuroimaging findings of apathy in Alzheimer's disease. Int Psychogeriatr. 2014;26(2):195–207.
9. Stella F, Radanovic M, Aprahamian I, Canineu PR, de Andrade LP, Forlenza OV. Neurobiological correlates of apathy in Alzheimer's disease and mild cognitive impairment: a critical review. J Alzheimers Dis. 2014;39(3):633–48.
10. Starkstein SE, Brockman S. The neuroimaging basis of apathy: empirical findings and conceptual challenges. Neuropsychologia. 2018;118(Pt B):48–53.
11. Roberts RO, Knopman DS, Mielke MM, Cha RH, Pankratz VS, Christianson TJ, et al. Higher risk of progression to dementia in mild cognitive impairment cases who revert to normal. Neurology. 2014;82(4):317–25.
12. Tabert MH, Manly JJ, Liu X, Pelton GH, Rosenblum S, Jacobs M, et al. Neuropsychological prediction of conversion to Alzheimer disease in patients with mild cognitive impairment. Arch Gen Psychiatry. 2006;63(8):916–24.
13. Qin R, Li M, Luo R, Ye Q, Luo C, Chen H, et al. The efficacy of gray matter atrophy and cognitive assessment in differentiation of aMCI and naMCI. Appl Neuropsychol Adult. 2020 Jan 16:1–7. doi: 10.1080/23279095.2019.1710509. Epub ahead of print.
14. Zandifar A, Fonov VS, Ducharme S, Belleville S, Collins DL, Alzheimer's disease neuroimaging I. MRI and cognitive scores complement each other to accurately predict Alzheimer's dementia 2 to 7 years before clinical onset. Neuroimage Clin. 2020;25:102121.
15. Gao Y, Nie K, Huang B, Mei M, Guo M, Xie S, et al. Changes of brain structure in Parkinson's disease patients with mild cognitive impairment analyzed via VBM technology. Neurosci Lett. 2017;658:121–32.
16. Chen F, Wu T, Luo Y, Li Z, Guan Q, Meng X, et al. Amnestic mild cognitive impairment in Parkinson's disease: white matter structural changes and mechanisms. PLoS One. 2019;14(12):e0226175.
17. Kunst J, Marecek R, Klobusiakova P, Balazova Z, Anderkova L, Nemcova-Elfmarkova N, et al. Patterns of grey matter atrophy at different stages of Parkinson's and Alzheimer's diseases and relation to cognition. Brain Topogr. 2019;32(1):142–60.
18. Braak H, Del Tredici K, Rub U, de Vos RA, Jansen Steur EN, Braak E. Staging of brain pathology related to sporadic Parkinson's disease. Neurobiol Aging. 2003;24(2):197–211.
19. Helmich RC, Vaillancourt DE, Brooks DJ. The future of brain imaging in Parkinson's disease. J Parkinsons Dis. 2018;8(s1):S47–51.

20. Le Heron C, Apps MAJ, Husain M. The anatomy of apathy: a neurocognitive framework for amotivated behaviour. Neuropsychologia. 2018;118(Pt B):54–67.

21. Pagonabarraga J, Kulisevsky J, Strafella AP, Krack P. Apathy in Parkinson's disease: clinical features, neural substrates, diagnosis, and treatment. Lancet Neurol. 2015;14(5):518–31.

22. Zahodne LB, Young S, Kirsch-Darrow L, Nisenzon A, Fernandez HH, Okun MS, et al. Examination of the Lille Apathy Rating Scale in Parkinson disease. Mov Disord. 2009;24(5):677–83.

23. Martínez-Horta S, Sampedro F, Pagonabarraga J, Fernandez-Bobadilla R, Marin-Lahoz J, Riba J, et al. Non-demented Parkinson's disease patients with apathy show decreased grey matter volume in key executive and reward-related nodes. Brain Imaging Behav. 2017;11(5):1334–42.

24. Carriere N, Besson P, Dujardin K, Duhamel A, Defebvre L, Delmaire C, et al. Apathy in Parkinson's disease is associated with nucleus accumbens atrophy: a magnetic resonance imaging shape analysis. Mov Disord. 2014;29(7):897–903.

25. Baggio HC, Segura B, Garrido-Millan JL, Marti MJ, Compta Y, Valldeoriola F, et al. Resting-state frontostriatal functional connectivity in Parkinson's disease-related apathy. Mov Disord. 2015;30(5):671–9.

26. Reijnders JS, Scholtissen B, Weber WE, Aalten P, Verhey FR, Leentjens AF. Neuroanatomical correlates of apathy in Parkinson's disease: a magnetic resonance imaging study using voxel-based morphometry. Mov Disord. 2010;25(14):2318–25.

27. Lucas-Jiménez O, Ojeda N, Pena J, Cabrera-Zubizarreta A, Diez-Cirarda M, Gomez-Esteban JC, et al. Apathy and brain alterations in Parkinson's disease: a multimodal imaging study. Ann Clin Transl Neurol. 2018;5(7):803–14.

28. Yang J, Burciu RG, Vaillancourt DE. Longitudinal progression markers of Parkinson's disease: current view on structural imaging. Curr Neurol Neurosci Rep. 2018;18(12):83.

29. Niccolini F, Politis M. Neuroimaging in Huntington's disease. World J Radiol. 2014;6(6):301–12.

30. Gregory S, Scahill RI. Functional magnetic resonance imaging in Huntington's disease. Int Rev Neurobiol. 2018;142:381–408.

31. Harris GJ, Pearlson GD, Peyser CE, Aylward EH, Roberts J, Barta PE, et al. Putamen volume reduction on magnetic resonance imaging exceeds caudate changes in mild Huntington's disease. Ann Neurol. 1992;31(1):69–75.

32. Zhang J, Gregory S, Scahill RI, Durr A, Thomas DL, Lehericy S, et al. In vivo characterization of white matter pathology in premanifest Huntington's disease. Ann Neurol. 2018;84(4):497–504.

33. Gregory S, Scahill RI, Seunarine KK, Stopford C, Zhang H, Zhang J, et al. Neuropsychiatry and white matter microstructure in Huntington's disease. J Huntingtons Dis. 2015;4(3):239–49.

34. Delmaire C, Dumas EM, Sharman MA, van den Bogaard SJ, Valabregue R, Jauffret C, et al. The structural correlates of functional deficits in early Huntington's disease. Hum Brain Mapp. 2013;34(9):2141–53.

35. Baake V, Coppen EM, van Duijn E, Dumas EM, van den Bogaard SJA, Scahill RI, et al. Apathy and atrophy of subcortical brain structures in Huntington's disease: a two-year follow-up study. Neuroimage Clin. 2018;19:66–70.

36. McColgan P, Razi A, Gregory S, Seunarine KK, Durr A, Roos RAC, et al. Structural and functional brain network correlates of depressive symptoms in premanifest Huntington's disease. Hum Brain Mapp. 2017;38(6):2819–29.

37. Thomalla G, Glauche V, Weiller C, Rother J. Time course of Wallerian degeneration after ischaemic stroke revealed by diffusion tensor imaging. J Neurol Neurosurg Psychiatry. 2005;76(2):266–8.

38. Brodaty H, Sachdev PS, Withall A, Altendorf A, Valenzuela MJ, Lorentz L. Frequency and clinical, neuropsychological and neuroimaging correlates of apathy following stroke—the Sydney Stroke Study. Psychol Med. 2005;35(12):1707–16.

39. Douven E, Kohler S, Rodriguez MMF, Staals J, Verhey FRJ, Aalten P. Imaging markers of post-stroke depression and apathy: a systematic review and meta-analysis. Neuropsychol Rev. 2017;27(3):202–19.

40. van Dalen JW, Moll van Charante EP, Nederkoorn PJ, van Gool WA, Richard E. Poststroke apathy. Stroke. 2013;44(3):851–60.

41. Matsuoka K, Yasuno F, Taguchi A, Yamamoto A, Kajimoto K, Kazui H, et al. Delayed atrophy in posterior cingulate cortex and apathy after stroke. Int J Geriatr Psychiatry. 2015;30(6):566–72.

42. Yang S, Hua P, Shang X, Cui Z, Zhong S, Gong G, et al. Deficiency of brain structural subnetwork underlying post-ischaemic stroke apathy. Eur J Neurol. 2015;22(2):341–7.

43. Cuadrado-Godia E, Dwivedi P, Sharma S, Ois Santiago A, Roquer Gonzalez J, Balcells M, et al. Cerebral small vessel disease: a review focusing on pathophysiology, biomarkers, and machine learning strategies. J Stroke. 2018;20(3):302–20.

44. Hollocks MJ, Lawrence AJ, Brookes RL, Barrick TR, Morris RG, Husain M, et al. Differential relationships between apathy and depression with white matter microstructural changes and functional outcomes. Brain. 2015;138(Pt 12):3803–15.

45. Lisiecka-Ford DM, Tozer DJ, Morris RG, Lawrence AJ, Barrick TR, Markus HS. Involvement of the reward network is associated with apathy in cerebral small vessel disease. J Affect Disord. 2018;232:116–21.

46. Schizophrenia Working Group of the Psychiatric Genomics Consortium. Biological insights from 108 schizophrenia-associated genetic loci. Nature. 2014;511(7510):421–7.

47. van Erp TG, Hibar DP, Rasmussen JM, Glahn DC, Pearlson GD, Andreassen OA, et al. Subcortical brain volume abnormalities in 2028 individuals with schizophrenia and 2540 healthy controls via the ENIGMA consortium. Mol Psychiatry. 2016;21(4):547–53.

48. van Erp TGM, Walton E, Hibar DP, Schmaal L, Jiang W, Glahn DC, et al. Cortical brain abnormalities in 4474 individuals with schizophrenia and 5098 control subjects via the Enhancing Neuro Imaging Genetics through Meta Analysis (ENIGMA) Consortium. Biol Psychiatry. 2018;84(9):644–54.

49. Kelly S, Jahanshad N, Zalesky A, Kochunov P, Agartz I, Alloza C, et al. Widespread white matter microstructural differences in schizophrenia across 4322 individuals: results from the ENIGMA Schizophrenia DTI Working Group. Mol Psychiatry. 2018;23(5):1261–9.

50. Bortolon C, Macgregor A, Capdevielle D, Raffard S. Apathy in schizophrenia: a review of neuropsychological and neuroanatomical studies. Neuropsychologia. 2018;118(Pt B):22–33.

51. Roth RM, Flashman LA, Saykin AJ, McAllister TW, Vidaver R. Apathy in schizophrenia: reduced frontal lobe volume and neuropsychological deficits. Am J Psychiatry. 2004;161(1):157–9.

52. Morch-Johnsen L, Nesvag R, Faerden A, Haukvik UK, Jorgensen KN, Lange EH, et al. Brain structure abnormalities in first-episode psychosis patients with persistent apathy. Schizophr Res. 2015;164(1-3):59–64.

53. Roth RM, Garlinghouse MA, Flashman LA, Koven NS, Pendergrass JC, Ford JC, et al. Apathy is associated with ventral striatum volume in schizophrenia spectrum disorder. J Neuropsychiatry Clin Neurosci. 2016;28(3):191–4.

54. Caravaggio F, Fervaha G, Menon M, Remington G, Graff-Guerrero A, Gerretsen P. The neural correlates of apathy in schizophrenia: an exploratory investigation. Neuropsychologia. 2018;118(Pt B):34–9.

55. Chuang JY, Murray GK, Metastasio A, Segarra N, Tait R, Spencer J, et al. Brain structural signatures of negative symptoms in depression and schizophrenia. Front Psychiatry. 2014;5:116.

56. Ohtani T, Bouix S, Hosokawa T, Saito Y, Eckbo R, Ballinger T, et al. Abnormalities in white matter connections between orbitofrontal cortex and anterior cingulate cortex and their associations with negative symptoms in schizophrenia: a DTI study. Schizophr Res. 2014;157(1–3):190–7.

57. Nakamura K, Kawasaki Y, Takahashi T, Furuichi A, Noguchi K, Seto H, et al. Reduced white matter fractional anisotropy and clinical symptoms in schizophrenia: a voxel-based diffusion tensor imaging study. Psychiatry Res. 2012;202(3):233–8.

58. Amodio A, Quarantelli M, Mucci A, Prinster A, Soricelli A, Vignapiano A, et al. Avolition-apathy and white matter connectivity in schizophrenia: reduced fractional anisotropy between amygdala and insular cortex. Clin EEG Neurosci. 2018;49(1):55–65.

59. Hu Y, Salmeron BJ, Gu H, Stein EA, Yang Y. Impaired functional connectivity within and between frontostriatal circuits and its association with compulsive drug use and trait impulsivity in cocaine addiction. JAMA Psychiatry. 2015;72(6):584–92.

60. Richard JM, Castro DC, Difeliceantonio AG, Robinson MJ, Berridge KC. Mapping brain circuits of reward and motivation: in the footsteps of Ann Kelley. Neurosci Biobehav Rev. 2013;37(9 Pt A):1919–31.

61. Kos C, van Tol MJ, Marsman JB, Knegtering H, Aleman A. Neural correlates of apathy in patients with neurodegenerative disorders, acquired brain injury, and psychiatric disorders. Neurosci Biobehav Rev. 2016;69:381–401.

62. Levy R, Dubois B. Apathy and the functional anatomy of the prefrontal cortex-basal ganglia circuits. Cereb Cortex. 2006;16(7):916–28.

63. Wolfers T, Doan NT, Kaufmann T, Alnaes D, Moberget T, Agartz I, et al. Mapping the heterogeneous phenotype of schizophrenia and bipolar disorder using normative models. JAMA Psychiatry. 2018;75(11):1146–55.

64. Alnaes D, Kaufmann T, van der Meer D, Cordova-Palomera A, Rokicki J, Moberget T, et al. Brain heterogeneity in schizophrenia and its association with polygenic risk. JAMA Psychiatry. 2019;76(7):739–48.

11
Brain Reward Systems and Apathy

Stefan Kaiser and Florian Schlagenhauf

Introduction

Apathy can be defined as a loss of motivation and/or a quantitative reduction of goal-directed behaviour (1, 2). The latter definition has the advantage of describing apathy in terms of observable behaviour and avoids the psychological term motivation. Nevertheless, there is a broad consensus that impaired motivation is a major cause for reduced goal-directed behaviour in patients with apathy. A link between clinical apathy and neurobiological systems underlying motivational and reward processes has high face validity and has been proposed for several years (3).

Motivated behaviour is strongly related to the attainment of rewards (4–6). In other words, an agent will engage in motivated behaviour in order to obtain a reward, even though the reward might not be direct and immediate. The relevant processes include the appreciation of reward before a decision is made, the integration of reward value and costs to make a decision on an action, and processes after the action has been implemented (reward consumption and reward learning).

These core functions of the reward system have been shown to be associated with apathy across neuropsychiatric disorders. However, results vary to some extent across disorders and there is also an important inter-individual variability within disorders. In the following, we give a brief overview of the structure and function of the reward system and then specifically address the functions that have most consistently been associated with apathy.

We focus mostly on studies conducted in patients with schizophrenia, but refer to other disorders to point out certain mechanisms and give a transdiagnostic appreciation at the end of this chapter. In patients with schizophrenia, apathy is considered to be part of the negative symptoms which can be structured into two factors (7). A motivational factor includes the items avolition, asociality and anhedonia, while the expression factor includes blunted affect and alogia. For practical purposes, we consider the motivational factor to be equivalent to apathy.

Reward Processing

What Is a Reward?

There is a consensus that reward is essential for goal-directed behaviour. However, a simple definition of the term is difficult because rewards vary across different dimensions (6). First, rewards can be of different natures (8). Primary rewards such as food and water directly fulfil the organism's needs necessary for survival, while secondary rewards such as money fulfil higher-order needs or are interchangeable for primary rewards. Rewards can also be more abstract, such as social or cultural approval. Second, rewards show variable quantitative properties, for example, with respect to magnitude, probability, and uncertainty (9). Furthermore, what is rewarding can vary depending on the current homeostatic state, for example, food is no longer rewarding in satiety. These parameters need to be integrated in order to obtain the value of a reward. Third, reward has different functions in the context of goal-directed behaviour (10). The classical notion of liking, wanting, and learning as reward functions is still relevant, but has been refined and extended, as we will outline later (see 'Functions of the Reward System').

Anatomical Structures of the Reward System

The brain reward system comprises anatomical structures which process reward-related information (Fig. 11.1). Reward information is widely represented in cortical and subcortical structures and there are no reward sensors nor primary sensory reward areas. However, early observations (e.g. by Olds and Milner (11)) showed that electrical self-stimulation was repeated by animals if electrodes were placed in certain areas, suggesting the existence of a definable reward system. Preclinical studies later identified a close overlap with the dopaminergic system, with nucleus accumbens and the ventral tegmental area as central structures.

The axons of midbrain dopaminergic neurons reach the striatum in a topographical organized pattern (12). Mesolimbic dopaminergic projections target the ventral striatum, which receives strong cortical inputs from anterior cingulate and orbitofrontal areas. The efferent output of the ventral striatum reaches the ventral pallidum and ventral tegmental area, which in turn innervate the thalamus from where cortical areas are innervated, closing the frontostriatothalamic circuit (12). Multiple parallel and partially overlapping loops have been proposed with the limbic loop being particularly important for reward-related processing and the associative and sensorimotor loop more related to cognitive and sensorimotor processing, respectively. Within this loop, a direct pathway originates from D_1-containing medium spiny neurons in the striatum and achieves positive feedback to the cortex, while the indirect pathway leads to negative feedback to the cortex via D_2 containing medium spiny neurons (13).

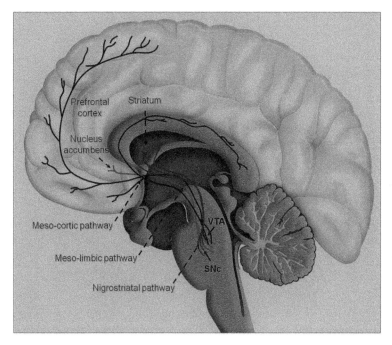

Fig. 11.1 Structures of the reward system. Dopaminergic neurons located in the ventral tegmental area (VTA) and the substantia nigra (SNc) project to the striatum (caudate nucleus, putamen, and ventral striatum including nucleus accumbens) and the prefrontal cortex (dorsal prefrontal and orbito-frontal cortex).

Reproduced from Arias-Carrión O, Stamelou M, Murillo-Rodriguez E, Menendez-Gonzalez M, Poppel E. Dopaminergic reward system: a short integrative review. Int Arch Med. 2010;3:24.

Other important structures include, for example, the amygdala, which projects to the ventral striatum and has been involved in Pavlovian (fear) learning, as well as structures regulating the activity of midbrain dopamine neurons such as pedunculopontine nucleus or lateral habenula (12).

Functions of the Reward System

Multiple processes use reward signals to guide behaviour. A classical organization is the distinction of liking, wanting, and learning, as key functions of the reward system (10). In this concept 'liking' designates the conscious pleasure associated with receipt of a reward. 'Wanting' corresponds to the desire to obtain a reward, also termed incentive salience. Finally, 'learning' uses reward information to optimize attainment of rewards in the future.

This approach is still of importance but has been developed and updated as new observations were integrated. The most important modifications emerge from the development of formal models for decision-making that subserve goal-directed behaviour

Table 11.1 Functions of the reward system following the RDoC framework

Construct	Subconstruct
Reward responsiveness	**Reward anticipation**
	Reward consumption
	Reward satiation
Reward learning	Habit
	Probabilistic and reinforcement learning
	Prediction error
Reward valuation	**Reward (magnitude, probability)**
	Delay
	Effort

Functions which have been proposed to be associated with apathy are shown in **bold** font.

(14), for example, concerning integration of reward magnitude and probability as well as effort and delay costs. In addition, concepts of reward-based learning have evolved with respect to model-free and model-based learning (15). There is currently no universally accepted structure of the different functions of the reward system. Here we use the organization in constructs and sub-constructs proposed in the most recent update of the National Institute of Mental Health (NIMH) Research Domain Criteria (RDoC) (Table 11.1) (16, 17).

Functions that Can Go Wrong

Reward Anticipation

Concept

Reward anticipation is an important function that guides behaviour. Originally, reward anticipation has been related to the 'wanting' or incentive salience function of reward that promotes approach to and consumption of rewards (10). This function can be distinguished from 'liking' and hedonic impact as well as the learning about rewards. These distinctions have been observed on the levels of subjective experience, behaviour, and neurophysiology.

In the recent update of the RDoC, reward anticipation has been defined more broadly as 'processes associated with the ability to anticipate and/or represent a future incentive—as reflected in language expression, behavioural responses, and/or engagement of the neural systems to cues about a future positive reinforcer' (16). This broader definition covers all the tasks commonly used to assess reward anticipation. However, with this broader definition there is obviously some overlap with other functions of the reward system. Reward anticipation is difficult to disentangle from the expected reward necessary to calculate a reward prediction error. In addition, it can be argued that reward anticipation in this broader sense requires some form of value representation, although reward values may be represented without being directly consciously accessible.

Measures

It has proven difficult to measure reward anticipation by *self-report* or by *clinician assessment*. Considerable effort has been put into the distinction of anticipatory from consummatory anhedonia (18). These two components can be assessed, for example, with the Temporal Experiences of Pleasure Scale (TEPS) (19). Anticipatory anhedonia refers to a lack of pleasure to anticipated pleasurable events or activities. The link between anticipatory anhedonia and reward anticipation seems straightforward and the terms have sometimes been used interchangeably in the literature. However, the empirical evidence of the association between anticipatory anhedonia assessed with a scale and behavioural and neural markers of reward anticipation has not been consistent. Thus, the assessment of reward anticipation on the level of self-rating and clinician assessment remains an important area of research.

On the level of *observable behaviour* in humans, the most commonly used parameter in humans is the acceleration of responses to a conditioned stimulus triggering reward anticipation in comparison to a conditioned stimulus not associated with reward anticipation. This effect has been termed reward-related speeding. In neuroimaging research, the monetary incentive delay (MID) task is frequently employed (see Fig. 11.2 for one example of this task) (20). In most versions of this task, participants show reward-related speeding, that is, faster reaction times after a reward-indicating cue than to a cue not indicating a potential reward (21). Other tasks such as cued reinforcement reaction time task have yielded similar results (22). It has to be acknowledged that in the animal literature the behavioural signatures of 'wanting' have been conceptualized differently.

The *neural correlates of reward anticipation* have been extensively studied with the MID task (20, 23, 24). Reward anticipation elicits a robust increase of the blood oxygen level-dependent signal in the ventral striatum, in particular the nucleus accumbens (Fig. 11.2). However, striatal activation has also been observed in the dorsal striatum, in particular the caudate nucleus and the putamen. In addition, numerous extrastriatal areas show increased activation during reward anticipation, for example, in the anterior cingulate gyrus, the superior frontal gyrus, the amygdala, the insula, and the thalamus. The recruitment of this broad range of regions in the MID task might reflect the fact that the task does not allow isolating reward anticipation. For example, the anticipation phase also requires the preparation of a motor response to the target. It has to be kept in mind that functional imaging using the MID task is only one of the possible approaches for identifying the neural correlates of reward anticipation, other tasks and other imaging modalities can be employed. The use of electrophysiological imaging techniques might allow the temporal dynamics of reward

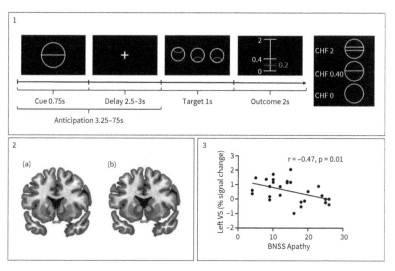

Fig. 11.2 Upper panel—trial structure of the monetary incentive delay task as employed by Kirschner et al. (34). A cue signals the maximum amount of reward that can be won during the trial. Following a delay, the participant has to respond to a target by pressing a button on the side of the deviant stimulus (in this case, left). During the outcome phase, the participant receives a feedback on the amount of money won (which is calculated based on the response time). Left lower panel—the ventral striatum (VS) region of interest is indicated in red. Panel (A) shows healthy participant's VS activation during reward anticipation in orange. Panel (B) shows the activation in patients with schizophrenia. Right lower panel—correlation plot with the Brief Negative Symptom Scale. Apathy on the x-axis and left VS signal change in the VS region of interest on the y-axis indicating a highly significant negative correlation of medium effect size.

Adapted with permission from Kirschner M, Hager OM, Bischof M, Hartmann MN, Kluge A, Seifritz E, et al. Ventral striatal hypoactivation is associated with apathy but not diminished expression in patients with schizophrenia. J Psychiatry Neurosci. 2016;41(3):152–61.

anticipation to be specified (25). However, functional imaging of the MID task is by far the most commonly employed approach in the study of apathy.

Association with Apathy

Some studies have suggested that self-reported anticipatory anhedonia might be specifically associated with clinician-rated apathy in patients with schizophrenia (26, 27). However, several recent studies have suggested that both anticipatory and consummatory anhedonia are correlated with apathy assessed by clinician and observer ratings (28, 29). In addition, anticipatory and consummatory anhedonia as assessed with the TEPS questionnaire do not seem to be specifically associated with their counterparts assessed with recently developed negative symptom scales (26, 30). This is not surprising as the latter are highly correlated. Overall, these findings suggest that it might be difficult to disentangle dysfunctional reward anticipation as a specific mechanism for apathy on the clinical level. However, this might depend on the underlying disorder as, for example, in Parkinson's disease anticipatory anhedonia has been suggested to be specifically associated with apathy (31).

In the MID task, reward-related speeding has been observed in patients with schizophrenia to be comparable to controls. Importantly, no study has so far reported a significant association of reward-related speeding with apathy or anticipatory anhedonia. It seems that these behavioural effects of reward anticipation are not sensitive to the effects of clinical psychopathology.

In patients with schizophrenia, functional neuroimaging studies have shown ventral striatal activation during reward anticipation to be consistently associated with broadly defined negative symptoms (32, 33). Increasing evidence shows that this association is essentially driven by apathy in contrast to diminished expression independent of the specific scale applied to measure psychopathology (Fig. 11.2) (34–36). Recent studies have also found dorsal caudate activity during reward anticipation to be specifically related to apathy (37, 38). Although an association of extrastriatal, in particular, prefrontal, regions with apathy has been suggested (39), results are less consistent.

Reduced striatal activation during reward anticipation is not a finding specific to schizophrenia, but has been observed, for example, in patients with depression and Parkinson's disease (40, 41). However, in these populations a link between reduced striatal activation and apathy (or anticipatory anhedonia) has not yet been clearly established.

Reward Consumption

Concept

The hedonic impact or 'liking' often associated with reward consumption is perhaps the most intuitive function of the reward system (10). Aside from the subjective experience of pleasure, 'liking' is associated with behavioural responses such as changes in facial expression. In the recent update of the RDoC, the broader concept of initial response to reward (or reward consumption) is defined as 'processes evoked by the initial presentation of a positive reinforcer as reflected by indices of neuronal activity and verbal or behavioural responses' (16).

Intuitively, one would expect people to engage less in behaviour if they do not experience pleasure resulting from its outcome. In other words, reduced 'liking' would result in apathy. However, this association has mostly not been empirically confirmed as we will outline later, supporting the differentiation between the hedonic and the motivational roles of the reward system.

Measures

The distinction of consummatory from anticipatory anhedonia has been discussed previously. In the present context, consummatory anhedonia as evaluated with the TEPS can be conceived of as the clinical symptom associated with impaired initial responses to rewards or the hedonic impact during reward consumption (27).

Hedonic impact of rewarding stimuli in the laboratory setting can be assessed by questionnaires and simple visual analogue scales that can be coupled with measures of arousal (42). In the animal literature, the sucrose preference test is the most commonly used measure for anhedonia. The development of a translational test in humans has proven to be difficult. The sweet taste has face validity but an association with consummatory anhedonia has so far not been established (43).

A large variety of functional neuroimaging paradigms have been used to investigate the hedonic impact of rewards and initial responsiveness to reward, but there is currently no established standard paradigm (44). It has to be noted that the MID task also allows the neural response to rewarding outcomes to be investigated in addition to reward anticipation (20). However, it is unclear whether the observed neural response reflects hedonic impact or another type of signal such as value updating or reward prediction error.

Association with Apathy

There is now solid experimental evidence showing that patients with schizophrenia are generally not impaired with respect to in-the-moment pleasure (45). This is consistent with the notion that anticipatory but not consummatory anhedonia is present, although this distinction has not been found in all studies. There is less evidence regarding a potential association of experimental measures of in-the-moment pleasure and apathy, but most studies did not find such an association in patients with schizophrenia.

It is important to note that impairment of the in-the-moment experience of pleasure has been observed across the schizophrenia spectrum in high-risk and first-episode populations as well as other psychiatric disorders such as major depression (46). However, a clear link between these impairments and clinical apathy has so far not been established.

On the neural level, some studies have showed reduced activation of the reward system during reward outcomes to be associated with apathy (36). However, these findings are not consistent (35). In this context, it is important to keep in mind that the MID task does not allow the initial neural response to reward consumption to be fully disentangled from other reward processes.

In summary, although an association of apathy with the initial response to reward may have face validity, the experimental evidence so far does not support a major role for this function of the reward system in the pathophysiology of apathy.

Reward Learning and Prediction Error

Concept

Reward learning describes the basic process of an individual adapting his/her behaviour based on rewarding (or punishing) feedback from the environment. As noted earlier, the NIMH RDoC matrix conceptualizes reward learning as part of the positive valence system and defines reward learning as a 'process by which organisms acquire information about stimuli, actions, and contexts that predict positive outcomes, and by which behaviour is modified when a novel reward occurs, or outcomes are better than expected' (16). Individuals learn from interacting with the environment and form associations between certain stimuli or actions and the availability of rewards. The process of acquiring new information about the reward value of stimuli or actions can be achieved by comparing the expected reward value with the actual experienced reward. The mismatch between expectation and experience can be quantified as a reward prediction error. A positive reward prediction error signals that the received reward is larger than expected and a negative reward prediction error signal indicates a less-than-expected reward. This process can be described by reinforcement learning (RL) algorithms, which offer a computational description of learning from interacting with the environment (47, 48). Reward learning encompasses appetitive Pavlovian learning where environmental stimuli or contexts are associated with reward delivery as well as instrumental learning processes where, according to Thorndike's law of effect, rewarded actions are more frequently performed than actions resulting in unpleasant feedback.

Measures

Experimental setups can be used to measure reward learning. In reward learning tasks, participants are presented with stimuli or several choice options, which are associated with rewarding outcomes with varying schedules. Measures of reward learning quantify the ability of a participant to acquire such new information by experience on the behavioural level and describe the underlying neural learning signals. There is a large variety of paradigms measuring reward learning. In Pavlovian conditioning experiments, such measures include implicit physiological responses towards appetitive conditioned stimulus (CS)+ stimulus compared to a control CS− stimulus, explicit ratings, or neural responses. In instrumental conditioning paradigms, choosing a more rewarding over a less rewarding option over time serves as a behavioural measure of the acquisition. The rewards utilized can range from primary rewards such as food or liquid to secondary rewards such as money. Both Pavlovian and instrumental tasks can differ in a variety of aspects, for example, deterministic versus probabilistic feedback, stable associations between stimuli/choice options with reward versus changing associations (volatile environments), gradual versus abrupt changes in those associations, as well as the number of choice options.

In probabilistic stimulus selection tasks, participants are presented with three pairs of stimuli each with different reward probabilities (e.g. 90/10, 80/20, and 60/40) and learn by trial and error to select the more rewarded option, which stays stable over time (49). In probabilistic reversal learning tasks (50), reward associations undergo sudden changes so that the previously more often rewarded choice option is now disadvantages and participants have to shift their responses. Reward learning tasks with probabilistic feedback, that is, being rewarded only 80% of choosing the better option, require participants integrating the experienced rewards over time in order to differentiate informative from noisy feedback. This function shows considerable overlap with other cognitive functions besides reward processing such as working memory. Reversals of reward contingencies require rapid adaptation of behaviour, which taps into multiple cognitive domains such as cognitive flexibility and inhibition of previously valid responses.

On the neural level, model-based functional magnetic resonance imaging (fMRI) during RL tasks measures underlying neural learning signatures such as prediction errors, which signal the difference between expected and received rewards and are used as teaching signals to update expected values at the time when the reward is received. Meta-analysis of human imaging model-based studies showed that reward prediction errors are coded in the bilateral ventral striatum, bilateral amygdala, midbrain, thalamus, frontal operculum, and insula with the amygdala being more active during Pavlovian learning and the dorsal striatal areas more during instrumental learning (51). Thus, human imaging studies confirm animal findings of reward prediction error coding in midbrain and dopaminergic target areas including the ventral and dorsal striatum.

Association with Apathy

On the behavioural level, patients with schizophrenia show deficits in instrumental reward learning tasks, that is, they chose the more rewarded stimulus less often, especially with probabilistic reward contingencies as well as with sudden reversals of reward contingencies (52), while simple deterministic discrimination learning seems to be unimpaired (53). In first-episode schizophrenia patients, deficits in flexible behavioural adaptation were stable over a 6-year follow-up period and independent of general IQ (54). Several studies suggested that patients with schizophrenia display selective impairments in learning from positive outcomes while learning from negative outcomes was unimpaired and that impaired learning from positive outcomes is specifically linked to apathy (55, 56), although not all studies have been fully consistent (57, 58). There is large variability in the performance of patients with schizophrenia, potentially suggesting neurocognitively distinct subgroups, related to more general cognitive capacities such as working memory (59).

On the neural level, during an appetitive Pavlovian conditioning, patients with schizophrenia showed attenuated blood oxygen level-dependent responses towards unexpected reward delivery, interpreted as reduced coding of positive prediction errors (60). During instrumental tasks, findings in patients with schizophrenia regarding reward prediction error coding in the ventral striatum have been mixed with reduced signal in unmedicated patients (61–63) and no overall group difference in medicated and more chronic patient groups (33, 64). Associations with negative symptoms have been described in some studies (64), but results are not conclusive (65). Due to the absence of a consistent association between apathy and neural reward prediction error coding, it was suggested that apathy may be more related to alterations in the generation and utilization of expected reward values as will be discussed in the next section.

A reduced representation of reward prediction error signals suggests alterations in basic reward learning mechanism potentially leading to reduced value representation of relevant and rewarding events and decreased motivational behaviour and experiences. This might be a transdiagnostic mechanism, as reduced striatal reward prediction error signalling in patients with major depression has also been shown to correlate with higher levels of anhedonia (65, 66).

Representation of Value

Concept
The ability to assign reward values to environmental stimuli or actions and to form a mental and neuronal representation of those values is central for predicting future outcomes and for using those predictions to generate appropriate behavioural responses. In order to decide between different choice options, subjective values for different types of rewards need to be mapped on a common scale. A dysfunction in the representation of reward values or in using those values has been suggested as a key mechanism of apathy in schizophrenia as well as other neuropsychiatric disorders (67, 68).

Measures
Reward value representation is a hypothetical (latent) construct, not directly observable, which has to be inferred from behaviour. Furthermore, it is challenging to isolate the representation of reward value from other processes of RL. In a reinforcement-learning framework, where reward prediction errors update expected value, reward learning and the representation of value are closely linked.

A suggested behavioural readout regards the choice preferences between previously conditioned stimuli in extinction. After participants have learned the reward values of different stimuli, they have to choose between novel combinations of those stimuli in a so-called transfer phase. During this transfer phase, participants do not receive feedback to prevent confounding the readout by new learning. This is implemented, for example, in the probabilistic stimulus selection task (56), where participants have to choose the more frequently rewarded stimulus from new combinations of previously learned stimuli. If during the acquisition phase, gain and loss-avoidance conditions are used, a transfer phase can probe choosing the 'frequent winner' versus 'frequent loss-avoider' stimuli, both of which have been learned by similar prediction error processing during acquisition but differ in their expected value (55). If participants fail to choose the frequent winner over the frequent loss-avoider, this indicates a deficit in representation (or utilization) of expected reward values.

Using computational models of choice behaviour offers the possibility to compute values for choice options and prediction errors on a trial-by-trial basis in order to disentangle both aspects of RL. Trial-by-trial values can then be used for model-based fMRI in order to identify their neuronal representation and probe group differences and associations with apathy. Imaging paradigms have to utilize appropriate timing in order to differentiate the trial phase where choice options are displayed and value representation can be studied from the feedback phase where reward is received and prediction errors are computed.

Animal studies have shown that various brain regions represent estimates of expected reward values (69). Human neuroimaging studies have shown that reward values are coded in frontostriatal circuits particularly in ventromedial prefrontal cortex (PFC) and orbitofrontal cortex (51, 70).

Association with Apathy

On the behavioural level, measures of value representation probed by choices between previously learned stimuli in transfer phases revealed that patients with schizophrenia showed a selective deficit in selecting the frequent winner but were unimpaired in avoiding the least frequently rewarded stimulus (56), suggesting a failure to generalize reward value information. In an influential behavioural study, Gold and colleagues found that schizophrenia patients with high negative symptoms showed impaired learning from rewards but were unimpaired in loss-avoidance learning, and in the transfer phase showed no preference for the gain relative to the loss-avoider stimulus (55). These findings were interpreted as a deficit in representation (or utilization) of expected reward values, particularly in patients with high apathy, which was further underlined by application of computational modelling (see 'The Role of Computational Modelling'), although the results are in need of replication.

On the neural level, associations between expected reward values and psychopathology are not consistent. Patients with schizophrenia showed reduced reward-value coding compared to controls and patients with major depression in the amygdala–hippocampal complex and parahippocampal gyrus, but this was associated with positive psychotic rather than negative symptom severity (65). Waltz and colleagues found a negative association between apathy scores and neural activity related to expected value-related activity in ventral striatum and ventromedial PFC (71). In contrast, Dowd and colleagues found dorsolateral PFC and caudate activity to be negatively related to anhedonia/avolition (57). Thus, two different pathways may contribute to the apathy domain: one 'reward' circuit including ventral striatum and ventromedial PFC and one 'cognitive' circuit including caudate nucleus and dorsolateral PFC.

Integration of Effort Costs

Concept

Decision-making requires the integration of the reward value of an option with associated costs (14). These costs come in different forms and include, for example, a temporal delay until the reward is obtained, the effort required to obtain the reward, and the associated risk. The integration of rewards and costs results in a value of an option for action. The individual will only engage in an action when its value is positive. If there are several options available, the person will choose the option with the highest value.

The main focus with respect to apathy lies on the integration of effort costs in decision-making (4). If effort costs are overweighed in the decision-making process relative to the potential rewards, the value of the respective option will decrease. Thus, the individual will be less likely to engage in goal-directed behaviour which can manifest itself as apathy.

Theoretically, several problems can impact effort-based decision-making and will lead to a reduced willingness to work for a reward. First, there can be an underestimation of the reward value associated with an option (see 'Representation of Value'). Second, the required effort associated with an option can be overestimated. Finally, the integration of reward value and effort cost can be impaired, even if the latter is correctly estimated. In experimental tasks, it is often difficult to clearly disentangle these potential mechanisms.

Measures

Currently, a large array of tasks is available for assessing effort-based decision-making in humans on the behavioural level. These tasks can be organized along different dimensions—the type of effort to be invested and the task structure. Both physical and cognitive effort can be required for certain options for action. Within these domains there is considerably heterogeneity in the operationalization of effort, for example, button presses versus handgrip for physical effort.

There are different types of task structures for effort-based decision-making. In the non-human literature, *progressive ratio tasks* are most frequently used. In these tasks, the number of actions (for example, lever presses) required to obtain a reward increases throughout the task. At some point, the agent will stop responding as the effort increases and this point is referred to as the break point, which is considered as a measure of willingness to work for a reward. In the human literature, progressive ratio tasks have been less frequently employed, but there are examples of cognitive and physical progressive ratio tasks.

A second group of tasks require a *binary decision* between a low-effort/low-reward and high-effort/high-reward option. The analysis of these tasks focuses on the proportion of high-effort choices. Some tasks allow the modulation of subjective choices to be estimated as a function of the effort required. One example is the physical effort task by Hartmann and colleagues (Fig. 11.3), which requires exercising different levels of effort operationalized as a percentage of the individually calibrated maximum handgrip strength (72). Cognitive binary choice tasks are also available.

A final group of tasks allow investing effort along a continuous range and thus pose less constraints which might correspond better to real-world situations. At the same time, quantification of decision parameters is more complicated in this type of task.

Some of the above-mentioned tasks have been adapted for fMRI. Overall, it has been suggested that the dorsal anterior cingulate cortex is associated with cost–benefit

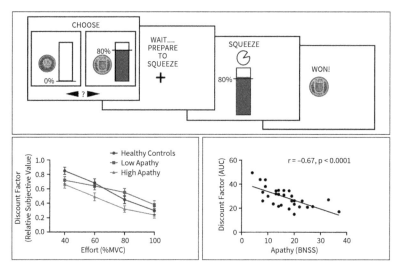

Fig. 11.3 Upper panel—trial structure of the physical effort-based decision-making task employed by Hartmann et al. (72). In each trial, the participant has to choose between a low-effort/low-reward option and a high-effort/high-reward option. In the latter, the effort varies between 40% and 100% of the participant's maximum strength and the reward between 1.5 and 5 Swiss Francs. This allows a discount factor for each individual to be calculated, reflecting the willingness to work for a reward. Left lower panel—the discount factor for healthy controls and patients with schizophrenia showing low or high apathy is plotted for each effort level. The figure shows that only the high-apathy patient consistently shows a lower discount factor than healthy controls. The discount factor across all effort levels can be calculated as the area under the curve in this figure. Right lower panel—the discount factor across all effort levels is strongly correlated with apathy as assessed with the Brief Negative Symptom Scale. In other words, the more apathetic a patient, the less willing they are to work for a reward.

Adapted with permission from Hartmann MN, Hager OM, Reimann AV, Chumbley JR, Kirschner M, Seifritz E, et al. Apathy but not diminished expression in schizophrenia is associated with discounting of monetary rewards by physical effort. Schizophr Bull. 2015;41(2):503–12.

integration and the calculation of a net option value, while physical effort has been shown to be represented in the anterior insula (4).

Association with Apathy

Several studies using binary choice physical effort tasks have shown that in patients with schizophrenia, negative symptoms are associated with fewer high-effort choices in order to obtain higher rewards (72–74). Hartmann and colleagues found a specific association of apathy with the discount factor, that is, the subjective value of options when handgrip effort has to be invested. In other words, more apathetic patients were less willing to work for a reward. However, not all studies found an association with negative symptoms of apathy (see (75) for a critical review). Only few studies in patients with schizophrenia have used progressive ratio tasks requiring a physical effort and only one study reported an association with apathy (76). The study of cognitive effort in patients with schizophrenia is complicated by the often coexisting cognitive impairment. Nevertheless, there are now several studies controlling for cognitive impairment that show that a reduction of high-effort choices is associated with negative symptoms and/or apathy (77, 78).

In these studies, it has so far proven difficult to unequivocally link the mechanism underlying dysfunctional choice patterns to negative symptoms and apathy. There is some evidence that impaired reward valuation and impaired cost–benefit integration are contributing factors, while the patients' estimation of the required effort seems to be less impaired (72). In addition, in more complex effort-based decision-making tasks, cognitive impairment has been shown to be a major determinant of performance (79). Functional neuroimaging could in principle contribute to disentangling the underlying processes, but very few studies have directly addressed the neural correlates of effort-based decision-making in schizophrenia and did not show brain regions consistently associated with apathy. However, in an important study, Wolf and colleagues have shown that hypoactivation of the ventral striatum during a monetary guessing task is associated with both apathy and reduced willingness to work for a reward on a progressive ratio task (80). This suggests that dysfunctional anticipation of a future reward as coded in the ventral striatum might be one key mechanism.

The role of dopamine neurotransmission in effort-based decision-making has received considerable interest. Rodent studies have consistently shown that the willingness to work is reduced by dopamine antagonism or depletion and is increased by agonistic dopaminergic drugs (5). In patients with schizophrenia, one would therefore expect a strong impact of the antipsychotic medication, but until now the association of effort-based decision-making with apathy has not consistently been shown to be linked to antipsychotic treatment. It has been suggested that a stronger focus should be on D_2 receptor affinity of antipsychotic drugs instead of classical equivalent doses, but other confounding factors are also important (81). In this context, the findings on effort-based decision-making in Parkinson's disease are of high interest. In these patients, higher dopamine levels have been shown to be associated with more high-reward/high-effort choices on physical and cognitive effort tasks (82, 83). However, it has not yet been fully established whether the effects of dopamine on clinical apathy are mediated by changes in effort-based decision-making.

Conclusion

The Role of Computational Modelling

Reward learning deficits may result from dysfunctions in reward anticipation, effort, or value representation. As we have discussed in the preceding sections, these different aspects may be difficult to disentangle on the behavioural level. Computational models of behavioural in combination with model-based imaging may help to dissect these different aspects.

Computational modelling can describe learning processes in a generative way on a trial-by-trial basis. The use of so-called generative models allows quantifying the mechanisms that have generated behavioural or neuronal data with a certain probability. By fitting different classes of models to the data in combination with model comparison, different learning strategies can be identified and parameters quantifying relevant inter-individual differences can be estimated. Standard RL models describe how individuals interact with the environment by assigning values to environmental stimuli and by using prediction errors as teaching signals to update the expected value (48). The prediction error δ on trial t is the difference between the received outcome R_t and the expected value $Q_{a,t}$ of the chosen action a according to the formula: $\delta_{Qa,t} = R_t - Q_{a,t}$. The prediction error is then used to update the expected value $Q_{a,t}$, where the learning rate α scales the influence of the prediction error: $Q_{a,t+1} = Q_{a,t} + \alpha\delta_{Qa,t}$. Choice probabilities are then generated using a softmax function where the likelihood of a subject choosing action a on trial t denoted as $p(a,t)$ is proportional to a value $Q_t(a)$ and which includes the so-called inverse temperature beta which gives an individual estimate of the balance between exploration and exploitation. A classical RL framework in which the influence of prediction errors on value updates is weighted by a learning rate can be extended by hierarchical Bayesian approaches where higher-level beliefs scale the influence of lower-level prediction errors.

A prominent example of applying computational modelling to understand apathy in patients with schizophrenia was the study by Gold et al. (55). They compared a Q-learning algorithm, where specific outcome values are learned for each stimulus, with a so-called actor-critic algorithm, which neglects the specific expected value of outcomes, so that the former but not the latter model can produce the observed pattern of 'choosing the frequent loss avoiders compared to infrequent winners' in the above-mentioned transfer phase. Controls and low-negative symptom patients showed a mixture of both learning mechanisms, but the influence of Q-learning was significantly reduced in patients with high negative symptoms compared to low negative symptom patients, suggesting that a different and more rigid learning strategy was applied by patients with apathy. This example shows the potential of computational modelling for developing a fine-grained approach to the association of specific reward system dysfunctions with apathy.

Reward System Dysfunction as a Transdiagnostic Mechanism of Apathy?

In this chapter, we have mainly provided examples from the schizophrenia literature that show an association between apathy and specific impairments in reward system functioning, in particular, reward anticipation, value representation, and integration of effort costs. However, the RDoC clearly aim to provide a transdiagnostic framework and we have pointed to some results that suggest that the association of reward system dysfunction with apathy cuts across disease categories. Nevertheless, it is surprising that there are very few truly transdiagnostic studies that have applied the same clinical and experimental measure to different populations. We advocate that future studies should use a fine-grained computational approach to the different functions of the reward system in order to explore shared mechanisms of apathy across disorders and distinct mechanisms within disorders.

References

1. Levy R, Dubois B. Apathy and the functional anatomy of the prefrontal cortex-basal ganglia circuits. Cereb Cortex. 2006;16(7):916–28.
2. Marin RS, Biedrzycki RC, Firinciogullari S. Reliability and validity of the Apathy Evaluation Scale. Psychiatry Res. 1991;38(2):143–62.
3. Wise RA. Dopamine and reward: the anhedonia hypothesis 30 years on. Neurotox Res. 2008;14(2–3):169–83.
4. Pessiglione M, Vinckier F, Bouret S, Daunizeau J, Le Bouc R. Why not try harder? Computational approach to motivation deficits in neuro-psychiatric diseases. Brain. 2018;141(3):629–50.
5. Salamone JD, Yohn SE, Lopez-Cruz L, San Miguel N, Correa M. Activational and effort-related aspects of motivation: neural mechanisms and implications for psychopathology. Brain. 2016;139(Pt 5):1325–47.
6. Schultz W. Multiple reward signals in the brain. Nat Rev Neurosci. 2000;1(3):199–207.
7. Kirkpatrick B. Developing concepts in negative symptoms: primary vs secondary and apathy vs expression. J Clin Psychiatry. 2014;75(Suppl 1):3–7.
8. Sescousse G, Caldu X, Segura B, Dreher JC. Processing of primary and secondary rewards: a quantitative meta-analysis and review of human functional neuroimaging studies. Neurosci Biobehav Rev. 2013;37(4):681–96.
9. Burke CJ, Tobler PN. Coding of reward probability and risk by single neurons in animals. Front Neurosci. 2011;5:121.
10. Berridge KC, Robinson TE. Parsing reward. Trends Neurosci. 2003;26(9):507–13.
11. Olds J, Milner P. Positive reinforcement produced by electrical stimulation of septal area and other regions of rat brain. J Comp Physiol Psychol. 1954;47(6):419–27.
12. Haber SN, Knutson B. The reward circuit: linking primate anatomy and human imaging. Neuropsychopharmacology. 2010;35(1):4–26.
13. Maia TV, Frank MJ. An integrative perspective on the role of dopamine in schizophrenia. Biol Psychiatry. 2017;81(1):52–66.
14. Bailey MR, Simpson EH, Balsam PD. Neural substrates underlying effort, time, and risk-based decision making in motivated behavior. Neurobiol Learn Mem. 2016;133:233–56.
15. O'Doherty JP, Cockburn J, Pauli WM. Learning, reward, and decision making. Annu Rev Psychol. 2017;68:73–100.
16. National Institute of Mental Health. RDoC Changes to the Matrix (CMAT) Workgroup Update: Proposed Positive Valence Domain Revisions. 2018. Available at: https://www.nimh.nih.gov/about/advisory-boards-and-groups/namhc/reports/cmat-pvs-report-508_157003.pdf.
17. Thant T, Yager J. Updating apathy: using Research Domain Criteria to inform clinical assessment and diagnosis of disorders of motivation. J Nerv Ment Dis. 2019;207(9):707–14.
18. Treadway MT, Zald DH. Reconsidering anhedonia in depression: lessons from translational neuroscience. Neurosci Biobehav Rev. 2011;35(3):537–55.

19. Gard DE, Gard MG, Kring AM, John OP. Anticipatory and consummatory components of the experience of pleasure: a scale development study. J Res Personal. 2006;40:1086–102.

20. Knutson B, Fong GW, Adams CM, Varner JL, Hommer D. Dissociation of reward anticipation and outcome with event-related fMRI. Neuroreport. 2001;12(17):3683–7.

21. Simon JJ, Walther S, Fiebach CJ, Friederich HC, Stippich C, Weisbrod M, et al. Neural reward processing is modulated by approach- and avoidance-related personality traits. Neuroimage. 2010;49(2):1868–74.

22. Cools R, Blackwell A, Clark L, Menzies L, Cox S, Robbins TW. Tryptophan depletion disrupts the motivational guidance of goal-directed behavior as a function of trait impulsivity. Neuropsychopharmacology. 2005;30(7):1362–73.

23. Oldham S, Murawski C, Fornito A, Youssef G, Yucel M, Lorenzetti V. The anticipation and outcome phases of reward and loss processing: a neuroimaging meta-analysis of the monetary incentive delay task. Hum Brain Mapp. 2018;39(8):3398–418.

24. Wilson RP, Colizzi M, Bossong MG, Allen P, Kempton M, Mtac, et al. The neural substrate of reward anticipation in health: a meta-analysis of fMRI findings in the monetary incentive delay task. Neuropsychol Rev. 2018;28(4):496–506.

25. Zhang Y, Li Q, Wang Z, Liu X, Zheng Y. Temporal dynamics of reward anticipation in the human brain. Biol Psychol. 2017;128:89–97.

26. Forbes C, Blanchard JJ, Bennett M, Horan WP, Kring A, Gur R. Initial development and preliminary validation of a new negative symptom measure: the Clinical Assessment Interview for Negative Symptoms (CAINS). Schizophr Res. 2010;124(1–3):36–42.

27. Gard DE, Kring AM, Gard MG, Horan WP, Green MF. Anhedonia in schizophrenia: distinctions between anticipatory and consummatory pleasure. Schizophr Res. 2007;93(1–3):253–60.

28. Da Silva S, Saperia S, Siddiqui I, Fervaha G, Agid O, Daskalakis ZJ, et al. Investigating consummatory and anticipatory pleasure across motivation deficits in schizophrenia and healthy controls. Psychiatry Res. 2017;254:112–7.

29. Simon JJ, Zimmermann J, Cordeiro SA, Maree I, Gard DE, Friederich HC, et al. Psychometric evaluation of the Temporal Experience of Pleasure Scale (TEPS) in a German sample. Psychiatry Res. 2018;260:138–43.

30. Bischof M, Obermann C, Hartmann MN, Hager OM, Kirschner M, Kluge A, et al. The brief negative symptom scale: validation of the German translation and convergent validity with self-rated anhedonia and observer-rated apathy. BMC Psychiatry. 2016;16(1):415.

31. Jordan LL, Zahodne LB, Okun MS, Bowers D. Hedonic and behavioral deficits associated with apathy in Parkinson's disease: potential treatment implications. Mov Disord. 2013;28(9):1301–4.

32. Juckel G, Schlagenhauf F, Koslowski M, Wustenberg T, Villringer A, Knutson B, et al. Dysfunction of ventral striatal reward prediction in schizophrenia. Neuroimage. 2006;29(2):409–16.

33. Radua J, Schmidt A, Borgwardt S, Heinz A, Schlagenhauf F, McGuire P, et al. Ventral striatal activation during reward processing in psychosis: a neurofunctional meta-analysis. JAMA Psychiatry. 2015;72(12):1243–51.

34. Kirschner M, Hager OM, Bischof M, Hartmann MN, Kluge A, Seifritz E, et al. Ventral striatal hypoactivation is associated with apathy but not diminished expression in patients with schizophrenia. J Psychiatry Neurosci. 2016;41(3):152–61.

35. Simon JJ, Biller A, Walther S, Roesch-Ely D, Stippich C, Weisbrod M, et al. Neural correlates of reward processing in schizophrenia—relationship to apathy and depression. Schizophr Res. 2010;118(1–3):154–61.

36. Waltz JA, Schweitzer JB, Ross TJ, Kurup PK, Salmeron BJ, Rose EJ, et al. Abnormal responses to monetary outcomes in cortex, but not in the basal ganglia, in schizophrenia. Neuropsychopharmacology. 2010;35(12):2427–39.
37. Mucci A, Dima D, Soricelli A, Volpe U, Bucci P, Frangou S, et al. Is avolition in schizophrenia associated with a deficit of dorsal caudate activity? A functional magnetic resonance imaging study during reward anticipation and feedback. Psychol Med. 2015;45(8):1765–78.
38. Stepien M, Manoliu A, Kubli R, Schneider K, Tobler PN, Seifritz E, et al. Investigating the association of ventral and dorsal striatal dysfunction during reward anticipation with negative symptoms in patients with schizophrenia and healthy individuals. PLoS One. 2018;13(6):e0198215.
39. Dowd EC, Barch DM. Pavlovian reward prediction and receipt in schizophrenia: relationship to anhedonia. PLoS One. 2012;7(5):e35622.
40. Keren H, O'Callaghan G, Vidal-Ribas P, Buzzell GA, Brotman MA, Leibenluft E, et al. Reward processing in depression: a conceptual and meta-analytic review across fMRI and EEG studies. Am J Psychiatry. 2018;175(11):1111–20.
41. du Plessis S, Bossert M, Vink M, van den Heuvel L, Bardien S, Emsley R, et al. Reward processing dysfunction in ventral striatum and orbitofrontal cortex in Parkinson's disease. Parkinsonism Relat Disord. 2018;48:82–8.
42. Kring AM, Elis O. Emotion deficits in people with schizophrenia. Annu Rev Clin Psychol. 2013;9:409–33.
43. Dichter GS, Smoski MJ, Kampov-Polevoy AB, Gallop R, Garbutt JC. Unipolar depression does not moderate responses to the Sweet Taste Test. Depress Anxiety. 2010;27(9):859–63.
44. Berridge KC, Kringelbach ML. Pleasure systems in the brain. Neuron. 2015;86(3):646–64.
45. Kring AM, Barch DM. The motivation and pleasure dimension of negative symptoms: neural substrates and behavioral outputs. Eur Neuropsychopharmacol. 2014;24(5):725–36.
46. Strauss GP, Cohen AS. A transdiagnostic review of negative symptom phenomenology and etiology. Schizophr Bull. 2017;43(4):712–9.
47. Dayan P, Daw ND. Decision theory, reinforcement learning, and the brain. Cogn Affect Behav Neurosci. 2008;8(4):429–53.
48. Sutton RS, Barto AG. Reinforcement Learning: An Introduction (2nd ed). Cambridge, MA: MIT Press; 2018.
49. Frank MJ, Seeberger LC, O'Reilly RC. By carrot or by stick: cognitive reinforcement learning in parkinsonism. Science. 2004;306(5703):1940–3.
50. Cools R, Clark L, Owen AM, Robbins TW. Defining the neural mechanisms of probabilistic reversal learning using event-related functional magnetic resonance imaging. J Neurosci. 2002;22(11):4563–7.
51. Chase HW, Kumar P, Eickhoff SB, Dombrovski AY. Reinforcement learning models and their neural correlates: an activation likelihood estimation meta-analysis. Cogn Affect Behav Neurosci. 2015;15(2):435–59.
52. Waltz JA. The neural underpinnings of cognitive flexibility and their disruption in psychotic illness. Neuroscience. 2017;345:203–17.
53. Barch DM, Pagliaccio D, Luking K. Mechanisms underlying motivational deficits in psychopathology: similarities and differences in depression and schizophrenia. Curr Top Behav Neurosci. 2016;27:411–49.
54. Leeson VC, Robbins TW, Matheson E, Hutton SB, Ron MA, Barnes TR, et al. Discrimination learning, reversal, and set-shifting in first-episode schizophrenia: stability over six years and specific associations with medication type and disorganization syndrome. Biol Psychiatry. 2009;66(6):586–93.

55. Gold JM, Waltz JA, Matveeva TM, Kasanova Z, Strauss GP, Herbener ES, et al. Negative symptoms and the failure to represent the expected reward value of actions: behavioral and computational modeling evidence. Arch Gen Psychiatry. 2012;69(2):129–38.

56. Waltz JA, Frank MJ, Robinson BM, Gold JM. Selective reinforcement learning deficits in schizophrenia support predictions from computational models of striatal-cortical dysfunction. Biol Psychiatry. 2007;62(7):756–64.

57. Dowd EC, Frank MJ, Collins A, Gold JM, Barch DM. Probabilistic reinforcement learning in patients with schizophrenia: relationships to anhedonia and avolition. Biol Psychiatry Cogn Neurosci Neuroimaging. 2016;1(5):460–73.

58. Hartmann-Riemer MN, Aschenbrenner S, Bossert M, Westermann C, Seifritz E, Tobler PN, et al. Deficits in reinforcement learning but no link to apathy in patients with schizophrenia. Sci Rep. 2017;7:40352.

59. Collins AG, Frank MJ. How much of reinforcement learning is working memory, not reinforcement learning? A behavioral, computational, and neurogenetic analysis. Eur J Neurosci. 2012;35(7):1024–35.

60. Waltz JA, Schweitzer JB, Gold JM, Kurup PK, Ross TJ, Salmeron BJ, et al. Patients with schizophrenia have a reduced neural response to both unpredictable and predictable primary reinforcers. Neuropsychopharmacology. 2009;34(6):1567–77.

61. Schlagenhauf F, Huys QJ, Deserno L, Rapp MA, Beck A, Heinze HJ, et al. Striatal dysfunction during reversal learning in unmedicated schizophrenia patients. Neuroimage. 2014;89:171–80.

62. Reinen JM, Van Snellenberg JX, Horga G, Abi-Dargham A, Daw ND, Shohamy D. Motivational context modulates prediction error response in schizophrenia. Schizophr Bull. 2016;42(6):1467–75.

63. Murray GK, Corlett PR, Clark L, Pessiglione M, Blackwell AD, Honey G, et al. Substantia nigra/ventral tegmental reward prediction error disruption in psychosis. Mol Psychiatry. 2008;13(3):239, 267–76.

64. Culbreth AJ, Westbrook A, Xu Z, Barch DM, Waltz JA. Intact ventral striatal prediction error signaling in medicated schizophrenia patients. Biol Psychiatry Cogn Neurosci Neuroimaging. 2016;1(5):474–83.

65. Gradin VB, Kumar P, Waiter G, Ahearn T, Stickle C, Milders M, et al. Expected value and prediction error abnormalities in depression and schizophrenia. Brain. 2011;134(Pt 6):1751–64.

66. Rothkirch M, Tonn J, Kohler S, Sterzer P. Neural mechanisms of reinforcement learning in unmedicated patients with major depressive disorder. Brain. 2017;140(4):1147–57.

67. Gold JM, Waltz JA, Prentice KJ, Morris SE, Heerey EA. Reward processing in schizophrenia: a deficit in the representation of value. Schizophr Bull. 2008;34(5):835–47.

68. Barch DM, Dowd EC. Goal representations and motivational drive in schizophrenia: the role of prefrontal-striatal interactions. Schizophr Bull. 2010;36(5):919–34.

69. Lee D, Seo H, Jung MW. Neural basis of reinforcement learning and decision making. Annu Rev Neurosci. 2012;35:287–308.

70. Levy DJ, Glimcher PW. The root of all value: a neural common currency for choice. Curr Opin Neurobiol. 2012;22(6):1027–38.

71. Waltz JA, Xu Z, Brown EC, Ruiz RR, Frank MJ, Gold JM. Motivational deficits in schizophrenia are associated with reduced differentiation between gain and loss-avoidance feedback in the striatum. Biol Psychiatry Cogn Neurosci Neuroimaging. 2018;3(3):239–47.

72. Hartmann MN, Hager OM, Reimann AV, Chumbley JR, Kirschner M, Seifritz E, et al. Apathy but not diminished expression in schizophrenia is associated with discounting of monetary rewards by physical effort. Schizophr Bull. 2015;41(2):503–12.

73. Fervaha G, Graff-Guerrero A, Zakzanis KK, Foussias G, Agid O, Remington G. Incentive motivation deficits in schizophrenia reflect effort computation impairments during cost-benefit decision-making. J Psychiatr Res. 2013;47(11):1590–6.

74. Gold JM, Strauss GP, Waltz JA, Robinson BM, Brown JK, Frank MJ. Negative symptoms of schizophrenia are associated with abnormal effort-cost computations. Biol Psychiatry. 2013;74(2):130–6.

75. Hartmann-Riemer MN, Kirschner M, Kaiser S. Effort-based decision-making paradigms as objective measures of apathy in schizophrenia? Curr Opin Behav Sci. 2018;22:70–5.

76. Strauss GP, Whearty KM, Morra LF, Sullivan SK, Ossenfort KL, Frost KH. Avolition in schizophrenia is associated with reduced willingness to expend effort for reward on a progressive ratio task. Schizophr Res. 2016;170(1):198–204.

77. Culbreth A, Westbrook A, Barch D. Negative symptoms are associated with an increased subjective cost of cognitive effort. J Abnorm Psychol. 2016;125(4):528–36.

78. Chang WC, Westbrook A, Strauss GP, Chu AOK, Chong CSY, Siu CMW, et al. Abnormal cognitive effort allocation and its association with amotivation in first-episode psychosis. Psychol Med. 2020;50(15):2599–609.

79. Cooper JA, Barch DM, Reddy LF, Horan WP, Green MF, Treadway MT. Effortful goal-directed behavior in schizophrenia: computational subtypes and associations with cognition. J Abnorm Psychol. 2019;128(7):710–22.

80. Wolf DH, Satterthwaite TD, Kantrowitz JJ, Katchmar N, Vandekar L, Elliott MA, et al. Amotivation in schizophrenia: integrated assessment with behavioral, clinical, and imaging measures. Schizophr Bull. 2014;40(6):1328–37.

81. Gold JM, Waltz JA, Frank MJ. Effort cost computation in schizophrenia: a commentary on the recent literature. Biol Psychiatry. 2015;78(11):747–53.

82. Le Heron C, Plant O, Manohar S, Ang YS, Jackson M, Lennox G, et al. Distinct effects of apathy and dopamine on effort-based decision-making in Parkinson's disease. Brain. 2018;141(5):1455–69.

83. McGuigan S, Zhou SH, Brosnan MB, Thyagarajan D, Bellgrove MA, Chong TT. Dopamine restores cognitive motivation in Parkinson's disease. Brain. 2019;142(3):719–32.

12

Neural Basis of Apathy

Functional Imaging Studies

André Aleman

Introduction

Apathy is a behavioural condition that arises from dysfunction of brain systems necessary for goal-directed behaviour. These can be described in structural terms, that is, changes in structure of brain regions, such as reductions in grey matter density (as reviewed in Chapter 10). In addition, alterations to neural systems can also be described in functional terms, for example, less activation of certain brain regions, or a change in connectivity patterns. This chapter will address such changes by reviewing recent functional neuroimaging studies (see Box 12.1 for a brief explanation of functional magnetic resonance imaging (fMRI) (1–4)).

The literature regarding neuroimaging correlates of apathy has been reviewed by Kos et al. (5), who identified 99 studies reporting on the association between a neuroimaging measure and an apathy scale in different disorders, varying from neurodegenerative diseases to acquired brain injury and psychiatric disorders. The neuroimaging techniques used encompassed both structural and functional neuroimaging. The review of all these studies suggested abnormalities within frontostriatal circuits to be most consistently associated with apathy across the different pathological conditions. Besides consistency across disorders and techniques, there also was considerable variance in brain regions implicated in apathy. This could suggest that different routes towards apathy are possible or that the concept of apathy may need to be 'deconstructed' into several different aspects with a unique neuroanatomical signature.

Apathy concerns a reduction of goal-directed behaviour and it may be instructive to examine the different processing features that underlie goal-directed behaviour. It has been argued that goal-directed behaviour requires several different processes, involving reward and effort processing, executive functioning (e.g. selecting and setting a goal), and self-initiation of behaviour, among others. Levy and Dubois (6) have noted that disruptions in any of these processes may lead to reductions in goal-directed behaviour and thus apathy. Other authors have echoed this in a similar way, such as Tumati et al. (7). Fig. 12.1 depicts a schematic model derived from their

Box 12.1   Functional magnetic resonance imaging

Functional magnetic resonance imaging (fMRI) allows for the assessment of brain activation, including the involvement of certain regions or the contribution of certain brain networks associated with specific conditions or states. Indeed, fMRI enables the measurement of neural correlates underlying relevant cognitive and emotional processes. The technique of fMRI is based on the (confirmed) assumption that neuronal activity induces an increase in oxygenated blood flow to the active region. This is referred to as the haemodynamic response. The resulting change in relative levels of oxyhaemoglobin and deoxyhaemoglobin (oxygenated or deoxygenated blood) can be detected due to their differential magnetic susceptibility. This effect is referred to as the blood oxygen level-dependent (BOLD) contrast. It is important to note that the BOLD contrast, as measured using fMRI, is not a direct measure of neuronal activity, but is nonetheless a good proxy of neural activation (1). For a recent introduction into human neuroimaging methods, see Op de Beeck and Nakatani (2).

Two main applications of fMRI paradigms can be distinguished: task-evoked fMRI and resting-state fMRI paradigms. During task-evoked fMRI paradigms, participants are asked to perform a task and task-related changes in BOLD signal are assessed to investigate which areas of the brain are active, or which interactions between regions are involved, during a specific mental operation (e.g. working memory). In resting-state paradigms, no particular task is performed and participants are asked to lie still and stay awake.

Using resting-state paradigms has several advantages (3). First, it circumvents the problem that differences in task performance between groups may influence fMRI results, a problem that is often encountered in task-based fMRI studies. Second, it reflects intrinsic connectivity patterns. That is, during wakeful rest, the brain shows intrinsic (or task-unrelated) ongoing neural and metabolic activity, reflected by spontaneous low-frequency fluctuations of the BOLD signal. In resting-state studies, these spontaneous fluctuations are examined. Interestingly, these fluctuations have been shown to correlate between spatially remote but functionally similar brain areas. Third, as there are no task demands (that can be too challenging for certain patient groups), resting-state measurements can easily be performed in a reliable way across different patient groups.

Several distinct resting-state networks have been identified including the somatomotor network, primary visual and auditory networks, default mode network, executive cognitive control network, dorsal and ventral attention networks, and salience network. Of note, resting-state networks been shown to reflect the underlying structural connections between brain areas, and have been shown to correspondent closely with BOLD dynamics during tasks and to correlate with cognitive performance (cf. Sporns (4) for an overview), which underscores their utility in studying the neural underpinnings of psychopathology.

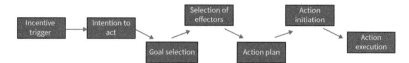

Fig. 12.1 Breakdown of possible component processes underlying goal-directed behaviour. An incentive trigger (e.g. anticipating praise or obtaining a monetary reward) gives rise to an intention to act, which translates into a final execution of an action pattern through goal selection, selection of action effectors, substantiation of an action plan, and the initiation of the action. For a more extensive model, see Tumati et al. (7). See text for description of neural systems involved.

proposal of relevant component processes. We will discuss these in turn and the neuroimaging evidence that bears upon each functional process.

As a general framework, reward value assignment is thought to be processed by the subgenual anterior cingulate cortex (ACC). Dopamine-innervated areas such as the ventral tegmental area (VTA)/substantia nigra and ventral striatum may play a driving role in addition to the orbitofrontal cortex. Based on the reward value and its self-relevance, which is processed in the posterior cingulate cortex, an intention to act is generated (volition) through the dynamic interaction of the dorsolateral prefrontal cortex (DLPFC) and the inferior parietal lobule. The intent to act triggers preparation for movement, where caudate and premotor cortex play a role. Selection of goals to be achieved in the external world and assessment of different paths to goal attainment are processed by the DLPFC and dorsal ACC. In parallel, an internally directed process contributes to the selection of the appropriate external goal based on the body schema and achievable motor plans, with the caudate (8) and cerebellum (9) playing a role. Once a movement is selected, coordination is processed from the broader lateral parietal cortex, which regulates fine control of the selected movement and necessary adjustments during its execution. Tumati et al. (7) have pointed to a further role of the parietal cortex in evaluating actual outcome with expected outcome based on visual input and changes in body schema. Whenever the two outcomes match, the likelihood that the outcome was produced due to actions of oneself is greater (sense of agency). The dorsal anterior cingulate assesses the outcome with respect to the original goal.

We will now review these component processes underlying goal-directed behaviour in more detail, taking into account neuroimaging evidence with respect to apathy.

It has been noted that goal-directed behaviour requires association of positive affective and emotional associations with ongoing and forthcoming behaviour (6). More specifically, Kring and Barch (10) have indicated that this relies on reward-related processes such as reward anticipation and the anticipation of a favourable outcome of an action, as well as intact emotional memory. Reward processing has been associated with a variety of brain regions within mesocorticolimbic networks, most notably the ventral striatum, orbitofrontal cortex, and anterior and posterior cingulate cortex (11). Indeed, negative symptoms have been found to be related to reduced activation of the ventral striatum during reward processing (12) and the ACC during processing of positive emotional stimuli (13). More specifically to negative symptoms in schizophrenia, ventral striatal activation during reward processing has been found in relation to apathy/amotivation, but not to expressive deficits (14, 15). Chapter 11 further discusses studies into the role of the reward system.

Reward Value

In order to engage with active behaviour, reward value is weighed against necessary effort. Consequently, studies have also paid attention to the computation of the effort needed to execute the action, as well as the willingness to expend that effort needed to initiate (and persevere with) goal-directed behaviour (10). In case the expected benefit of an action exceeds the expected effort, there is sufficient approach motivation needed to prepare and execute the action. Regarding the neural level, effort computation and expenditure is thought to involve the striatum, ventromedial prefrontal cortex, and insula (16). Difficulties in computing effort cost and expenditure have been reported in relation to negative symptoms (17, 18). Furthermore, in patients with schizophrenia, difficulties in effort expenditure have been related to reduced activation of the nucleus accumbens, the posterior cingulate gyrus, and the medial frontal gyrus (19). However, how this relates to apathy remains to be investigated. Stepien et al. (20) reported an association between apathy and reduced dorsal striatal activity during reward anticipation in patients with schizophrenia (which was not found in healthy comparison subjects). They suggest that this finding may imply that impaired action-outcome selection is involved in the pathophysiology of motivational deficits in schizophrenia.

The relevance of reward processing for apathy has also been reported in patients with disorders other than schizophrenia. For example, Martínez-Horta et al. (21) found neurophysiological evidence of impaired incentive processing in patients with Parkinson's disease (PD). They measured the amplitude of the feedback-related negativity, an event-related brain potential associated with performance outcome valence, following monetary gains and losses in PD patients and healthy controls performing a gambling task. The results revealed that feedback-related negativity was significantly reduced in PD patients with apathy, as compared to non-apathetic patients and healthy controls. The authors conclude that their findings are indicative of impaired incentive processing and suggest a compromised mesocorticolimbic pathway in cognitively intact PD patients with apathy. It is of interest, in this regard, whether and how the nature of dopaminergic abnormalities contributes to apathy. A study by Chung et al. (22) using dopamine transporter positron emission tomography scans in 108 non-demented patients with PD (34 with apathy and 74 without) reported that the pattern of striatal dopamine depletion did not contribute to apathy. The authors suggested that apathy in PD may be associated with extrastriatal lesions that accompany PD rather than striatal dopaminergic deficits.

Executive Functioning

Another important component process involved in goal-directed action concerns executive functioning. When the reward/effort ratio is such that one is inclined to engage in the action, intact executive functioning (including processes such as allocation of attention, rule finding, set-shifting, and the maintenance of goals and subgoals) is needed to plan the action (4). These processes have often been associated with activation and connectivity in a network of frontal, striatal, and parietal regions (23). In patients with schizophrenia, disturbances in executive functioning have been found (see Chapter 7 for further discussion in relationship to apathy) and have been associated with activation and network connectivity (24, 25).

In relation to negative symptoms, reduced activation has been found in the left DLPFC, left premotor cortex, and bilateral nucleus accumbens during processing of novel stimuli (26) and to reduced activation in the right hippocampus, amygdala, superior temporal cortex, fusiform gyrus, and thalamus, the left middle frontal gyrus and lateral parietal cortex, and the bilateral insula, cuneus, and posterior cingulate cortex during the processing of target stimuli (27) during auditory oddball paradigms.

Moreover, stronger severity of amotivation has been found in association with reduced activation in the thalamus and parietal cortex during planning behaviour (28).

Klaasen et al. (29) examined the neural correlates of apathy during set-shifting in a healthy sample of participants selected for high and low levels of apathy using the Apathy Evaluation Scale (AES). Set-shifting relates to cognitive flexibility and is of importance for goal-directed behaviour. It has been noted that goal-directed actions require a balance between flexible shifting between behaviours and maintaining current behaviour despite distractions or competing behaviours (30). Reduced cognitive flexibility may thus contribute to apathy.

Cognitive flexibility concerns the ability to switch between cognitive processes in response to a changing environment or internal goals and relies on intact salience detection and attention, working memory, inhibition, and shifting (31). Shafritz et al. (32) developed a task to measure specific behavioural properties of cognitive flexibility, namely maintenance of a rule in mind, inhibition of an initial response, and periodically (overtly) changing the response rule. This task distinguishes behavioural switches (a change in response to different stimuli) from cognitive switches (a change in response rule) and salience decoupling (detecting a change in relevant stimuli). Klaasen et al. (29) used this task to contrast neural activation patterns of subjects with high versus low levels of apathy on the AES.

Results showed an association between apathy and reduced activation in the (medial) superior frontal gyrus and crus I/II of the cerebellum during cognitive set-shifting, the switching of a response rule. This suggests a possible involvement of these areas and cognitive set-shifting in the occurrence of apathy. More specifically, they may point to a possible disruption of action plan construction due to deficits in executive functioning. Naturally, caution is needed in interpreting these findings, as results in healthy individuals may not translate one-to-one to psychiatric or neurological populations. Nonetheless, these results may be a starting point for further research. Of note, a study measuring electroencephalography during a set-shifting task has shown an association between apathy and the strength of an event-related potential that has been associated with shifting of attention to novel stimuli (the P3a), both in healthy controls and PD patients (33). Future studies on the association between (neural correlates of) executive functioning and apathy in patients with schizophrenia may shed more light on this topic.

Self-Initiation

Finally, the initiation or auto-activation of thoughts or behaviour is imperative to execute goal-directed action (4). Indeed, such intentional behaviour is of critical importance for normal daily functioning. It comprises multiple components, including deciding whether to act, what action to perform, and when to execute it (34).

Difficulties in action initiation are reflected in reduced activation of mental set and emotional response, and lack of self-generated thoughts (mental emptiness) and self-generated actions. In patients with reduced thought or action initiation, there may be a clear contrast between an obvious reduction of self-generated actions and a normal production of actions in response to external demands. Self-initiation of behaviour is thought to rely on the anterior midcingulate cortex and (pre-)supplementary motor area, SMA (35, 36) and disruptions in these areas may lead to reduced goal-directed behaviour and therefore to amotivation (6).

Previous research on self-initiated behaviour in healthy individuals suggested that self-initiated behaviour is associated with the recruitment of fronto-parieto-striatal regions (34). Separate components of self-initiated behaviour have been studied, including a selection component (i.e. deciding what action to perform), and a timing component (i.e. deciding on when to initiate a prespecified or self-chosen action). Using fMRI, what and when components of action execution have been studied in healthy individuals employing a task that evoked either self-initiated, or externally triggered finger movements (36). In this study, selecting which action to perform was associated with activation in medial frontal regions including the bilateral pre-supplementary motor cortex extending to the anterior midcingulate cortex, in addition to DLPFC, dorsal premotor cortices, and inferior parietal lobules. Deciding on the timing of action, execution was associated with largely overlapping regions, however with additional recruitment of the bilateral anterior insula, anterior putamen, globus pallidi, and left cerebellum (36). Taken together, primary and supplementary motor regions, the DLPFC, ACC, inferior parietal lobules, and (parts of) the striatum have been consistently related to selection and timing components of action and therefore may have high relevance for disturbances in self-initiated behaviour underpinning apathy. Indeed, substantial evidence was found for consistent involvement of the ACC and inferior parietal lobules in a dysfunctional fronto-parieto-striatal network, in relation to apathy across disorders (5). These results suggest that regions that were associated with apathy are largely in accordance with those involved in self-initiation of actions.

Kos et al. (37) investigated whether levels of apathy in a healthy population were associated with neural correlates of action initiation of self-selected behaviour. To this end, they employed an event-related fMRI paradigm adapted from Hoffstaedter et al. (36) that allowed us to investigate both the action selection and timing components of self-initiated action. Activation of fronto-parieto-striatal regions during self-initiation was replicated. However, the neural correlates of self-initiated action did not explain variance in the different levels of apathy between participants. This was not the case when mass univariate analysis was used, nor when multivariate patterns of brain activation were evaluated. The authors therefore suggested that other hypotheses, for example, regarding a putative role of deficits in reward anticipation, effort expenditure, or executive difficulties, deserve further investigation as they may have more explanatory power. On the other hand, they acknowledge the limitations of studying varying levels of apathy in healthy individuals. Impaired self-initiation may be more readily apparent in patient samples, with more severe levels of apathy.

Unfortunately, there is a lack of studies investigating the neural correlates of self-initiation in relationship to apathy in patient samples. A study by Bonnelle et al. (38) investigated an important underlying mechanism for self-initiated actions, that is, the translation of intentions into actions using an effort and reward-based decision-making task during fMRI. They studied healthy participants with varying levels of apathy and hypothesized that apathy in otherwise healthy people might be associated with differences in brain systems underlying either motivation to act (specifically in effort and reward-based decision-making) or in action processing (transformation of an intention into action). Apathy was associated with increased effort sensitivity as well as greater recruitment of neural systems involved in action anticipation: SMA and cingulate motor zones. Notably, decreased structural and functional connectivity between ACC and SMA were associated with increased apathy. The results can be taken to support the hypothesis that effort sensitivity and translation of intentions into actions might contribute to apathy. More specifically, the authors hypothesize that inefficient communication between ACC and SMA might lead to increased physiological cost—and greater effort sensitivity—for action initiation in more apathetic people.

Neural Correlates of Other Cognitive Processes Relevant to Apathy

A number of studies have been published that use fMRI to investigate functional brain connectivity in the resting state, that is, without a cognitive task. The differences in intrinsic functional connectivity can nonetheless point to the contribution of specific brain networks and cognitive functions subserved by those networks.

Servaas et al. (39) investigated dynamic functional connectivity (DFC) in the resting state in relationship to apathy in patients with schizophrenia. The aim of this study was to investigate whether apathy in schizophrenia is associated with rigidity (lack of variability) in behaviour and brain functioning. To this end, they investigated associations between variability in the DFC in relevant functional brain networks, apathy, and variability in physical activity in 31 patients with schizophrenia. Based on actigraphy (each patient wore a watch-like device for a period of time), activity variability was calculated on the activity counts using the root of the mean squared successive difference (MSSD). Variability (MSSD) in dynamic functional brain connectivity was calculated for three networks, including the default-mode network, frontoparietal network, and salience-reward network. As expected, the results confirmed that lower activity variability was associated with higher levels of apathy. Furthermore, higher levels of apathy were associated with lower brain variability in DFC in the default-mode network and salience-reward network. In addition, higher activity variability was associated with higher variability in DFC in the salience-reward network. Thus, levels of apathy were associated with less variability in physical activity and more rigid functional brain network behaviour in the default-mode network and salience-reward network. Although resting-state network analysis does not provide direct evidence of cognitive processes involved, it is of interest to note that these networks have been shown relevant for self-related processing, mental simulation, and reward processing, which are pivotal for self-initiated goal-directed behaviour. The investigators suggest that functional rigidity of these networks may contribute to reduced goal-directed behaviour, characteristic of apathy. This hypothesis deserves further investigation using task-based paradigms.

Two other studies of resting-state connectivity and apathy in schizophrenia patients focused on the VTA, a key node in the dopamine system (40, 41). Giordano et al. (40) investigated the association between resting-state functional connectivity (RS-FC) of the VTA and avolition in 26 subjects with schizophrenia, compared to 22 healthy controls. Compared to the control subjects, patients showed significantly reduced RS-FC of the VTA with bilateral ventrolateral prefrontal cortex, bilateral insular cortex (IC) and right lateral occipital complex. They also showed increased RS-FC of the VTA with bilateral DLPFC. Significant negative correlations were found between avolition and RS-FC of the VTA with bilateral insular cortex, right ventrolateral prefrontal cortex, and right lateral occipital complex. From these findings, the investigators conclude that avolition is linked to a disconnectivity of the VTA from several key cortical regions involved in the integration of value information with action selection.

Xu et al. (41) examined the association between apathy or 'social amotivation' (four items of the Positive and Negative Syndrome Scale that correlate highly with the AES, see Chapter 7) and VTA-seeded intrinsic connectivity in 84 people with schizophrenia using RS-FC. In line with a previous study in healthy participants, they report spontaneous fluctuations of midbrain dopaminergic regions to be positively associated with striatal and prefrontal fluctuations in people with schizophrenia. Concerning apathy, social amotivation was negatively associated with functional connectivity between the VTA and medial- and lateral prefrontal cortex, the temporoparietal junction, and dorsal and ventral striatum. These associations were observed independently of depressive and positive symptoms.

Although the results of this study do not fully concur with the results from Giordano et al. (40), which may be due to differences in samples and apathy measures, both studies imply that apathy in people with schizophrenia is associated with altered intrinsic connectivity of mesocorticolimbic pathways linked to cognitive control and reward processing. Thus, dysconnectivity of dopaminergic neuronal ensembles that are fundamental to approach behaviour and motivation deserves further investigation, as it may help explain the lack of initiative in people with avolition and social amotivation.

A different approach to the analysis of resting-state fMRI data was taken by Sun et al. (42), who investigated regional homogeneity of brain activity in patients with PD. Regional homogeneity refers to concurrent activity patterns of brain regions. Specifically, it reflects regions that are not only active at the same time frequency but are also active in sync with neighbouring voxels. Compared with both PD patients without apathy and healthy control subjects, patients with apathy showed significantly lower regional homogeneity values in the dorsal ACC and right caudate.

Conclusion

In conclusion, functional neuroimaging studies support the involvement of neural systems underlying goal-directed behaviour in apathy. According to Starkstein and Brockman (43), dysfunction of the ACC is the strongest anatomical correlate of apathy in Alzheimer's disease, whereas lesions of the basal ganglia are the most common correlates of apathy in cerebrovascular disorders. These regions may be regarded as key hubs in networks subserving goal selection, action initiation, and execution. Their involvement is also apparent in other disorders (e.g. schizophrenia). Indeed, neuroimaging findings support involvement of ACC and medial prefrontal cortex in addition to striatum and other regions important for salience/reward processing (e.g. insula and orbitofrontal cortex) and executive functioning (e.g. DLPFC). In addition to the forementioned circuits, the parietal cortex has recently been argued to be of relevance (7), though it can be considered to be part and parcel of the frontoparietal control network. Future research should focus on more precise measurement of component processes underlying goal-directed behaviour using refined tasks during fMRI.

References

1. Logothetis NK. The neural basis of the blood-oxygen-level-dependent functional magnetic resonance imaging signal. Philos Trans R Soc B Biol Sci. 2002;357(1424):1003–37.

2. Op de Beeck H, Nakatani C. Introduction to Human Neuroimaging. Cambridge: Cambridge University Press; 2019.
3. van den Heuvel MP, Hulshoff Pol HE. Exploring the brain network: a review on resting-state fMRI functional connectivity. Eur Neuropsychopharmacol. 2010;20(8):519–34.
4. Sporns O. Discovering the Human Connectome. Cambridge, MA: MIT Press; 2012.
5. Kos C, van Tol MJ, Marsman JBC, Knegtering H, Aleman A. Neural correlates of apathy in patients with neurodegenerative disorders, acquired brain injury, and psychiatric disorders. Neurosci Biobehav Rev. 2016;69:381–401.
6. Levy R, Dubois B. Apathy and the functional anatomy of the prefrontal cortex-basal ganglia circuits. Cereb Cortex. 2006;16(7):916–28.
7. Tumati S, Martens S, de Jong BM, Aleman A. Lateral parietal cortex in the generation of behavior: implications for apathy. Prog Neurobiol. 2019;175:20–34.
8. Haber SN. Corticostriatal circuitry. Dialogues Clin Neurosci. 2016;18(1):7–21.
9. Gao Z, Davis C, Thomas AM, Economo MN, Abrego AM, Svoboda K, et al. A cortico-cerebellar loop for motor planning. Nature. 2018;563(7729):113–6.
10. Kring AM, Barch DM. The motivation and pleasure dimension of negative symptoms: neural substrates and behavioral outputs. Eur Neuropsychopharmacol. 2014;24(5):725–36.
11. Liu X, Hairston J, Schrier M, Fan J. Common and distinct networks underlying reward valence and processing stages: a meta-analysis of functional neuroimaging studies. Neurosci Biobehav Rev. 2011;35(5):1219–36.
12. Radua J, Schmidt A, Borgwardt S, Heinz A, Schlagenhauf F, McGuire P, et al. Ventral striatal activation during reward processing in psychosis: a neurofunctional meta-analysis. JAMA Psychiatry. 2015;72(12):1243–51.
13. Nelson BD, Bjorkquist OA, Olsen EK, Herbener ES. Schizophrenia symptom and functional correlates of anterior cingulate cortex activation to emotion stimuli: an fMRI investigation. Psychiatry Res. 2015;234(3):285–91.
14. Hartmann MN, Hager OM, Reimann AV, Chumbley JR, Kirschner M, Seifritz E, et al. Apathy but not diminished expression in schizophrenia is associated with discounting of monetary rewards by physical effort. Schizophr Bull. 2015;41(2):503–12.
15. Simon JJ, Cordeiro SA, Weber MA, Friederich HC, Wolf RC, Weisbrod M, et al. Reward system dysfunction as a neural substrate of symptom expression across the general population and patients with schizophrenia. Schizophr Bull. 2015;41(6):1370–8.
16. Treadway M, Buckholtz J, Cowan R, Woodward N, Li R, Ansari M, et al. Dopaminergic mechanisms of individual differences in human effort-based decision-making. J Neurosci. 2012;32(18):6170–6.
17. Fervaha G, Foussias G, Agid O, Remington G. Neural substrates underlying effort computation in schizophrenia. Neurosci Biobehav Rev. 2013;37(10 Pt 2):2649–65.
18. Gold JM, Waltz JA, Frank MJ. Effort cost computation in schizophrenia: a commentary on the recent literature. Biol Psychiatry. 2015;78(11):747–53.
19. Huang J, Yang XH, Lan Y, Zhu CY, Liu XQ, Wang YF, et al. Neural substrates of the impaired effort expenditure decision making in schizophrenia. Neuropsychology. 2016;30(6):685–96.
20. Stepien M, Manoliu A, Kubli R, Schneider K, Tobler PN, Seifritz E, et al. Investigating the association of ventral and dorsal striatal dysfunction during reward anticipation with negative symptoms in patients with schizophrenia and healthy individuals. PLoS One. 2018;13(6):e0198215.
21. Martínez-Horta S, Riba J, de Bobadilla RF, Pagonabarraga J, Pascual-Sedano B, Antonijoan RM, et al. Apathy in Parkinson's disease: neurophysiological evidence of impaired incentive processing. J Neurosci. 2014;34(17):5918–26.

22. Chung SJ, Lee JJ, Ham JH, Lee PH, Sohn YH. Apathy and striatal dopamine defects in non-demented patients with Parkinson's disease. Parkinsonism Relat Disord. 2016;23:62–5.
23. Leh SE, Petrides M, Strafella AP. The neural circuitry of executive functions in healthy subjects and Parkinson's disease. Neuropsychopharmacology. 2010;35(1):70–85.
24. Minzenberg MJ, Laird AR, Thelen S, Carter CS, Glahn DC. Meta-analysis of 41 functional neuroimaging studies of executive function in schizophrenia. Arch Gen Psychiatry. 2009;66(8):811–22.
25. Deserno L, Sterzer P, Wüstenberg T, Heinz A, Schlagenhauf F. Reduced prefrontal-parietal effective connectivity and working memory deficits in schizophrenia. J Neurosci. 2012;32(1):12–20.
26. Wolf DH, Turetsky BI, Loughead J, Elliott MA, Pratiwadi R, Gur RE, et al. Auditory oddball fMRI in schizophrenia: association of negative symptoms with regional hypoactivation to novel distractors. Brain Imaging Behav. 2008;2:132–45.
27. Shaffer JJ, Peterson MJ, McMahon MA, Bizzell J, Calhoun V, van Erp TGM, et al. Neural correlates of schizophrenia negative symptoms: distinct subtypes impact dissociable brain circuits. Mol Neuropsychiatry. 2015;1(4):191–200.
28. Liemburg EJ, Dlabac-De Lange JJ, Bais L, Knegtering H, van Osch MJ, Renken RJ, et al. Neural correlates of planning performance in patients with schizophrenia—relationship with apathy. Schizophr Res. 2015;161(2–3):367–75.
29. Klaasen NG, Kos C, Aleman A, Opmeer EM. Apathy is related to reduced activation in cognitive control regions during set-shifting. Hum Brain Mapp. 2017;38(5):2722–33.
30. Goschke T, Bolte A. Emotional modulation of control dilemmas: the role of positive affect, reward, and dopamine in cognitive stability and flexibility. Neuropsychologia. 2014;62:403–23.
31. Dajani DR, Uddin LQ. Demystifying cognitive flexibility: implications for clinical and developmental neuroscience. Trends Neurosci. 2015;38(9):571–8.
32. Shafritz KM, Kartheiser P, Belger A. Dissociation of neural systems mediating shifts in behavioral response and cognitive set. Neuroimage. 2005;25(2):600–6.
33. Seer C, Lange F, Georgiev D, Jahanshahi M, Kopp B. Event-related potentials and cognition in Parkinson's disease: an integrative review. Neurosci Biobehav Rev. 2016;71:691–714.
34. Haggard P. Human volition: towards a neuroscience of will. Nat Rev Neurosci. 2008;9(12):934–46.
35. Jenkins IH, Jahanshahi M, Jueptner M, Passingham RE, Brooks DJ. Self-initiated versus externally triggered movements. II. The effect of movement predictability on regional cerebral blood flow. Brain. 2000;123(Pt 6):1216–28.
36. Hoffstaedter F, Grefkes C, Zilles K, Eickhoff SB. The 'what' and 'when' of self-initiated movements. Cereb Cortex. 2013;23(3):520–30.
37. Kos C, Klaasen NG, Marsman JC, Opmeer EM, Knegtering H, Aleman A, et al. Neural basis of self-initiative in relation to apathy in a student sample. Sci Rep. 2017;7(1):3264.
38. Bonnelle V, Manohar S, Behrens T, Husain M. Individual differences in premotor brain systems underlie behavioral apathy. Cereb Cortex. 2016;26(2):807–19.
39. Servaas MN, Kos C, Gravel N, Renken RJ, Marsman JC, van Tol MJ, et al. Rigidity in motor behavior and brain functioning in patients with schizophrenia and high levels of apathy. Schizophr Bull. 2019;45(3):542–51.
40. Giordano GM, Stanziano M, Papa M, Mucci A, Prinster A, Soricelli A, et al. Functional connectivity of the ventral tegmental area and avolition in subjects with schizophrenia: a resting state functional MRI study. Eur Neuropsychopharmacol. 2018;28(5):589–602.

41. Xu P, Klaasen NG, Opmeer EM, Pijnenborg GHM, van Tol MJ, Liemburg EJ, et al. Intrinsic mesocorticolimbic connectivity is negatively associated with social amotivation in people with schizophrenia. Schizophr Res. 2019;208:353–9.
42. Sun HH, Pan PL, Hu JB, Chen J, Wang XY, Liu CF. Alterations of regional homogeneity in Parkinson's disease with "pure" apathy: a resting-state fMRI study. J Affect Disord. 2020;274:792–8.
43. Starkstein SE, Brockman S. The neuroimaging basis of apathy: empirical findings and conceptual challenges. Neuropsychologia. 2018;118(Pt B):48–53.

13

Pharmacology of Apathy

Lisa Nobis and Masud Husain

Introduction

With increasing awareness of the high prevalence of apathy across brain disorders and its impact on quality of life for patients and caregivers (1), there is considerable interest in developing effective therapies for the condition. While there are currently no guidelines for drug treatment of apathy, theories on the underlying pathology of motivational deficits have inspired several pharmacological approaches. Much of this work on humans has built on conceptual frameworks that have developed from extensive research on animal models of motivational deficits (2). Studies in both healthy humans and patients with brain disorders have revealed that there might be different domains of motivation and apathy: behavioural, cognitive, emotional, and social (3). Understandably, most of the animal work on motivational deficits has focused on the behavioural axis, as the others are more challenging to measure. Bearing this caveat in mind, here we consider both the foundational basic studies performed in animals as well as application to emerging treatment approaches for behavioural apathy in neurological disorders.

Pharmacology of Motivation and Apathy

Dopamine

A key process that is considered to be dysfunctional in apathy is cost–benefit analysis of whether to engage in a potentially rewarding behaviour, given the effort required to obtain a particular reward (4). The extent to which the potential reward and associated effort impact cost–benefit analysis will influence an individual's motivation to perform an action. Moreover, this sensitivity to reward has been shown to rely heavily on the mesocorticolimbic dopamine system (5, 6), which is why dopamine is considered to play such an essential role in motivated behaviour and apathy. In the mesocorticolimbic system, dopamine neurons project from the ventral tegmental area to subcortical and cortical areas (Fig. 13.1a), including the ventral striatum/

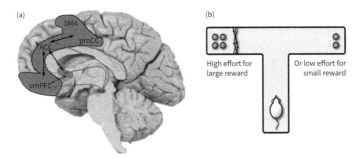

Fig. 13.1 Dopamine and motivation. (a) Mesocorticolimbic system. Dopamine originating in the VTA projects to the ventral striatum (VS), ventromedial prefrontal cortex, and anterior cingulate cortex (ACC). (b) Example of a T-maze task in which an animal chooses between a high-reward, high-effort cost option and a low-reward, lower-effort cost option. pmCC, posterior mid-cingulate cortex; SMA, supplementary motor area; vmPFC, ventromedial prefrontal cortex; VTA, ventral tegmental area.

Adapted with permission from Le Heron C, Holroyd CB, Salamone J, Husain M. Brain mechanisms underlying apathy. J Neurol Neurosurg Psychiatry. 2019;90(3):302–12. CC-BY-4.0.

nucleus accumbens (NAc), amygdala, hippocampus, and prefrontal areas such as anterior cingulate cortex (ACC).

Rodent studies in which the dopaminergic system of the animal has been disrupted or lesioned, provide striking evidence for its fundamental role in effort-based decision-making for rewards (2). Typically, in many such studies, an animal is given a choice between a preferred, high-reward food option that can be obtained with high effort such as scaling a wall, or a less preferred but low-effort food option which requires no climbing over obstacles (Fig. 13.1b). Alternatively, the high-effort option might require an increasing number of lever presses to obtain and it is possible to measure at which 'breakpoint' of presses an animal is no longer willing to exert effort for a particular level of reward.

The dopamine system has been manipulated by effectively lesioning or depleting key areas of dopamine transmission, or by systemic or local administration of drugs which bind to dopamine receptors. Using these methods, several investigations have reported that depletion of NAc/ventral striatal dopamine or administration of dopamine receptor antagonists leads to a shift in choice behaviour such that animals are more likely to select the low-effort option over the high-effort option (reviewed in (2, 6)). In addition, excitotoxic lesions of the core region of the NAc, or connections between this area and the ACC (7), lead to a similar shift in preference towards low-effort/low-reward options. In contrast, administration of a selective dopamine reuptake (dopamine transporter) inhibitor can shift responses toward high-effort/high-reward options (8).

Aside from these shifts in effort-related reward discounting, dopamine has been implicated in temporal discounting of rewards, too. For example, methylphenidate, which is thought to increase tonic dopamine levels by blocking reuptake of dopamine

(9), improved the ability to wait for a larger reward rather than choose an immediate smaller reward (10). However, methylphenidate is not selective for dopamine. It also acts as a noradrenaline reuptake inhibitor, thereby increasing noradrenergic tone. In line with this, methylphenidate increases firing rates in the locus coeruleus and ventral tegmental area, which is likely due to the increased stimulation of noradrenaline and dopamine receptors in these nuclei (11). Methylphenidate also increases dopamine and noradrenaline levels in prefrontal cortex (12). Due to a likely interaction between noradrenaline and dopamine release, effects of methylphenidate on decision-making may be caused by the manipulation of both these neurotransmitter systems (12).

There are several types of dopamine receptors in the brain. As a result of their expression in areas implicated in reward processing (Fig. 13.1a), D_1–D_3 dopamine receptors are considered to be especially important for motivated behaviour (13). For example, overexpression of postsynaptic D_2 receptors in the NAc, but not in the dorsal striatum, specifically reduced the sensitivity to effort in rodents (14). However, the role of different dopamine receptors in motivated behaviour is complex. For example, modulation of *either* D_1 or D_2 receptor systems by systemic administration of drugs that are either antagonists or agonists have produced similar effects on effort-based decision-making (reviewed in (6)). Highly selective D_1 or D_2 antagonists shift choice behaviour towards less-effort options in rats, with these effects being attenuated by their respective agonists. Intriguingly though, local infusion of a D_1 receptor antagonist—but not a D_2 antagonist—into the ACC led to a behavioural shift in choice to the low-effort option (15).

Another study tested the utility of D_1, D_2, and D_3 receptor agonists in reversing the motivation deficit induced by dopaminergic neuron loss in the substantia nigra compacta (SNc) (16). Rats were first given lesions in the SNc to mimic the dopaminergic neuron loss in Parkinson's disease. They then received one of three dopamine agonists selective for each of the receptor types. Motivational deficits were assessed before and after treatment. Only a D_3-specific dopamine agonist could improve motivation. In addition, this effect could be blocked by administering a D_3 antagonist, but not a D_2 antagonist (16). Thus, the results of this investigation might suggest that specifically D_3 dopamine receptors could be an important target for pharmacological treatment of apathy in Parkinson's disease.

Indeed, evidence for a *causal* role of dopamine depletion in the development of apathy in humans comes mostly from Parkinson's disease and to some extent Huntington's disease (17, 18). In both disorders, dopaminergic dysfunction is considered a core pathological feature, and both diseases are associated with a high prevalence of loss of motivation and apathy (17, 19). In Parkinson's disease, degeneration of dopamine neurons in the midbrain is considered to cause dysfunction in the mesocorticolimbic dopamine system, leading to reduced willingness to allocate effort for reward (19, 20). In humans, this is typically assessed by examining people's willingness to exert an effort for a monetary reward. For example, one study found that patients with Parkinson's disease (without clinical apathy) were less willing to exert effort by squeezing a handle for a given monetary reward than healthy controls (21). However, patients were more willing to exert effort for the same rewards when tested *on* their regular dopaminergic medication compared to when tested *off* their medication. Thus, the dopaminergic dysfunction in Parkinson's disease may cause motivational deficits even in the absence of clinical apathy, and this might be improved with dopaminergic medication.

Intriguingly though, when Parkinson's patients with apathy were compared to those without apathy on this paradigm, the effects of apathy and of being *on* dopaminergic medication were found to affect different aspects of reward-effort processing (20). While apathetic patients were less willing to allocate effort for low rewards, the effects of dopamine were distinctly different: increasing the likelihood of all patients— with and without apathy—exerting effort for high-reward–high-effort options. Thus, although dopamine modulates effort-based decision-making for rewards, dopamine depletion might *not* necessarily be the primary cause of apathy, even in Parkinson's disease. As discussed in later sections, non-dopaminergic drugs also can have significant effects on apathy in this condition.

More indirect evidence for the involvement of dopamine in human decision-making comes from rare patients with bilateral focal lesions of the basal ganglia or the ACC, such as after stroke, who can develop sudden-onset clinical apathy (22, 23). In some cases, dopamine agonists (mainly affecting D_2/D_3 receptors) have proven effective in improving reward sensitivity and reversing clinical apathy (23). In Alzheimer's disease, apathy correlates with decreased activity in ACC, possibly the result of dysfunctional dopaminergic input from the midbrain (24). Dopaminergic dysfunction is further supported by reports of decreased dopaminergic receptor density (25) and dopamine transporter availability (26) in Alzheimer's disease.

In summary, both animal and human studies point to a potential contributory role of dopaminergic disruption in the development of apathy by affecting effort-based decision-making for obtaining rewards. Several investigations have examined therapies targeted at the dopamine system for improvement of motivational deficits in apathy.

Noradrenaline

Noradrenergic neurons originate in the locus coeruleus, and project to a wide variety of cortical and subcortical regions (27). Traditionally, the noradrenergic system has been understood mainly as a mediator of attention and arousal. However, a growing body of evidence from single-neuron recordings in animals suggests a role in motivational processes. For example, activity of locus coeruleus neurons increased not only with reward cue onset, but also before an animal exerts effort to obtain a reward (28). Intriguingly, this activity could predict the amount of force the animal exerted, independent of the effort level. In line with the theory that dopaminergic activity encodes decisions about the value of a reward given its associated cost, the authors also reported increased dopamine neuron responses in the SNc with increased reward size and reduced effort level (28). However, there was no correlation between force production and SNc activity. Thus, while dopamine neurons may encode whether an action is worth performing given its cost–benefit trade-off, noradrenergic activity might support energization of behaviour by allocation of resources needed to overcome action cost (29).

These complementary roles of dopamine and noradrenergic transmission in decision-making have also been observed in pharmacological studies. For example, in a study using a rodent model of the Iowa Gambling Task, rats were offered a number of response options with different probabilities of reward and punishment. In order to maximize their total food, the animals had to learn to avoid large reward options that were more frequently paired with longer punishment timeouts. A decrease in advantageous choice behaviour was found only with simultaneous administration of dopamine and noradrenaline reuptake inhibitors, but not with either one compound alone (30). In addition, although effects of methylphenidate on decision-making are often attributed to a change in dopaminergic tone, the drug inhibits reuptake of both dopamine and noradrenaline (11, 12). Thus, the beneficial effect of methylphenidate on decision-making processes may be partly due to its influence on the noradrenergic system. This is important when considering clinical trials that have used methylphenidate for the treatment of apathy, discussed later in this chapter.

Serotonin

The serotonergic system has received much attention in research on anxiety and depression, mostly because of the antidepressant effects of selective serotonin reuptake inhibitors (SSRIs) (31). However, there is increasing evidence that serotonin plays an important role in reward processing, and thus may be crucial in the development of treatments for apathy. The dorsal raphe nucleus in the midbrain is the main source of serotonin in the forebrain, and projects to reward-processing related areas such as the basal ganglia and ACC (32). Dorsal raphe nucleus neurons that contain serotonin signal both reward magnitude and likelihood (33–35). They also increase activity both during consumption of rewarding food, and while waiting for reward (36). This suggests that serotonin may mediate control over behaviour while anticipating future rewards. However, the effects of serotonergic modulation are far less consistent than with dopamine, and many other theories of serotonergic function have been proposed.

For example, one investigation raised the possibility that serotonergic neurons encode the overall 'beneficialness' of the current motivational state, taking into account reward probability, reward value, and associated cost (35). However, another strand of research suggested that it has opposite functions to that of dopamine (37), involving punishment rather than reward processing. In humans, lowering serotonergic activity by acute tryptophan depletion reduced the sensitivity to punishment (38), while increasing serotonergic activity by administration of an SSRI increased sensitivity (39). Overall, there is support for serotonin's role in reward processing (40), in punishment processing (41), and in the interplay of both (42, 43). In addition, a recent report also proposed serotonergic modulation of effort sensitivity (44). The authors demonstrated that humans treated with the SSRI escitalopram produced more effort without experiencing any change in their sensitivity to reward compared to a control group (44). Thus, escitalopram, which increases the level of serotonin in the brain, reduced participants' effort sensitivity, but had no impact on reward sensitivity.

Some data from several clinical studies also suggest that serotonergic degeneration is linked to apathy (45, 46). For example, in patients with Parkinson's disease, more pronounced serotonergic degeneration in the basal ganglia was present in apathetic compared to non-apathetic patients, as indexed by a positron emission tomography presynaptic serotoninergic ligand (45). Interestingly, in this study apathy was not associated with dopaminergic cell loss, as measured by a positron emission tomography ligand for the presynaptic dopamine transporter. Reduced levels of serotonin, but not dopamine, were also associated with apathy in patients with rapid eye movement sleep behaviour disorder, a prodromal form of Parkinson's disease (47). In summary, evidence of serotonin's role in motivated behaviour, as well as the association of serotonergic degeneration with apathy in Parkinson's disease, indicate the potential for pharmacologically targeting the serotonergic system for the treatment of apathy.

Acetylcholine

Since the dopaminergic system has been considered to be relatively preserved in Alzheimer's disease, but motivational deficits are still a common symptom of the condition, another line of research on the pharmacology of apathy has focused on acetylcholine (48), a neurotransmitter implicated in the memory dysfunction of Alzheimer's disease. However, cholinergic interneurons are also present in brain regions areas that have been implicated in motivation, such as the NAc (49). As central acetylcholine does not have direct excitatory or inhibitory effects, it is considered a neuromodulator, rather than neurotransmitter, in the brain (50).

Investigations on acetylcholine typically involve administering agonists or antagonists of the two receptor types: muscarinic and nicotinic (50). In one rodent study, blockade of muscarinic acetylcholine receptor activity in the NAc decreased reward-seeking behaviour, while blocking nicotinic receptor activity increased it (51). The authors further demonstrated that this effect was due to secondary modulation of dopamine release. The muscarinic receptor antagonists caused a suppression, while the nicotinic receptor antagonists caused an increase in dopamine release related to reward-predictive cues. Thus, cholinergic receptors in the NAc may be involved in motivated behaviour by modulating dopamine release. Pharmacological therapies that have antagonistic effects on nicotinic receptors, or agonistic effects on muscarinic acetylcholine receptors, might therefore be potentially useful for the treatment of apathy.

In humans, several investigations have reported more severe cholinergic disruption in frontal areas in Alzheimer's disease, with reduced frontal brain activity correlating with severity of apathy (52, 53). However, apathy is more common in those patients who also have extrapyramidal symptoms, such as postural instability, rigidity, and abnormal gait, all of which are core symptoms of Parkinson's disease (54). Thus, the additional involvement of dopaminergic dysfunction may increase the risk of apathy in Alzheimer's disease, consistent with the modulating effect of acetylcholine on dopamine release. Conversely, in Parkinson's disease, there is evidence of cholinergic dysfunction in addition to dopaminergic depletion. The cholinesterase inhibitor rivastigmine, often prescribed in Parkinson's disease dementia and the related condition of dementia with Lewy bodies, has been shown to be effective in improving apathy even in non-demented Parkinson's disease patients (55).

Adenosine

Another neuromodulator that affects dopamine transmission in the striatum is adenosine. Through activation of adenosine receptors, adenosine can induce the release of acetylcholine, glutamate, gamma-aminobutyric acid (GABA), and dopamine (56). The receptor subtypes A_1 and A_{2A} are the most abundant receptors in the brain, with high expression of A_{2A} receptors in dopamine-rich areas such as the striatum (57). As the dopamine D_2 and adenosine A_{2A} receptors interact on a cellular level, A_{2A} receptor antagonists have been investigated as antiparkinsonian medication in animals (58). In addition, effects of adenosine A_{2A} receptor agonists acting at the NAc resemble those produced by dopamine receptor antagonism (59), increasing effort sensitivity and reducing reward sensitivity. In turn, the increase in effort sensitivity caused by administration of dopamine D_2 antagonists such as haloperidol could be reversed by administration of adenosine A_{2A} receptor antagonists, but not by adenosine A_1 receptor antagonists (60, 61). Consistent with this, mice without A_{2A} receptors did not show the changes in motivation typically induced by the dopamine D_2 antagonist haloperidol (62).

Thus, adenosine A_{2A} receptor antagonists may be useful to reverse the effect of dopamine depletion on motivated behaviour in apathy.

Pharmacological Treatments of Apathy in Neurological Disorders

Drug treatments for apathy in neurological disorders are at a relatively early stage. Many studies have reported effects on small numbers; some are case series or reports. Larger trials have been performed in Parkinson's disease and the related condition of dementia with Lewy bodies, as well as in Alzheimer's disease, but the instruments used to assess apathy have varied widely, with some relying only on self-report questionnaires. This understandably makes evaluation difficult, but it is nevertheless encouraging to see new trials in development that might use more sensitive measures in large groups of patients. One other important concern is about the dose of medication and individual variation in response. As yet, these issues have not been systematically addressed. In the following sections, we review the current state of the field by considering some important conditions in which treatments have been attempted.

Parkinson's Disease

Unsurprisingly, most pharmacological treatment approaches for apathy in Parkinson's disease have targeted the dopaminergic system. The most direct, but least specific approach to increase the level of dopamine is by administering levodopa, the precursor of dopamine, which is also commonly used for the treatment of motor symptoms in Parkinson's disease. Generally, the severity of motivational deficits and apathy tends to be lower in patients treated with dopaminergic drugs, in a dose-dependent manner (63). In addition, patients with Parkinson's disease score lower on behavioural measures of apathy while *on* compared to *off* their medication (21).

Dopamine agonists such as pramipexole (64), piribedil (65), and rotigotine (66), as well as the monoamine oxidase inhibitor rasagiline (67), have also been associated with improvements in motivated behaviour in Parkinson's disease (19). Pramipexole, piribedil, and ropinirole primarily target the D_2 and/or D_3 receptors and are thought not to interfere, directly at least, with the serotonergic system (68). Among the different dopaminergic agents, a large study comparing levodopa, pramipexole, and ropinirole reported pramipexole to be the most effective for the treatment of apathy in Parkinson's disease (64). Clinical apathy was present in 11.2% of patients in the pramipexole group, compared to 20.3% and 23.8% in the ropinirole and levodopa groups, respectively. However, patients were recruited based on their current medications, and thus were not randomly assigned to the three treatments. Although the groups were matched for demographics, there may have been differences in frequency of clinically significant apathy at baseline.

Other compounds that have been tested for their efficacy in treating apathy in Parkinson's disease include methylphenidate and rivastigmine. Methylphenidate blocks reuptake of both dopamine and noradrenaline, increasing levels of both neurotransmitters. Only one investigation has reported an improvement of apathy in a case study of Parkinson's disease after treatment with methylphenidate, but not with the SSRI paroxetine (69). A clinical trial investigating the usefulness of the cholinesterase inhibitor rivastigmine for the treatment of apathy in Parkinson's disease also reported a significant improvement in patients who did not suffer from dementia or depression (55). In this study, patients received either placebo or rivastigmine for 6 months. Although the sample size was small, with only 14 and 16 patients in the placebo and rivastigmine groups, respectively, the authors reported a significant improvement in the rivastigmine group, with large effect size, using the Lille Apathy Rating Scale. While 81% of patients in the treated group experienced a decrease in apathy as measured by the Lille Apathy Rating Scale, only 25% in the placebo group improved.

Positive effects on apathy were also observed in a pivotal early trial of rivastigmine in dementia with Lewy bodies (70). Not only was there an improvement in cognitive function, but the authors also reported significant amelioration of apathy as assessed on the Neuropsychiatric Inventory (NPI). Similarly, a case series using the cholinesterase inhibitor donepezil in dementia with Lewy bodies found a decrease in apathy in five of the seven patients treated (71). These data suggest that it is possible to obtain some benefit from modulating the cholinergic system.

Despite the apparent association between apathy and the serotonergic system in Parkinson's disease, there have been no controlled studies on the effectiveness of SSRI treatment for apathy. In fact, some have argued that SSRIs may worsen apathy (67, 72). For example, one observational study examined the association between Apathy Scale scores and antidepressant use in 181 Parkinson's patients and found that SSRIs, but not other types of antidepressants, were associated with greater apathy. In contrast, use of monoamine oxidase B inhibitors, which increase availability of dopamine, was related to less apathy (67). Because of the observational nature of this study, however, a causal effect of SSRI treatment on increased apathy cannot be established.

In summary, dopaminergic therapy for apathy in Parkinson's disease shows some promise, but there is also evidence for positive effects of cholinesterase inhibitors. However, interactions with other neurotransmitters and neuromodulators have not been sufficiently studied to provide general treatment guidelines.

Alzheimer's Disease

Several groups have investigated whether cholinesterase inhibitors, such as donepezil, have an impact on apathy in Alzheimer's disease. The results from these studies are inconsistent. For example, two trials assessing the efficacy of donepezil on apathy in large groups did not find any significant differences after either 24 weeks or 1 year of treatment (73, 74). However, change in apathy was included as a secondary outcome, and patients were not selected based on the presence of clinical apathy at baseline. In contrast, another 24-week study tested the efficacy of donepezil on NPI scores as a primary outcome measure. Apathy was reported in 67% of patients at baseline, and improved significantly in about 83% of patients in the treatment group, compared to 70% in the placebo group (75). Other differences such as dementia type, severity, and duration may also be reasons for the inconsistency across studies, with some authors suggesting that donepezil would be most beneficial in early Alzheimer's disease (76).

Galantamine, another cholinesterase inhibitor which also acts as an allosteric potentiating ligand at nicotinic receptors, had no effect on apathy in a large study with mild Alzheimer's patients, although there was a worsening of neuropsychiatric symptoms in the untreated group (77). Similarly, a large study using galantamine for treatment of apathy in moderate to severe Alzheimer's disease did not find a significant improvement in NPI scores on the drug compared to placebo (78). In contrast, rivastigmine reduced apathy in an open-label study in Alzheimer's disease, with 48% of patients who were newly prescribed rivastigmine showing improvements in apathy (79).

While some of these studies show promising effects of cholinergic treatment of apathy in dementia, an estimated 60% of Alzheimer's disease patients do not respond to it (80). Dopaminergic treatment may be useful in these cases, but few studies have pursued this. Herrmann and colleagues performed a double-blind, placebo-controlled trial in 13 patients with Alzheimer's disease and apathy. Every patient received either methylphenidate or placebo for a period of 2 weeks each in a cross-over, within-subject design. Treatment success was measured with total change on the Apathy Evaluation Scale, between baseline and the end of treatment. Total change scores indicated slightly, but significantly, greater improvement with methylphenidate compared to placebo (81). However, the small sample size and relatively short treatment period of 2 weeks limit interpretation. Nevertheless, a between-subjects trial with a larger sample size ($n = 60$) and a 12-week treatment duration provides further positive evidence for an effect of methylphenidate on apathy (82). Scores on the Apathy Evaluation Scale were significantly reduced in the methylphenidate group at 8 and 12 weeks by about 30%, compared to 20% in the placebo group (Fig. 13.2).

In contrast, in the Apathy in Dementia Methylphenidate Trial (ADMET), 60 patients with Alzheimer's disease were randomly assigned to a 6-week treatment with

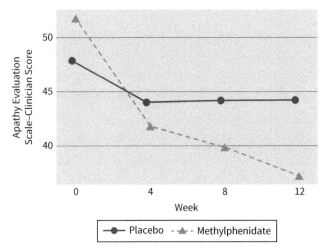

Fig. 13.2 Methylphenidate for the treatment of apathy in Alzheimer's disease. Apathy Evaluation Scale-Clinician scores over time in groups of patients with Alzheimer's disease decreasing 20% in placebo and 30% in methylphenidate groups.

methylphenidate or placebo. The primary outcome was change in the informant version of the Apathy Evaluation Scale, which did not significantly differ between the two groups after treatment (83). A larger, phase III trial, ADMET 2, will report on a 6-month randomized controlled intervention involving 200 cases.

Another approach that has been tried is treatment with the SSRI citalopram. A retrospective analysis of data from a previous observational trial with 34 patients was performed to assess the effects of citalopram on the apathy domain of the NPI. No statistically significant difference in apathy scores was found, although scores were low at baseline (84). Similarly, a meta-analysis of 11 studies investigating treatment with the N-methyl-D-aspartate receptor antagonist memantine in Alzheimer's disease reported significant effects for agitation, delusions, disinhibition, and night-time disturbances, but not for apathy (85).

Overall, evidence for effective treatment of apathy in Alzheimer's disease is limited. A meta-analysis of 21 studies, with a total of 6384 participants, reported a potential benefit of both methylphenidate and donepezil (86). However, the authors concluded that quality of evidence is low, based on the current lack of studies which have examined apathy as a primary outcome measure, and which recruited patients exhibiting clinically significant apathy at baseline.

Huntington's Disease

Although apathy is one of the most common neuropsychiatric symptoms in Huntington's disease, which involves dysfunction within the mesocorticolimbic system, only one trial has investigated pharmacological treatment (87). Gelderblom and colleagues used the atypical antidepressant bupropion, a noradrenaline–dopamine reuptake inhibitor and nicotinic receptor antagonist (88). They did not find a difference between placebo and bupropion in apathy after treatment of 10 weeks. Intriguingly, simply participating in the trial improved apathy, as a reduction in motivational deficits was observed in both groups compared to baseline.

Frontotemporal Dementia

Only one study has tested the pharmacological treatment of apathy in frontotemporal dementia. The authors aimed to establish whether increasing prefrontal dopaminergic function using agomelatine could improve apathy in 24 patients with frontotemporal dementia. Agomelatine's mechanism of action is complex, as it binds to both melatonergic, and serotonergic (5-HT_{2C}) receptors. Its antagonism to 5-HT_{2C} receptors is thought to increase dopaminergic and noradrenergic tone in prefrontal cortex. Thus, to separate the melatonergic from the dopaminergic/noradrenergic effects of agomelatine, patients were randomized in a within-subject, cross-over design to receive agomelatine and melatonin in two phases of 10 weeks. The authors reported a significant improvement of apathy after treatment with agomelatine, but not melatonin (89). Thus, the beneficial effect on apathy is likely due to the dopaminergic/noradrenergic effects, rather than involvement of the melatonergic system.

Stroke and Traumatic Brain Injury

Research on pharmacological treatment for apathy after stroke or traumatic brain injury mostly consists of case studies. For example, a number of reports suggest the usefulness of dopaminergic therapy for the treatment of apathy after stroke, such as the D_2/D_3 receptor agonist ropinirole (90). After a frontal lobe stroke, an 80-year-old man developed severe apathy, which improved considerably after administration of ropinirole. Blood flow was measured before and after treatment, and the authors found an increase in blood flow in the frontal lobe and basal ganglia with ropinirole. While the increase in blood flow could reflect natural recovery, the behavioural response co-incided relatively immediately following the administration of ropinirole (90).

In addition, a patient with considerable apathy after bilateral basal ganglia infarcts was successfully treated with ropinirole and showed improvement on behavioural measures of reward sensitivity (23). Other dopaminergic agents that were successfully used in single-case studies are methylphenidate (91), pramipexole (92), rotigotine (92), bromocriptine (93), and bupropion (94). Apart from dopaminergic therapy, two studies using GABA receptor agonists zolpidem and nefiracetam have also reported improvement of post-stroke apathy (95, 96). Nefiracetam improved apathy, but not depression, in a trial in which 48 patients were treated with 12 weeks of either 600 mg or 900 mg of nefiracetam, and 22 patients were assigned to placebo. However, only the group which received the larger dose of 900 mg of nefiracetam was significantly different to placebo (95). Case series with patients who developed apathy after traumatic brain injury support the possible use of selegiline (97), amantadine (98, 99), and bromocriptine (93), all of which affect the dopaminergic system. For example, in a case series of four patients that had developed apathy, but not depression, after traumatic brain injury, selegiline significantly improved scores on the Apathy Evaluation Scale (97). However, follow-up periods differed between patients, so that some improvements could be related to spontaneous recovery.

Conclusion

In this chapter we have reviewed neurotransmitter systems associated with motivated behaviour and apathy. Many lines of evidence point to a critical role of the mesocorticolimbic dopaminergic system in the development and treatment of apathy. However, little is known about potential dose-dependent effects of dopaminergic treatment. Dopaminergic function has been hypothesized to follow an inverted U-shape, with both under- and overdosing of dopamine having detrimental effects to cognition and behaviour (100). Thus, over- or undermedication may play a role in inconsistent results across studies. This may be especially relevant when treating apathy in disorders that involve more or less dopaminergic dysfunction, such as Parkinson's disease and stroke, respectively.

While effects of dopaminergic treatment on effort- and reward-based decision-making have been characterized fairly well, this needs to be performed in more detail for treatments targeting other neurotransmitter systems. In addition, there is considerable evidence for an interaction between dopamine, noradrenaline, serotonin, acetylcholine, adenosine, and likely other neuromodulators in the brain. As apathy is a common symptom in many different underlying disorders which involve dysfunction across a variety of neurotransmitter systems, future research might profitably focus on the difficult area of interplay between these systems. This may inform how and whether treatment for apathy could be tailored to the underlying disorder and individual patients.

References

1. Husain M, Roiser JP. Neuroscience of apathy and anhedonia: a transdiagnostic approach. Nat Rev Neurosci. 2018;19(8):470–84.
2. Salamone JD, Correa M. Neurobiology and pharmacology of activational and effort-related aspects of motivation: rodent studies. Curr Opin Behav Sci. 2018;22:114–20.
3. Robert P, Lanctôt KL, Agüera-Ortiz L, Aalten P, Bremond F, Defrancesco M, et al. Is it time to revise the diagnostic criteria for apathy in brain disorders? The 2018 international consensus group. Eur Psychiatry. 2018;54:71–6.
4. Le Heron C, Holroyd CB, Salamone J, Husain M. Brain mechanisms underlying apathy. J Neurol Neurosurg Psychiatry. 2019;90(3):302–12.
5. Walton ME, Bouret S. What is the relationship between dopamine and effort? Trends Neurosci. 2019;42(2):79–91.
6. Salamone JD, Correa M, Ferrigno S, Yang JH, Rotolo RA, Presby RE. The psychopharmacology of effort-related decision making: dopamine, adenosine, and insights into the neurochemistry of motivation. Pharmacol Rev. 2018;70(4):747–62.
7. Hauber W, Sommer S. Prefrontostriatal circuitry regulates effort-related decision making. Cereb Cortex. 2009;19(10):2240–7.
8. Sommer S, Danysz W, Russ H, Valastro B, Flik G, Hauber W. The dopamine reuptake inhibitor MRZ-9547 increases progressive ratio responding in rats. Int J Neuropsychopharmacol. 2014;17(12):2045–56.
9. Sagvolden T, Aase H, Zeiner P, Berger D. Altered reinforcement mechanisms in attention-deficit/hyperactivity disorder. Behav Brain Res. 1998;94(1):61–71.
10. Rajala AZ, Jenison RL, Populin LC. Decision making: effects of methylphenidate on temporal discounting in nonhuman primates. J Neurophysiol. 2015;114(1):70–9.
11. Karim TJ, Reyes-Vazquez C, Dafny N. Comparison of the VTA and LC response to methylphenidate: a concomitant behavioral and neuronal study of adolescent male rats. J Neurophysiol. 2017;118(3):1501–14.
12. Koda K, Ago Y, Cong Y, Kita Y, Takuma K, Matsuda T. Effects of acute and chronic administration of atomoxetine and methylphenidate on extracellular levels of noradrenaline, dopamine and serotonin in the prefrontal cortex and striatum of mice. J Neurochem. 2010;114(1):259–70.

13. Beaulieu JM, Gainetdinov RR. The physiology, signaling, and pharmacology of dopamine receptors. Pharmacol Rev. 2011;63(1):182–217.
14. Trifilieff P, Feng B, Urizar E, Winiger V, Ward RD, Taylor KM, et al. Increasing dopamine D2 receptor expression in the adult nucleus accumbens enhances motivation. Mol Psychiatry. 2013;18(9):1025–33.
15. Schweimer J, Hauber W. Dopamine D1 receptors in the anterior cingulate cortex regulate effort-based decision making. Learn Mem. 2006;13(6):777–82.
16. Carnicella S, Drui G, Boulet S, Carcenac C, Favier M, Duran T, et al. Implication of dopamine D3 receptor activation in the reversal of Parkinson's disease-related motivational deficits. Transl Psychiatry. 2014;4(6):e401.
17. Craufurd D, Thompson JC, Snowden JS. Behavioral changes in Huntington disease. Neuropsychiatry Neuropsychol Behav Neurol. 2001;14(4):219–26.
18. Pedersen KF, Larsen JP, Alves G, Aarsland D. Prevalence and clinical correlates of apathy in Parkinson's disease: a community-based study. Parkinsonism Relat Disord. 2009;15(4):295–9.
19. Chong TTJ, Husain M. The role of dopamine in the pathophysiology and treatment of apathy. Prog Brain Res. 2016;229:389–426.
20. Le Heron C, Plant O, Manohar S, Ang YS, Jackson M, Lennox G, et al. Distinct effects of apathy and dopamine on effort-based decision-making in Parkinson's disease. Brain. 2018;141(5):1455–69.
21. Chong TTJ, Bonnelle V, Manohar S, Veromann KR, Muhammed K, Tofaris GK, et al. Dopamine enhances willingness to exert effort for reward in Parkinson's disease. Cortex. 2015;69:40–6.
22. Schmidt L, d'Arc BF, Lafargue G, Galanaud D, Czernecki V, Grabli D, et al. Disconnecting force from money: effects of basal ganglia damage on incentive motivation. Brain. 2008;131(5):1303–10.
23. Adam R, Leff A, Sinha N, Turner C, Bays P, Draganski B, et al. Dopamine reverses reward insensitivity in apathy following globus pallidus lesions. Cortex. 2013;49(5):1292–303.
24. Theleritis C, Politis A, Siarkos K, Lyketsos CG. A review of neuroimaging findings of apathy in Alzheimer's disease. Int Psychogeriatrics. 2014;26(2):195–207.
25. Mitchell RA, Herrmann N, Lanctot KL. The role of dopamine in symptoms and treatment of apathy in Alzheimer's disease. CNS Neurosci Ther. 2011;17(5):411–27.
26. David R, Koulibaly M, Benoit M, Garcia R, Caci H, Darcourt J, et al. Striatal dopamine transporter levels correlate with apathy in neurodegenerative diseases. A SPECT study with partial volume effect correction. Clin Neurol Neurosurg. 2008;110(1):19–24.
27. Berridge CW, Waterhouse BD. The locus coeruleus–noradrenergic system: modulation of behavioral state and state-dependent cognitive processes. Brain Res Rev. 2003;42(1):33–84.
28. Arazzani C, San-Galli A, Gilardeau S, Bouret S. Noradrenaline and dopamine neurons in the reward/effort trade-off: a direct electrophysiological comparison in behaving monkeys. J Neurosci. 2015;35(20):7866–77.
29. Floresco SB. Noradrenaline and dopamine: sharing the workload. Trends Neurosci. 2015;38(8):465–7.
30. Baarendse PJJ, Winstanley CA, Vanderschuren LJMJ. Simultaneous blockade of dopamine and noradrenaline reuptake promotes disadvantageous decision making in a rat gambling task. Psychopharmacology (Berl). 2013;225(3):719–31.
31. Willner P, Scheel-Krüger J, Belzung C. The neurobiology of depression and antidepressant action. Neurosci Biobehav Rev. 2013;37(10 Pt 1):2331–71.
32. Jacobs BL, Azmitia EC. Structure and function of the brain serotonin system. Physiol Rev. 1992;72(1):165–229.
33. Nakamura K, Matsumoto M, Hikosaka O. Reward-dependent modulation of neuronal activity in the primate dorsal raphe nucleus. J Neurosci. 2008;28(20):5331–43.

34. Liu Z, Zhou J, Li Y, Hu F, Lu Y, Ma M, et al. Dorsal raphe neurons signal reward through 5-HT and glutamate. Neuron. 2014;81(6):1360–74.

35. Luo M, Li Y, Zhong W. Do dorsal raphe 5-HT neurons encode "beneficialness"? Neurobiol Learn Mem. 2016;135:40–9.

36. Li Y, Zhong W, Wang D, Feng Q, Liu Z, Zhou J, et al. Serotonin neurons in the dorsal raphe nucleus encode reward signals. Nat Commun. 2016;7:10503.

37. Daw ND, Kakade S, Dayan P. Opponent interactions between serotonin and dopamine. Neural Networks. 2002;15(4–6):603–16.

38. Crockett MJ, Apergis-Schoute A, Herrmann B, Lieberman MD, Lieberman M, Müller U, et al. Serotonin modulates striatal responses to fairness and retaliation in humans. J Neurosci. 2013;33(8):3505–13.

39. Fischer AG, Endrass T, Reuter M, Kubisch C, Ullsperger M. Serotonin reuptake inhibitors and serotonin transporter genotype modulate performance monitoring functions but not their electrophysiological correlates. J Neurosci. 2015;35(21):8181–90.

40. Seymour B, Daw ND, Roiser JP, Dayan P, Dolan R. Serotonin selectively modulates reward value in human decision-making. J Neurosci. 2012;32(17):5833–42.

41. Faulkner P, Deakin JFW. The role of serotonin in reward, punishment and behavioural inhibition in humans: insights from studies with acute tryptophan depletion. Neurosci Biobehav Rev. 2014;46(3):365–78.

42. McCabe C, Mishor Z, Cowen PJ, Harmer CJ. Diminished neural processing of aversive and rewarding stimuli during selective serotonin reuptake inhibitor treatment. Biol Psychiatry. 2010;67(5):439–45.

43. Palminteri S, Clair AH, Mallet L, Pessiglione M. Similar improvement of reward and punishment learning by serotonin reuptake inhibitors in obsessive-compulsive disorder. Biol Psychiatry. 2012;72(3):244–50.

44. Meyniel F, Goodwin GM, William Deakin JF, Klinge C, Macfadyen C, Milligan H, et al. A specific role for serotonin in overcoming effort cost. eLlife. 2016;5:1–18.

45. Maillet A, Krack P, Lhommée E, Météreau E, Klinger H, Favre E, et al. The prominent role of serotonergic degeneration in apathy, anxiety and depression in de novo Parkinson's disease. Brain. 2016;139(9):2486–502.

46. Schrag A, Politis M. Serotonergic loss underlying apathy in Parkinson's disease. Brain. 2016;139(9):2338–9.

47. Barber TR, Griffanti L, Muhammed K, Drew DS, Bradley KM, McGowan DR, et al. Apathy in rapid eye movement sleep behaviour disorder is associated with serotonin depletion in the dorsal raphe nucleus. Brain. 2018;141(10):2848–54.

48. Nobis L, Husain M. Apathy in Alzheimer's disease. Curr Opin Behav Sci. 2018;22:7–13.

49. Zhou FM, Wilson CJ, Dani JA. Cholinergic interneuron characteristics and nicotinic properties in the striatum. J Neurobiol. 2002;53(4):590–605.

50. Picciotto MR, Higley MJ, Mineur YS. Acetylcholine as a neuromodulator: cholinergic signaling shapes nervous system function and behavior. Neuron. 2012;76(1):116–29.

51. Collins AL, Aitken TJ, Greenfield VY, Ostlund SB, Wassum KM. Nucleus accumbens acetylcholine receptors modulate dopamine and motivation. Neuropsychopharmacology. 2016;41(12):2830–8.

52. Theleritis C, Politis A, Siarkos K, Lyketsos CG. A review of neuroimaging findings of apathy in Alzheimer's disease. Int Psychogeriatrics. 2014;26(2):195–207.

53. Sultzer DL, Mahler ME, Mandelkern MA, Cummings JL, Van Gorp WG, Hinkin CH, et al. The relationship between psychiatric symptoms and regional cortical metabolism in Alzheimer's disease. J Neuropsychiatry Clin Neurosci. 1995;7(4):476–84.

54. Starkstein SE, Petracca G, Chemerinski E, Kremer J. Syndromic validity of apathy in Alzheimer's disease. Am J Psychiatry. 2001;158(6):872–7.

55. Devos D, Moreau C, Maltete D, Lefaucheur R, Kreisler A, Eusebio A, et al. Rivastigmine in apathetic but dementia and depression-free patients with Parkinson's disease: a double-blind, placebo-controlled, randomised clinical trial. J Neurol Neurosurg Psychiatry. 2014;85(6):668–74.
56. Sebastião AM, Ribeiro JA. Adenosine A2 receptor-mediated excitatory actions on the nervous system. Prog Neurobiol. 1996;48(3):167–89.
57. Schiffmann SN, Fisone G, Moresco R, Cunha RA, Ferré S. Adenosine A2A receptors and basal ganglia physiology. Prog Neurobiol. 2007;83(5):277–92.
58. Pinna A. Adenosine A2A receptor antagonists in Parkinson's disease: progress in clinical trials from the newly approved istradefylline to drugs in early development and those already discontinued. CNS Drugs. 2014;28(5):455–74.
59. Mingote S, Font L, Farrar AM, Vontell R, Worden LT, Stopper CM, et al. Nucleus accumbens adenosine A2A receptors regulate exertion of effort by acting on the ventral striatopallidal pathway. J Neurosci. 2008;28(36):9037–46.
60. Mott AM, Nunes EJ, Collins LE, Port RG, Sink KS, Hockemeyer J, et al. The adenosine A2A antagonist MSX-3 reverses the effects of the dopamine antagonist haloperidol on effort-related decision making in a T-maze cost/benefit procedure. Psychopharmacology (Berl). 2009;204(1):103–12.
61. Farrar AM, Segovia KN, Randall PA, Nunes EJ, Collins LE, Stopper CM, et al. Nucleus accumbens and effort-related functions: behavioral and neural markers of the interactions between adenosine A2A and dopamine D2 receptors. Neuroscience. 2010;166(4):1056–67.
62. Pardo M, Lopez-Cruz L, Valverde O, Ledent C, Baqi Y, Müller CE, et al. Adenosine A2A receptor antagonism and genetic deletion attenuate the effects of dopamine D2 antagonism on effort-based decision making in mice. Neuropharmacology. 2012;62(5–6):2068–77.
63. Skorvanek M, Rosenberger J, Gdovinova Z, Nagyova I, Saeedian RG, Groothoff JW, et al. Apathy in elderly nondemented patients with Parkinson's disease. J Geriatr Psychiatry Neurol. 2013;26(4):237–43.
64. Pérez-Pérez J, Pagonabarraga J, Martínez-Horta S, Fernández-Bobadilla R, Sierra S, Pascual-Sedano B, et al. Head-to-head comparison of the neuropsychiatric effect of dopamine agonists in Parkinson's disease: a prospective, cross-sectional study in non-demented patients. Drugs Aging. 2015;32(5):401–7.
65. Thobois S, Lhommée E, Klinger H, Ardouin C, Schmitt E, Bichon A, et al. Parkinsonian apathy responds to dopaminergic stimulation of D2/D3 receptors with piribedil. Brain. 2013;136(5):1568–77.
66. Wang H, Wang L, He Y, Yu G. Rotigotine transdermal patch for the treatment of neuropsychiatric symptoms in Parkinson's disease: a meta-analysis of randomized placebo-controlled trials. J Neurol Sci. 2018;393:31–8.
67. Zahodne LB, Bernal-Pacheco O, Bowers D, Ward H, Oyama G, Limotai N, et al. Are selective serotonin reuptake inhibitors associated with greater apathy in Parkinson's disease? J Neuropsychiatry Clin Neurosci. 2012;24(3):326–30.
68. Piercey MF. Pharmacology of pramipexole, a dopamine D3-preferring agonist useful in treating Parkinson's disease. Clin Neuropharmacol. 1998;21(3):141–51.
69. Chatterjee A, Fahn S. Methylphenidate treats apathy in Parkinson's disease. J Neuropsychiatry Clin Neurosci. 2002;14(4):461–2.
70. McKeith I, Del Ser T, Spano P, Emre M, Wesnes K, Anand R, et al. Efficacy of rivastigmine in dementia with Lewy bodies: a randomised, double-blind, placebo-controlled international study. Lancet. 2000;356(9247):2031–6.
71. Lanctôt KL, Herrmann N. Donepezil for behavioural disorders associated with Lewy bodies: a case series. Int J Geriatr Psychiatry. 2000;15(4):338–45.

72. Wongpakaran N, van Reekum R, Wongpakaran T, Clarke D. Selective serotonin reuptake inhibitor use associates with apathy among depressed elderly: a case-control study. Ann Gen Psychiatry. 2007;6:7.

73. Seltzer B, Zolnouni P, Nunez M, Goldman R, Kumar D, Ieni J, et al. Efficacy of donepezil in early-stage Alzheimer disease. Arch Neurol. 2004;61(12):1852–6.

74. Winblad B, Engedal K, Soininen H, Verhey F, Waldemar G, Wimo A, et al. A 1-year, randomized, placebo-controlled study of donepezil in patients with mild to moderate AD. Neurology. 2001;57(3):489–95.

75. Gauthier S, Feldman H, Hecker J, Vellas B, Ames D, Subbiah P, et al. Efficacy of donepezil on behavioral symptoms in patients with moderate to severe Alzheimer's disease. Int Psychogeriatrics. 2002;14(4):389–404.

76. Tariot PN, Cummings JL, Katz IR, Mintzer J, Perdomo CA, Schwam EM, et al. A randomized, double-blind, placebo-controlled study of the efficacy and safety of donepezil in patients with Alzheimer's disease in the nursing home setting. J Am Geriatr Soc. 2001;49(12):1590–9.

77. Cummings JL, Schneider L, Tariot PN, Kershaw PR, Yuan W. Reduction of behavioral disturbances and caregiver distress by galantamine in patients with Alzheimer's disease. Am J Psychiatry. 2004;161(3):532–8.

78. Rockwood K, Mintzer J, Truyen L, Wessel T, Wilkinson D. Effects of a flexible galantamine dose in Alzheimer's disease: a randomised, controlled trial. J Neurol Neurosurg Psychiatry. 2001;71(5):589–95.

79. Gauthier S, Juby A, Morelli L, Rehel B, Schecter R, EXTEND Investigators. A large, naturalistic, community-based study of rivastigmine in mild-to-moderate AD: the EXTEND Study. Curr Med Res Opin. 2006;22(11):2251–65.

80. Tanaka M, Namiki C, Thuy DHD, Yoshida H, Kawasaki K, Hashikawa K, et al. Prediction of psychiatric response to donepezil in patients with mild to moderate Alzheimer's disease. J Neurol Sci. 2004;225(1–2):135–41.

81. Herrmann N, Rothenburg LS, Black SE, Ryan M, Liu BA, Busto UE, et al. Methylphenidate for the treatment of apathy in Alzheimer disease: prediction of response using dextroamphetamine challenge. J Clin Psychopharmacol. 2008;28(3):296–301.

82. Padala PR, Padala KP, Lensing SY, Ramirez D, Monga V, Bopp MM, et al. Methylphenidate for apathy in community-dwelling older veterans with mild Alzheimer's disease: a double-blind, randomized, placebo-controlled trial. Am J Psychiatry. 2018;175(2):159–68.

83. Rosenberg PB, Lanctôt KL, Drye LT, Herrmann N, Scherer RW, Bachman DL, et al. Safety and efficacy of methylphenidate for apathy in Alzheimer's Disease: a randomized, placebo-controlled trial. J Clin Psychiatry. 2013;74(8):810–6.

84. Siddique H, Hynan LS, Weiner MF. Effect of a serotonin reuptake inhibitor on irritability, apathy, and psychotic symptoms in patients with Alzheimer's disease. J Clin Psychiatry. 2009;70(6):915–8.

85. Kishi T, Matsunaga S, Iwata N. The effects of memantine on behavioral disturbances in patients with Alzheimer's disease: a meta-analysis. Neuropsychiatr Dis Treat. 2017;13:1909–28.

86. Ruthirakuhan MT, Herrmann N, Abraham T, Chan S, Lanctôt K. Pharmacological interventions for apathy in Alzheimer's disease. Cochrane Database Syst Rev. 2016;5:CD012197.

87. Gelderblom H, Wü Stenberg T, Mclean T, Mü Tze L, Fischer W, Saft C, et al. Bupropion for the treatment of apathy in Huntington's disease: a multicenter, randomised, double-blind, placebo-controlled, prospective crossover trial. PLoS One. 2017;12(3):e0173872.

88. Stahl SM, Pradko JF, Haight BR, Modell JG, Rockett CB, Learned-Coughlin S. A review of the neuropharmacology of bupropion, a dual norepinephrine and dopamine reuptake inhibitor. Prim Care Companion J Clin Psychiatry. 2004;6(4):159–66.

89. Callegari I, Mattei C, Benassi F, Krueger F, Grafman J, Yaldizli Ö, et al. Agomelatine improves apathy in frontotemporal dementia. Neurodegener Dis. 2016;16(5–6):352–6.

90. Kohno N, Abe S, Toyoda G, Oguro H, Bokura H, Yamaguchi S. Successful treatment of post-stroke apathy by the dopamine receptor agonist ropinirole. J Clin Neurosci. 2010;17(6):804–6.

91. Spiegel DR, Kim J, Greene K, Conner C, Zamfir D. Apathy due to cerebrovascular accidents successfully treated with methylphenidate: a case series. J Neuropsychiatry Clin Neurosci. 2009;21(2):216–9.

92. Blundo C, Gerace C. Dopamine agonists can improve pure apathy associated with lesions of the prefrontal-basal ganglia functional system. Neurol Sci. 2015;36(7):1197–201.

93. Powell JH, al-Adawi S, Morgan J, Greenwood RJ. Motivational deficits after brain injury: effects of bromocriptine in 11 patients. J Neurol Neurosurg Psychiatry. 1996;60(4):416–21.

94. Aragona B, De Luca R, Piccolo A, Le Cause M, Destro M, Casella C, et al. Is bupropion useful in the treatment of post-stroke thalamic apathy? A case report and considerations. Funct Neurol. 2018;33(4):213–6.

95. Robinson RG, Jorge RE, Clarence-Smith K, Starkstein S. Double-blind treatment of apathy in patients with poststroke depression using nefiracetam. J Neuropsychiatry Clin Neurosci. 2009;21(2):144–51.

96. Autret K, Arnould A, Mathieu S, Azouvi P. Transient improvement of poststroke apathy with zolpidem: a single-case, placebo-controlled double-blind study. BMJ Case Rep. 2013;2013:bcr2012007816.

97. Newburn G, Newburn D. Selegiline in the management of apathy following traumatic brain injury. Brain Inj. 2005;19(2):149–54.

98. Kraus MF, Maki PM. Effect of amantadine hydrochloride on symptoms of frontal lobe dysfunction in brain injury: case studies and review. J Neuropsychiatry Clin Neurosci. 1997;9(2):222–30.

99. Van Reekum R, Bayley M, Garner S, Burke IM, Fawcett S, Hart A, et al. N of 1 study: amantadine for the amotivational syndrome in a patient with traumatic brain injury. Brain Inj. 1995;9(1):49–54.

100. Cools R, D'Esposito M. Inverted-U shaped dopamine actions on human working memory and cognitive control. Biol Psychiatry. 2011;69(12):e113–25.

14

Psychosocial Approaches to the Treatment of Apathy

Marcel Riehle, Zuzana Kasanova, and Tania M. Lincoln

Defining Apathy as a Treatment Target for Psychological Interventions

Apathy has been defined as a marked reduction in goal-directed activity in at least two of three dimensions of activity: behaviour and cognition, emotion, and social interaction (1) (for details on the definition, see Chapter 1 of this volume). As such, apathy is a transdiagnostic concept and interventions need to target its underlying psychological processes rather than any specific disorder. In this chapter we therefore adopt a translational approach, in which we draw on evidence from specific disorders to review different types of psychological interventions for apathy as a transdiagnostic concept. In a first step, we show how apathy overlaps with the concepts of negative symptoms in schizophrenia and amotivation in depression. We then present available treatment options for reduced goal-directed activity within these disorders, discuss their mechanisms of change as well as their similarities and differences, and review their evidence base. At the end of the chapter, we present promising advances in theory and technology that have the potential to shape psychological interventions for apathy in the future. It is important to note that we refer to the impairments defined as apathy by Robert et al. (1) in the following sections, even when the respective field's literature usually uses different terminology.

Apathy in Mental Disorders

A lack of goal-directed behaviour is a recurrent concept in mental disorders, even though different terminology is often used. Concept-wise, the closest approximation to apathy is what has been defined as negative symptoms in schizophrenia. As does apathy, negative symptoms include a lack of expressive behaviour, of goal-directed behaviour, and of motivation to engage or persist in such behaviour (cf. Chapter 7 in this volume (2, 3)). The two concepts primarily differ in whether to emphasize the role of internal motivational states over outwardly observable goal-directed behaviour (i.e. negative symptoms (4, 5)) or vice versa (i.e. apathy (1)).

Furthermore, the expressive and motivational deficits that define negative symptoms in schizophrenia can be found in various mental disorders and, recently, transdiagnostic conceptualizations have shed light on similarities and differences across diagnostic boundaries (6–8). For example, apathy can be found in varying degrees of severity in roughly one-third to one-half of all patients with schizophrenia (6) and to a similar extent in mood and anxiety disorders (7). In terms of severity, however, patients with schizophrenia seem to present with a more prominent and more diversified symptom profile of apathy than those with mood and anxiety disorders (6). Additionally, the reduced goal-directed activity that defines apathy can be caused by different psychological processes, some of which are more prominent in one and less prominent in another diagnostic category (6).

Psychological Processes Involved in Apathy

Goal-directed behaviour is thought to be the result of a cost–benefit calculation in which a behaviour's assumed benefits outweigh its assumed costs. In apathy, the assumed costs seem to outweigh the assumed benefits too often, and behaviour is not initiated (8). A comprehensive review of all involved psychological processes is beyond the scope of this chapter and has been provided elsewhere (6, 8). Instead, we highlight four key concepts that influence the cost–benefit calculation and that should be considered during treatment planning because each of them may lead to apathy— on their own or in combination.

Neuropsychological Impairments

Many patients experiencing apathy also show impairments in neuropsychological areas such as attention, long- and short-term memory, and executive functions (6). Broadly speaking, these impairments toughen the cost–benefit calculation at several points, raising the burden to initiate behaviour. For example, impaired retrieval of past rewards impedes the anticipation of pleasure for future events (9), impaired working memory impedes selecting an action from several alternatives (6), and difficulties in cognitive control make the organization and planning of activities highly effortful (6, 8). It is therefore advisable to obtain patients' neuropsychological profiles before treatment, and to examine whether any impairments are functionally tied to the patient's apathy.

Demotivating Beliefs

In light of imperfect information to predict the outcomes of our actions, sets of core beliefs exert top-down influence to guide our actions. In apathy, demotivating beliefs such as 'I don't have what it takes, so why bother at all?' are frequently incorporated into this set of guiding beliefs (10). They devalue the potential merits of behaviour initiation (e.g. 'I will not enjoy this anyway') or emphasize the costs (e.g. 'It will take too much energy to do this') (10, 11). The beliefs are thought to form as a response to repeated failure experiences in order to protect the person from further harm, thus creating a mechanism maintaining apathy (11, 12). Knowing which demotivating beliefs a patient holds is therefore very valuable information that can be assessed using validated questionnaires (e.g. 10).

Anhedonia

Anhedonia, that is, a reduced 'in-the-moment' experience of pleasure, revokes the reinforcing quality of pleasurable activities and by this reduces persistence and engagement in these activities (8, 13). Therefore, anhedonia is a very potent agent in creating and maintaining apathy. Accordingly, whether or not a patient experiences anhedonia should be clarified when interventions are planned to reduce apathy (7). Unfortunately, the retrospective assessment of anhedonia is highly prone to bias due to the combination of demotivating beliefs and imperfect memory (9). Options for the momentary assessment of pleasure are behavioural experiments (see 'Interventions') or mobile-based monitoring (see 'Future Directions in the Psychological Treatment of Apathy').

Impaired Anticipation of Pleasure

Some patients present with an impairment in feeling pleasure in anticipation of an activity. In people with schizophrenia, it has been repeatedly shown that the 'in-the-moment' experience of pleasure is intact whereas the levels of anticipated pleasure are reduced (6, 8). Thus, goal-directed activity emerges in these patients because the experience of future pleasure is not expected to be relevant enough to prompt behaviour. Neuropsychological impairments and demotivating beliefs are important contributors to this mechanism. It is nevertheless worth noting that the lowered expectation of pleasure to be received from an activity can also coincide with or may even be caused by anhedonia. Thus, even though apathy in people with schizophrenia may involve intact hedonic responding but impaired anticipation of pleasure, apathy in depression typically involves both anhedonia and impaired anticipation of pleasure (6–8). Comparing anticipated and 'in-the-moment' levels of pleasure, for example, via behavioural experiments (see 'Interventions'), can help to distinguish anhedonia from impaired anticipation of pleasure.

Individualizing Treatment Targets

It is important to keep in mind that apathy is usually multicausal, with several impairments coexisting or interacting within a single individual. Therefore, different individuals will present with different sets of impairments that require different therapeutic approaches. Based on these considerations, there will be no one-size-fits-all approach to the psychological treatment of apathy. Instead, accurate diagnostic assessment is needed to identify potential areas of impairment in need of intervention.

A framework has been proposed for how to use functional analysis to individualize negative symptom treatment in schizophrenia (14) that can also be applied to apathy. The basic premise of functional analysis is that for any problematic behaviour to become a persistent symptom, there need to be persistent impairments or there need to be reinforcing proximate consequences. The clinician therefore is trying to answer the question of what is causing and maintaining apathy for a particular person.

In the case of apathy, the problematic behaviour is a lack of goal-directed behaviour (e.g. staying in bed rather than getting up, staying at home doing nothing rather than going to the movies). We have outlined several persistent impairments in the previous section that give rise to apathy. Negative reinforcers of lack of goal-directed behaviour are—among others (14)—relief of tension (e.g. anxiety, worry) or of effort expenditure requirements (e.g. staying in bed has saved energy). Functional analysis may then reveal which of the potentially involved processes actually serves a function in the emergence and maintenance of the apathetic behaviour, and at the same time eliminate processes that are irrelevant for this patient. Ultimately, this helps to sort out which therapeutic approach is (or which approaches are) best suited for the patient. The following review of intervention strategies therefore includes sections on both the mechanisms targeted in the interventions and their efficacy.

Interventions

We selected the interventions for our review based on the available evidence mostly in research on the negative symptoms of schizophrenia and depression. As a minimum requirement for inclusion, we established that at least one sufficiently powered randomized controlled trial (RCT) testing the intervention's efficacy in reducing apathy or related constructs has been published. We then present evidence from such RCTs rather than from pilot trials, non-randomized, or non-controlled studies.

Cognitive Behavioural Therapy

Techniques and Proposed Mechanisms of Change
Cognitive behavioural therapy (CBT) is one of the most consistently used psychological approaches to the treatment of apathy. Cognitive and behavioural techniques are generally combined in a broader framework that emphasizes the triad of thought, action, and emotion. Nevertheless, we will highlight two types of interventions, one that targets demotivational beliefs and one that directly targets the behavioural deficits.

Treatment targets for the cognitive part of the therapy draw on the thought–action and thought–emotion connection represented in the cognitive triad. Thus, demotivating beliefs are the focus of this part of treatment. Cognitive therapy challenges these beliefs via techniques such as Socratic dialogue or weighing of pros and cons (for detailed descriptions, see (15, 16)). Ultimately, the aim of these cognitive interventions is to enable patients to generate alternative, more adaptive interpretations (e.g. 'I can't know whether or not I will enjoy this, so I should try it' rather than 'I won't enjoy this anyway, so why try it?'), which should then motivate goal-directed behaviour.

Behavioural techniques targeting apathy draw on the behaviour–emotion connection represented in the cognitive triad. The most common technique in this regard is behavioural activation. The basic premise of this technique is that patients' reduced activity leads to a lack of positive reinforcers with a common consequence being depressed mood (17). Behavioural techniques attempt to reverse this downward spiral by encouraging, scheduling, and monitoring daily activity plans that include potentially pleasurable activities. Classical behavioural activation includes activities taken from a nomothetic list of pleasurable activities (18), but some authors have proposed a more idiosyncratic approach (e.g. (19)), drawing on activities that the patient remembers to have enjoyed at some point in life.

Behavioural activation and cognitive therapy can be merged in behavioural experiments, where patients try out an activity and compare their anticipated pleasure with their actual level of pleasure when engaging in these activities. Therapists are then able to point out mismatches, and direct attention to the cognitive triad of thought, action, and emotion in order to encourage the patient to re-evaluate previously held dysfunctional beliefs (cf. (20)).

In sum, the goal of CBT is to enhance goal-directed activity by deploying the positive reinforcement qualities of pleasurable activities, and by lifting belief-related barriers to volition. We can therefore expect that CBT interventions work for patients who show apathy in the dimensions of behaviour and cognition and in social interaction. On the other side, patients with severe levels of anhedonia (as part of the emotion dimension of the apathy criteria) may need additional elements augmenting the experience of positive emotions (cf. (7, 20, 21)).

Evidence

We will primarily present evidence for CBT for reducing apathy in negative symptoms of schizophrenia. Although there is an extant literature on how CBT (including behavioural activation) is effective in patients with major depression (e.g. (22, 23)), the primary outcome in this literature is generally the level of depressive symptoms rather than level of goal-directed behaviour (24). Studies reporting on the negative symptoms of schizophrenia as an outcome thus provide a better estimate of the efficacy of CBT for apathy.

So far, there is good reason to assume that CBT is suited to reduce negative symptoms in schizophrenia. The largest and highest-quality trial of CBT specifically for negative symptoms in schizophrenia ($N = 198$) (25) found significant improvements in negative symptoms following CBT, but these effects were no larger than for the control treatment, cognitive remediation (CR), which is described in the following subsection. Motivation, but not emotional expression, increased with medium effect size in an RCT that tested cognitive therapy according to Beck et al. (15) versus treatment as usual (TAU) ($N = 60$) (26). Another study combined motivational interviewing and behavioural activation for the treatment of negative symptoms in schizophrenia and found a large treatment effect compared to TAU ($N = 47$) (27). Meta-analyses have produced conflicting findings on whether or not CBT improves negative symptoms (28, 29). However, the interpretation of these meta-analyses is problematic because the vast majority of the included studies did not focus on negative symptom treatment (30, 31). In a systematic review, we found that in the very few trials explicitly focusing on the treatment of negative symptoms, CBT improves motivational impairments and social functioning, while the effect on reduced emotional expression is negligible (30). Thus, even though the evidence base is sparse, CBT seems to be effective for the treatment of several aspects of apathy.

Cognitive Remediation

Techniques and Proposed Mechanisms of Change

CR, also cognitive rehabilitation, seeks to enhance neuropsychological functions related to performance of activities of daily living such as attention, executive functions, or memory (32). It does so by presenting patients with tasks that enable the neuropsychological domain in question to be directly practised (e.g. sequence tapping to practise working memory and visuospatial skills). Task difficulty is set individually to enable errorless learning via repeated practice, scaffolding, and personalized feedback (33). Some CR programmes also include teaching of compensatory strategies for difficulties that do not respond to practice (32) or metacognitive strategies (33, 34). CR can be delivered via paper and pencil or computerized (including mobile and virtual reality applications), and is facilitated by a CR therapist, who selects tasks with appropriate difficulty, provides positive feedback, and encourages patients to engage in treatment.

There are two principal ways in which CR may help to reduce apathy (cf. (35)). Primarily, improving neuropsychological functions is assumed to help overcome some very basic obstacles for action initiation, which is a precondition for goal-directed behaviour (9). Another way that CR may help to reduce apathy is by indirectly affecting demotivating beliefs; errorless learning and the explication of success via positive feedback form a very potent refutation of these beliefs that are thought to form as a consequence of experiencing failure over and over again (e.g. (11)).

CR should thus be effective for apathy across all three domains included in the Robert et al. (1) apathy criteria, given that patients present with impairments in neuropsychological domains.

Evidence

We will again draw on the literature of CR as a treatment for the negative symptoms of schizophrenia, for which meta-analytic evidence is available (35). The CR literature relevant to apathy is less developed for other mental disorders such as major depressive disorder (36) and for traumatic brain injury or Parkinson's disease (37–39).

The largest study to have tested the effect of CR on negative symptoms in schizophrenia (N = 198) (25) found significant improvements in negative symptoms, with CR being as effective as CBT. Similar findings have been reported by one other study comparing CR to CBT (N = 40) (40). One recent study (N = 61) (34) showed superiority of a variant of CR over TAU in reducing negative symptoms. A recent meta-analysis estimated that the effect of CR on the negative symptoms of schizophrenia is small to moderate (g = −0.30 to −0.40) (35). Overall, the evidence currently suggests that CR is about as effective as CBT to reduce apathy.

Social Skills Training

Techniques and Proposed Mechanism of Action

Broadly speaking, social skills training (SST) targets deficits in an individual's capacity to successfully interact with other people. SST is routed in social learning theory (41) and so the most typical element of SST is guided role-play that is used to practise social behaviour (i.e. verbal and non-verbal communication) in different areas of social situations (e.g. (42)). Skills are usually taught in the areas of problem-solving, assertiveness, and, less often, affiliation. The commonly employed group format allows for model learning alongside the practice elements with positive and corrective feedback. Less frequently, SST is delivered in a one-on-one setting, limiting model learning and practice opportunities to the patient–therapist dyad for the benefit of a therapeutic environment that for some patients is less aversive than a group setting (for a thorough description of the one-on-one setting see (42)).

Several possible mechanisms of change are discussed via which SST could decrease apathy (cf. (43)). One premise of these proposed mechanisms of change is that people with apathy show deficits in social skills. Supporting evidence for this premise comes from studies suggesting that people with relevant negative symptoms of schizophrenia show less social affiliation skills (44) leading to rejection by others (45). However, it is unclear whether these people do not possess the skills, or are not motivated to act on them (cf. (46)). Accordingly, SST could lead to actual skill acquisition or could activate appropriate social behaviour that is already present but not regularly shown. Either way, patients would interact more successfully with others. Social learning theory predicts that this should lead to more social engagement (41), thus reducing apathy.

SST should, therefore, be primarily effective for those people who exhibit apathy in the social interaction domain *and* who have social skills deficits that would obstruct behavioural activation or refutation of demotivating beliefs.

Evidence

Akin to the other treatment approaches outlined in this chapter, research on SST in schizophrenia provides the broadest literature base. For example, a 2016 meta-analysis on the efficacy of psychological interventions for depression considered 198 treatment trials (23) but only seven small-scale trials (combined $N \approx 100$) tested SST. The meta-analysis found that SST significantly reduces depression, but it did not distinguish depressed mood from apathy symptoms.

In the schizophrenia literature, an influential meta-analysis (43) showed that SST can reduce negative symptoms in schizophrenia with a small to moderate effect size (no. of studies = 6; $N = 363$; effect size = −0.40) and also has similar positive effects on performance-based measures of social and daily-living skills (no. of studies = 7; $N = 481$; effect size = 0.52). More recently, a meta-analysis suggests that SST may even outperform other active psychological treatments in reducing negative symptoms (47). However, the interpretation of these effects is impaired by the fact that none of the studies considered has tested SST as a treatment specifically for people with negative symptoms (30). In sum, there is some evidence that SST could reduce apathy with a moderate effect size, but thorough tests in people with apathy are needed to confirm this.

Specific and Integrative Approaches and Treatment Programmes

In this section, we will present additional therapeutic approaches that have either been developed to specifically target aspects of apathy, or due to their scope are likely suited to target apathy. Some of these approaches are still in an experimental state and, for some, evidence is only available from small trials. This section thus aims to provide an overview of recent developments in the field.

We have already emphasized the importance of creating positive emotional experiences for patients with apathy. The Positive Emotions Program for Schizophrenia (PEPS) (21), is dedicated to achieving this goal. It combines elements of experiential learning, mindfulness practice (i.e. mediation/relaxation), behavioural exercises (such as expression imitation training), and cognitive therapy for defeatist beliefs (see earlier in chapter) in a group format. A first RCT ($N = 80$) in participants with schizophrenia and negative symptoms showed that PEPS compared to TAU reduced negative symptoms with a moderate effect post treatment and a moderate to large effect at 6-month follow-up (48).

Positive Affect Treatment (PAT) (7) also specifically aims at improving reward sensitivity and ultimately positive emotional experience to reduce anhedonia. This 'behavioural and cognitive treatment' (49, p. 458) includes—among other elements—behavioural activation augmented by specific 'in-the-moment' recounting of pleasurable activities, imagining future pleasant events, reframing of neutral or negative events, and compassion-focused training such as exercises on joy, loving-kindness, or gratitude (for a detailed description see (7)). In a first RCT ($N = 96$), PAT was compared to a treatment that solely focused on reducing negative affect in a sample of participants with depression or anxiety disorders. At 6-month follow-up, PAT was superior over the comparison treatment in increasing positive affect and in decreasing negative affect, depression, anxiety, stress, and suicidal ideation with moderate effect sizes (49). It is worth noting that the negative affect treatment was stripped of all elements that are used to enhance positive affect and as such was not state-of-the-art CBT. Nevertheless, these first results are promising in light of the fact that CBT for depression and anxiety often fails to improve positive affect (7).

Motivation and Enhancement (MOVE) (20) training takes a similar approach as PEPS and PAT in that it was developed as an integrative psychological approach to promote positive experiences in those with negative symptoms. This is achieved by 'emotional processing of success', creating and enhancing the experience and awareness of positive experiences through success in daily life. Additionally, MOVE involves the typical CBT elements outlined previously. That is, cognitive therapy for demotivating beliefs, behavioural experiments, and behavioural activation. It also includes a module for SST for patients with skills deficits, and is set up as a home-based/community-based treatment. Thus, practitioners engage with patients in their own environments, at home or in public (e.g. restaurants, parks, etc.). A first RCT ($N = 51$) has provided evidence for the utility of MOVE, and resulted in a moderate treatment effect after 9 months of treatment (20).

Another programme, Cognitive Behavioral Social Skills Training (CBSST) (50), combines group CBT with SST. CBSST includes a 'thought challenging' module for demotivating beliefs similar to the CBT approach delineated earlier. Its tenets are integrated into subsequent role play-based social skills and problem-solving modules in the safe environment of the therapy group. Granholm and colleagues have shown in a large RCT ($N = 149$) that CBSST is effective in reducing negative symptoms, with a moderate to large effect at follow-up 1 year post treatment (46). Moreover, a reduction in self-defeatist beliefs, but not asociality beliefs, served as a mediator for the reduction in negative symptoms (51). However, so far, no dismantling studies have segregated the effects of CBT and SST in CBSST. Thus, the contribution of the SST elements over the influence of CBT remains unknown. Also, negative symptom levels in the trial were low to moderate and it remains to be seen if patients with more severe symptomatology will also benefit.

Motivational interviewing employs specifically tailored dialogue to empower patients to actively engage in their behavioural change. Although this approach was originally designed to address substance abuse, its emphasis on fostering activation and agency renders it particularly suitable for targeting apathy. So far, motivational interviewing has not been specifically applied to apathy. In a cluster RCT, motivational interviewing proved to reduce depression ($N = 168$) (52), and in one small RCT ($N = 35$) was found to reduce the negative symptoms of schizophrenia, and to increasing self-reported motivation, interpersonal functioning and observer-rated personal care rate in the psychiatric ward (53).

Acceptance and commitment therapy (ACT) is a cognitive and behavioural therapy that tackles experiential avoidance, psychological rigidity, and undue attachment to maladaptive beliefs in order to enable goal-directed behaviour consistent with core values (54). Thus, ACT has clear potential to successfully address apathy. Meta-analyses of the effectiveness of ACT in reduction of depression have reported medium to large effects (55–57), positioning it as superior to TAU and equivalent to CBT. While also apt for reducing depressive and affective symptoms in the context of psychosis (58, 59), ACT compared to TAU reduced negative symptoms of psychosis in only one small RCT ($N = 27$) (60), whereas it did not in two other RCTs ($N = 29$ (58); $N = 96$ (61)).

Mindfulness-based interventions are an extension of ACT additionally including elements on self-compassion and mindfulness. As a whole, mindfulness-based interventions have been proposed to ameliorate internalized stigma and symptom-related distress that might show up as apathy (62). An RCT of a mindfulness-based intervention in individuals with psychosis reported a trend towards an improvement in negative symptoms ($N = 44$) (63). A moderate effect on negative symptoms was also detected using an acceptance-based CBT (64), which in practice heavily relies on mindfulness techniques.

Finally, the UK National Institute for Health and Care Excellence guidelines (65) recommended 'music and arts' therapy for the treatment of negative symptoms in schizophrenia. Among these approaches, and mostly driving this recommendation, was body-oriented psychotherapy that had shown promising results in a first RCT (66). However, a subsequently conducted, large-scale multicentre RCT ($N = 275$) found no effect of body-oriented psychotherapy on negative symptoms (67), thus questioning its utility as a treatment for apathy.

Future Directions in the Psychological Treatment of Apathy

We have shown that behavioural activation, enhancement of positive experience, cognitive therapy for demotivating beliefs, CR of executive function deficits, and SST are all viable psychological approaches that can ameliorate different aspects of apathy, respectively. However, their efficacy is largely in the small to moderate effect-size range. As shown in the previous section, CBT, CR, and SST are not mutually exclusive and researchers (and clinicians) have started to investigate whether combinations produce synergistic effects. So far, these efforts have produced larger effects. However, these effects are still only in the moderate effect-size range. Also, the more comprehensive treatment packages are longer, which increases the risk of treatment fatigue (68). This could be the reason for the higher drop-out rates for the comprehensive approaches, such as CBSST (69) and MOVE (20), compared to the other focused interventions for negative symptoms (30). Finally, the different psychological mechanisms that are involved in apathy and interact with various environmental influences (e.g.

childhood neglect) (70), call for personalized approaches to therapy that are likely to increase the efficacy compared to the 'one-size-fits-all approaches' presently available (14). Beyond the content, adjusting the dose of therapy to the severity, evolving needs, and challenges of each patient is also a promising way of increasing efficiency and reducing drop-out. Finally, health behaviours such as treatment adherence and treatment seeking are in itself goal-directed behaviours (68), thus prone to be negatively affected by apathy. This is further compounded by statistics showing that despite universal insurance coverage, the vast majority of individuals suffering from mental illness go untreated (71).

It is therefore important to find ways to increase the engagement in treatments for apathy. This is why we end this chapter in laying out how emerging approaches and technological advances may improve access, engagement, personalization, and thus effectiveness of interventions targeting apathy.

The personalization of both treatment contents and dosage should include shared decision-making between therapists and patients. Shared decision-making is a cross-cutting treatment strategy that seeks to balance the power asymmetry between patients and clinicians by achieving consensus between the clinician and the patient in each decision about treatment. For example, more favourable outcomes of CBT for psychosis were associated with factors such as collaboratively agreed, individualized goals for therapy and tasks to practise between sessions (72). While not designed to target apathy nor negative symptoms per se, a meta-analysis revealed a small beneficial effect on empowerment of patients with psychosis involved in shared decision-making (73). We would expect that increasing empowerment helps to refute defeatist beliefs and, in turn, to diminish apathy.

Another way to actively engage patients in their therapy process is to allow them to gain insight into their own symptom dynamics and behaviour patterns through technology. The rapid advancement and proliferation of digital technology has enabled the development of mobile-based digital health apps and web-based programmes. These digital health interventions feature versatility, ecological validity, and personalization potential that is forging a novel model of mental healthcare. In addition to the potential to close the gap between the therapist office and daily life, computer and mobile technology features good availability, affordability, engagement in treatment, and reduced stigma of 'seeing a therapist' (74). Likely because of this combination, these technologies have shown high acceptability and feasibility in those with severe mental illness (75), which makes them attractive media for psychological therapies for apathy. For example, computerized CBT was shown to be feasible and effective in targeting depression (76), and a mobile-based add-on to ACT therapy, ACT in Daily Life in early stages of psychosis (77, 78), are among the growing body of evidence for the therapeutic potential of digital technology when used in conjunction to traditional care. We will highlight two approaches that have shown promising first results, and that seem to be particularly relevant to the treatment of apathy.

In an RCT of behavioural activation in daily life (79), participants with remitted depression or residual depressive symptoms ($N = 102$) performed ecological momentary assessments for 8 weeks (for more information on ecological momentary assessment as a method of data collection see (80)). Thus, all participants tracked their mood, mental state, and activity several times a day throughout the trial and one-half of them received additional weekly personalized feedback on how much time they had allocated to different activities, and how much positive affect they had experienced during each activity. Over time, both groups improved in positive affect (81) and depression scores (79), but only the group that had received feedback continued improving up to 6 months after the intervention (79). A somewhat different approach was favoured in the personalized real-time intervention for motivational enhancement (PRIME) intervention in early psychosis (82). This mobile-based digital health app employs a community of peers also participating in the intervention and motivational coaches to support each individual in attainment of self-identified goals, in their own environment and on-demand. The participants were prompted by the app to break down their longer-term goals to smaller, actionable ones to be performed on a daily basis. The progress was visible to the peers who offered their encouragement in online fora, while coaches were supporting the participants via text messages. In a pilot RCT of PRIME versus TAU ($N = 38$), social motivation, anticipated pleasure, effort expenditure, and self-efficacy increased following 12 weeks of PRIME, while defeatist beliefs and self-reported depression symptoms diminished, an effect that was retained after 3 months post intervention (82). The intervention thus acted upon several psychological processes key to apathy.

Technology is also being used to innovate the non-pharmacological treatment of apathy in major neurocognitive and neurodegenerative disorders, such as Alzheimer's or Parkinson's disease (83). As these disorders have a high prevalence of apathy (83, 84), it is not surprising that initial evidence points towards a general efficacy of psychological approaches in reducing apathy in these disorders (e.g. (85, 86)) using similar approaches to those discussed within this chapter (e.g. behavioural activation, CR, social interaction enhancement; for an overview see (83)). Here, too, the development of effective digital health interventions using channels such as the aforementioned mobile-health applications, telemedicine, or virtual reality is hoped to further advance the field (83). Given promising first findings, interventions using these technologies will rise in acceptance levels over the next decades because more and more patients with neurocognitive disorders (and their practitioners) will become adept in using them.

Regardless of the modality of the delivery of any of the interventions in this section, they all converge on common therapeutic principles: personalization to the needs of the individual patient, attention to the environmental factors that exert influence on the patient, and treating the patient as an active partner in the therapy process. We may expect that emerging psychological treatments of apathy synergistically blend components of other interventions, include shared decision-making as well as options to personalize therapy contents and dosage, and use novel digital technologies.

References

1. Robert P, Lanctôt KL, Agüera-Ortiz L, Aalten P, Bremond F, Defrancesco M, et al. Is it time to revise the diagnostic criteria for apathy in brain disorders? The 2018 international consensus group. Eur Psychiatry. 2018;54:71–6.

2. Kirkpatrick B, Fenton WS, Carpenter WT, Marder SR. The NIMH-MATRICS consensus statement on negative symptoms. Schizophr Bull. 2006;32(2):214–9.

3. Marder SR, Galderisi S. The current conceptualization of negative symptoms in schizophrenia. World Psychiatry. 2017;16(1):14–24.

4. Blanchard JJ, Kring AM, Horan WP, Gur R. Toward the next generation of negative symptom assessments: the collaboration to advance negative symptom assessment in schizophrenia. Schizophr Bull. 2011;37(2):291–9.

5. Horan WP, Kring AM, Blanchard JJ. Anhedonia in schizophrenia: a review of assessment strategies. Schizophr Bull. 2006;32(2):259–73.

6. Strauss GP, Cohen AS. A transdiagnostic review of negative symptom phenomenology and etiology. Schizophr Bull. 2017;43(4):712–29.

7. Craske MG, Meuret AE, Ritz T, Treanor M, Dour HJ. Treatment for anhedonia: a neuroscience driven approach. Depress Anxiety. 2016;33(10):927–38.

8. Barch DM, Pagliaccio D, Luking K. Mechanisms underlying motivational deficits in psychopathology: similarities and differences in depression and schizophrenia. Curr Top Behav Neurosci. 2016;27:411–49.

9. Strauss GP, Gold JM. A new perspective on anhedonia in schizophrenia. Am J Psychiatry. 2012;169(4):364–73.

10. Pillny M, Krkovic K, Lincoln TM. Development of the Demotivating Beliefs Inventory and Test of the Cognitive Triad of Amotivation. Cognit Ther Res. 2018;42(6):867–77.

11. Beck AT, Rector NA, Stolar N, Grant P. A cognitive conceptualization of negative symptoms. In: Beck AT, Rector NA, Stolar N, Grant P (Eds), Schizophrenia Cognitive Theory, Research, and Therapy. New York: Guilford Press; 2011, pp. 142–58.

12. White RG, Laithwaite H, Gilbert P. Negative symptoms in schizophrenia. The role of social defeat. In: Gumley A, Gillham A, Taylor K, Schwannauer M (Eds), Psychosis and Emotion. London: Routledge; 2013, pp. 178–90.

13. Watson D, Naragon-Gainey K. On the specificity of positive emotional dysfunction in psychopathology: evidence from the mood and anxiety disorders and schizophrenia/schizotypy. Clin Psychol Rev. 2010;30(7):839–48.

14. Lincoln TM, Riehle M, Pillny M, Helbig-Lang S, Fladung A-K, Hartmann-Riemer M, et al. Using functional analysis as a framework to guide individualized treatment for negative symptoms. Front Psychol. 2017;8:2108.

15. Beck AT, Rector NA, Stolar N, Grant P. Cognitive assessment and therapy of negative symptoms. In: Beck AT, Rector NA, Stolar N, Grant P (Eds), Schizophrenia Cognitive Theory, Research, and Therapy. New York: Guilford Press; 2011, pp. 257–86.

16. Beck AT. Cognitive therapy: nature and relation to behavior therapy. Behav Ther. 1970;1(2):184–200.

17. Lewinsohn PM. A behavioral approach to depression. In: Friedman RJ, Katz MM (Eds), The Psychology of Depression: Contemporary Theory and Research. Oxford: John Wiley & Sons; 1974, pp. 157–78.

18. Lewinsohn PM, Graf M. Pleasant activities and depression. J Consult Clin Psychol. 1973;41(2):261–8.

19. Jacobson NS, Martell CR, Dimidjian S. Behavioral activation treatment for depression: returning to contextual roots. Clin Psychol Sci Pract. 2006;8(3):255–70.

20. Velligan DI, Roberts D, Mintz J, Maples N, Li X, Medellin E, et al. A randomized pilot study of MOtiVation and Enhancement (MOVE) training for negative symptoms in schizophrenia. Schizophr Res. 2015;165(2):175–80.
21. Nguyen A, Frobert L, McCluskey I, Golay P, Bonsack C, Favrod J. Development of the Positive Emotions Program for Schizophrenia: an intervention to improve pleasure and motivation in schizophrenia. Front Psychiatry. 2016;7:13.
22. Cuijpers P, Berking M, Andersson G, Quigley L, Kleiboer A, Dobson KS. A meta-analysis of cognitive-behavioural therapy for adult depression, alone and in comparison with other treatments. Can J Psychiatry. 2013;58(7):376–85.
23. Barth J, Munder T, Gerger H, Nüesch E, Trelle S, Znoj H, et al. Comparative efficacy of seven psychotherapeutic interventions for patients with depression: a network meta-analysis. Focus (Madison). 2016;14(2):229–43.
24. Ekers D, Webster L, Van Straten A, Cuijpers P, Richards D, Gilbody S. Behavioural activation for depression; an update of meta-analysis of effectiveness and sub group analysis. PLoS One. 2014;9(6):e100100.
25. Klingberg S, Wölwer W, Engel C, Wittorf A, Herrlich J, Meisner C, et al. Negative symptoms of schizophrenia as primary target of cognitive behavioral therapy: results of the randomized clinical TONES study. Schizophr Bull. 2011;37(Suppl 2):S98–110.
26. Grant PM, Huh GA, Perivoliotis D, Stolar NM, Beck AT. Randomized trial to evaluate the efficacy of cognitive therapy for low-functioning patients with schizophrenia. Arch Gen Psychiatry. 2012;69(2):121–7.
27. Choi KH, Jaekal E, Lee GY. Motivational and behavioral activation as an adjunct to psychiatric rehabilitation for mild to moderate negative symptoms in individuals with schizophrenia: a proof-of-concept pilot study. Front Psychol. 2016;7:1759.
28. Wykes T, Steel C, Everitt B, Tarrier N. Cognitive behavior therapy for schizophrenia: effect sizes, clinical models, and methodological rigor. Schizophr Bull. 2008;34(3):523–37.
29. Velthorst E, Koeter M, van der Gaag M, Nieman DH, Fett AKJ, Smit F, et al. Adapted cognitive–behavioural therapy required for targeting negative symptoms in schizophrenia: meta-analysis and meta-regression. Psychol Med. 2015;45(03):453–65.
30. Riehle M, Pillny M, Lincoln TM. Ist Negativsymptomatik bei Schizophrenie überhaupt behandelbar? Ein systematisches Literaturreview zur Wirksamkeit psychotherapeutischer Interventionen für Negativsymptomatik. Verhaltenstherapie. 2017;27(3):199–208.
31. Fusar-Poli P, Papanastasiou E, Stahl D, Rocchetti M, Carpenter W, Shergill S, et al. Treatments of negative symptoms in schizophrenia: meta-analysis of 168 randomized placebo-controlled trials. Schizophr Bull. 2015;41(4):892–9.
32. Novakovic-Agopians T, Abrams GM. Cognitive rehabilitation therapy. In: Encyclopedia of the Neurological Sciences. New York: Elsevier; 2014, pp. 824–6.
33. Wykes T, Reeder C, Corner J, Williams C, Everitt B. The effects of neurocognitive remediation on executive processing in patients with schizophrenia. Schizophr Bull. 1999;25(2):291–307.
34. Mueller DR, Khalesi Z, Benzing V, Castiglione CI, Roder V. Does Integrated Neurocognitive Therapy (INT) reduce severe negative symptoms in schizophrenia outpatients? Schizophr Res. 2017;188:92–7.
35. Cella M, Preti A, Edwards C, Dow T, Wykes T. Cognitive remediation for negative symptoms of schizophrenia: a network meta-analysis. Clin Psychol Rev. 2017;52:43–51.
36. Porter RJ, Bowie CR, Jordan J, Malhi GS. Cognitive remediation as a treatment for major depression: a rationale, review of evidence and recommendations for future research. Aust N Z J Psychiatry. 2013;47(12):1165–75.
37. Brett CE, Sykes C, Pires-Yfantouda R. Interventions to increase engagement with rehabilitation in adults with acquired brain injury: a systematic review. Neuropsychol Rehabil. 2017;27(6):959–82.

38. Calleo J, Burrows C, Levin H, Marsh L, Lai E, York MK. Cognitive rehabilitation for executive dysfunction in Parkinson's disease: application and current directions. Parkinsons Dis. 201;2012:512892.

39. Worthington A, Wood RL. Apathy following traumatic brain injury: a review. Neuropsychologia. 2018;118:40–7.

40. Penadés R, Catalán R, Salamero M, Boget T, Puig O, Guarch J, et al. Cognitive remediation therapy for outpatients with chronic schizophrenia: a controlled and randomized study. Schizophr Res. 2006;87(1–3):323–31.

41. Bandura A. Principles of Behavior Modification. Oxford: Holt, Rinehart, & Winston; 1969.

42. Bellack AS, Mueser KT, Gingerich S, Agresta J (Eds). Social Skills Training for Schizophrenia. New York: Guilford Press; 2004.

43. Kurtz MM, Mueser KT. A meta-analysis of controlled research on social skills training for schizophrenia. J Consult Clin Psychol. 2008;76(3):491–504.

44. Blanchard JJ, Park SG, Catalano LT, Bennett ME. Social affiliation and negative symptoms in schizophrenia: examining the role of behavioral skills and subjective responding. Schizophr Res. 2015;168(1–2):491–7.

45. Riehle M, Mehl S, Lincoln TM. The specific social costs of expressive negative symptoms in schizophrenia: reduced smiling predicts interactional outcome. Acta Psychiatr Scand. 2018;138(2):133–44.

46. Granholm E, Holden J, Link PC, McQuaid JR. Randomized clinical trial of cognitive behavioral social skills training for schizophrenia: improvement in functioning and experiential negative symptoms. J Consult Clin Psychol. 2014;82(116B):1173–85.

47. Turner DT, van der Gaag M, Karyotaki E, Cuijpers P. Psychological interventions for psychosis: a meta-analysis of comparative outcome studies. Am J Psychiatry. 2014;171(5):523–38.

48. Favrod J, Nguyen A, Chaix J, Pellet J, Frobert L, Fankhauser C, et al. Improving pleasure and motivation in schizophrenia: a randomized controlled clinical trial. Psychother Psychosom. 2019;88(2):84–95.

49. Craske MG, Treanor M, Dour H, Meuret A, Ritz T. Positive affect treatment for depression and anxiety: a randomized clinical trial for a core feature of anhedonia. J Consult Clin Psychol. 2019;87(5):457–71.

50. Holden J, Granholm E. Group cognitive behavioural social skills training for schizophrenia. In: Steel C (Ed), CBT for Schizophrenia: Evidence-Based Interventions and Future Directions. Chichester: Wiley-Blackwell; 2013, pp. 169–89.

51. Granholm E, Holden J, Worley M. Improvement in negative symptoms and functioning in cognitive-behavioral social skills training for schizophrenia: mediation by defeatist performance attitudes and asocial beliefs. Schizophr Bull. 2018;44(3):653–61.

52. Keeley RD, Engel M, Nordstrom K, Brody DS, Burke BL, Moralez E, et al. Motivational interviewing improves depression outcome in primary care: a cluster randomized trial. J Consult Clin Psychol. 2016;84(11):993–1007.

53. Cho JM, Lee K. Effects of motivation interviewing using a group art therapy program on negative symptoms of schizophrenia. Arch Psychiatr Nurs. 2018;32(6):878–84.

54. Hayes SC, Smith SX. Get Out of Your Mind & Into Your Life: The New Acceptance & Commitment Therapy. Oakland, CA: New Harbinger Publications; 2005.

55. Twohig MP, Levin ME. Acceptance and commitment therapy as a treatment for anxiety and depression: a review. Psychiatr Clin North Am. 2017;40(4):751–70.

56. Hacker T, Stone P, MacBeth A. Acceptance and commitment therapy—do we know enough? Cumulative and sequential meta-analyses of randomized controlled trials. J Affect Disord. 2016;190:551–65.

57. A-Tjak JGL, Davis ML, Morina N, Powers MB, Smits JAJ, Emmelkamp PMG. A meta-analysis of the efficacy of acceptance and commitment therapy for clinically relevant mental and physical health problems. Psychother Psychosom. 2015;84(1):30–6.

58. Gumley A, White RG, Briggs A, Ford I, Barry S, Stewart C, et al. A parallel group random-ised open blinded evaluation of acceptance and commitment therapy for depression after psychosis: pilot trial outcomes (ADAPT). Schizophr Res. 2017;183:143–50.

59. Gaudiano BA, Herbert JD. Acute treatment of inpatients with psychotic symptoms using acceptance and commitment therapy: pilot results. Behav Res Ther. 2006;44(3):415–37.

60. White RG, Gumley A, McTaggart J, Rattrie L, McConville D, Cleare S, et al. A feasibility study of acceptance and commitment therapy for emotional dysfunction following psych-osis. Behav Res Ther. 2011;49(12):901–7.

61. Shawyer F, Farhall J, Thomas N, Hayes SC, Gallop R, Copolov D, et al. Acceptance and commitment therapy for psychosis: randomised controlled trial. Br J Psychiatry. 2017;210(2):140–8.

62. Davis L, Kurzban S. Mindfulness-based treatment for people with severe mental illness: a literature review. Am J Psychiatr Rehabil. 2012;15(2):202–32.

63. López-Navarro E, Del Canto C, Belber M, Mayol A, Fernández-Alonso O, Lluis J, et al. Mindfulness improves psychological quality of life in community-based patients with severe mental health problems: a pilot randomized clinical trial. Schizophr Res. 2015;168(1–2):530–6.

64. Shawyer F, Farhall J, Mackinnon A, Trauer T, Sims E, Ratcliff K, et al. A randomised con-trolled trial of acceptance-based cognitive behavioural therapy for command hallucin-ations in psychotic disorders. Behav Res Ther. 2012;50(2):110–21.

65. National Institute for Health and Care Excellence. Psychosis and Schizophrenia in Adults: Treatment and Management. Clinical guideline [CG178]. Last updated 1 March 2014. Available at: https://www.nice.org.uk/guidance/cg178

66. Röhricht F, Priebe S. Effect of body-oriented psychological therapy on negative symptoms in schizophrenia: a randomized controlled trial. Psychol Med. 2006;36(5):669–78.

67. Priebe S, Savill M, Wykes T, Bentall RP, Reininghaus U, Lauber C, et al. Effectiveness of group body psychotherapy for negative symptoms of schizophrenia: multicentre random-ised controlled trial. Br J Psychiatry. 2016;209(1):54–61.

68. Heckman BW, Mathew AR, Carpenter MJ. Treatment burden and treatment fatigue as bar-riers to health. Curr Opin Psychol. 2015;5:31–6.

69. Granholm E, Holden J, Link PC, McQuaid JR, Jeste D V. Randomized controlled trial of cognitive behavioral social skills training for older consumers with schizo-phrenia: defeatist performance attitudes and functional outcome. Am J Geriatr Psychiatry. 2013;21(3):251–62.

70. Bailey T, Alvarez-Jimenez M, Garcia-Sanchez AM, Hulbert C, Barlow E, Bendall S. Childhood trauma is associated with severity of hallucinations and delusions in psych-otic disorders: a systematic review and meta-analysis. Schizophr Bull. 2018;44(5):1111–22.

71. Wittchen HU, Jacobi F, Rehm J, Gustavsson A, Svensson M, Jönsson B, et al. The size and burden of mental disorders and other disorders of the brain in Europe 2010. Eur Neuropsychopharmacol. 2011;21(9):655–79.

72. O'Keeffe J, Conway R, McGuire B. A systematic review examining factors predicting fa-vourable outcome in cognitive behavioural interventions for psychosis. Schizophr Res. 2017;183:22–30.

73. Stovell D, Morrison AP, Panayiotou M, Hutton P. Shared treatment decision-making and empowerment related outcomes in psychosis: systematic review and meta-analysis. Br J Psychiatry. 2016;209(1):23–8.

74. Sandoval LR, Torous J, Keshavan MS. Smartphones for smarter care? Self-management in schizophrenia. Am J Psychiatry. 2017;174(8):725–8.

75. Berry N, Lobban F, Emsley R, Bucci S. Acceptability of interventions delivered online and through mobile phones for people who experience severe mental health problems: a sys-tematic review. J Med Internet Res. 2016;18(5):e121.

76. Gilbody S, Littlewood E, Hewitt C, Brierley G, Tharmanathan P, Araya R, et al. Computerised cognitive behaviour therapy (cCBT) as treatment for depression in primary care (REEACT trial): large scale pragmatic randomised controlled trial. BMJ. 2015;351:h5627.

77. Vaessen T, Steinhart H, Batink T, Klippel A, Van Nierop M, Reininghaus U, et al. ACT in daily life in early psychosis: an ecological momentary intervention approach. Psychosis. 2019;11(2):93–104.

78. Batink T, Bakker J, Vaessen T, Kasanova Z, Collip D, van Os J, et al. Acceptance and commitment therapy in daily life training: a feasibility study of an mhealth intervention. JMIR mHealth uHealth. 2016;4(3):e103.

79. Kramer I, Simons CJP, Hartmann JA, Menne-Lothmann C, Viechtbauer W, Peeters F, et al. A therapeutic application of the experience sampling method in the treatment of depression: a randomized controlled trial. World Psychiatry. 2014;13(1):68–77.

80. Myin-Germeys I, Kasanova Z, Vaessen T, Vachon H, Kirtley O, Viechtbauer W, et al. Experience sampling methodology in mental health research: new insights and technical developments. World Psychiatry. 2018;17(2):123–32.

81. Hartmann JA, Wichers M, Menne-Lothmann C, Kramer I, Viechtbauer W, Peeters F, et al. Experience sampling-based personalized feedback and positive affect: a randomized controlled trial in depressed patients. PLoS One. 2015;10(6):e0128095.

82. Schlosser DA, Campellone TR, Truong B, Etter K, Vergani S, Komaiko K, et al. Efficacy of PRIME, a mobile app intervention designed to improve motivation in young people with schizophrenia. Schizophr Bull. 2018;44(5):1010–20.

83. Manera V, Abrahams S, Agüera-Ortiz L, Bremond F, David R, Fairchild K, et al. Recommendations for the nonpharmacological treatment of apathy in brain disorders. Am J Geriatr Psychiatry. 2020;28(4):410–20.

84. Manera V, Fabre R, Stella F, Loureiro JC, Agüera-Ortiz L, López-Álvarez J, et al. A survey on the prevalence of apathy in elderly people referred to specialized memory centers. Int J Geriatr Psychiatry. 2019;34(10):1369–77.

85. Mizrahi R, Starkstein SE. Epidemiology and management of apathy in patients with Alzheimer's disease. Drugs Aging. 2007;24:547–54.

86. Rajkumar AP, Ballard C, Fossey J, Corbett A, Woods B, Orrell M, et al. Apathy and its response to antipsychotic review and nonpharmacological interventions in people with dementia living in nursing homes: WHELD, a factorial cluster randomized controlled trial. J Am Med Dir Assoc. 2016;17(8):741–7.

15
Brain Stimulation

André Aleman, Jozarni J. Dlabac-De Lange, and Prasad Padala

Introduction

First, we will provide a short introduction to the two most commonly used and studied non-invasive brain stimulation techniques, repetitive transcranial magnetic stimulation (rTMS) and transcranial direct current stimulation (tDCS). Subsequently, an overview will be given of findings in neuropsychiatric conditions that have been studied. Finally, factors that are of importance to consider when designing or interpreting brain stimulation studies will be addressed. These concern frequency and intensity of stimulation, scalp location, duration of treatment, and blinding.

Transcranial Magnetic Stimulation

Brain stimulation with magnetic fields was introduced in 1985 by Barker and colleagues (1) and has since been increasingly applied in cognitive and clinical neuroscience. Indeed, it has been hailed as a novel technique for treatment of psychiatric and neurological symptoms. The underlying principle for stimulating the brain with rTMS is based on Faraday's law of induction for time-varying currents. More specifically, a time-varying magnetic field is generated by a current pulse through a stimulator coil placed over a specific scalp position (Fig. 15.1). The rapidly changing external magnetic field induces electric current intracranially. Thus, the rapid rise and fall of the magnetic field induces a flow of current in the underlying brain tissue, and hence neural activation. The diameter of the induced field is of approximately 2–3 cm, the same figure holds for the depth of stimulation. This means that only cortical regions can be stimulated directly. Indeed, several neuroimaging studies have confirmed activation of underlying brain areas after rTMS, for example over the motor cortex (2, 3) or over the prefrontal cortex. Using H_2O positron emission tomography, Speer et al. (4) observed increased blood flow after 10 Hz rTMS to the left dorsolateral prefrontal cortex (DLPFC), whereas 1 Hz stimulation decreased blood flow. It is well established (especially by measurements over the motor cortex) that low-frequency stimulation affects cortical excitability in a different way compared to high-frequency stimulation.

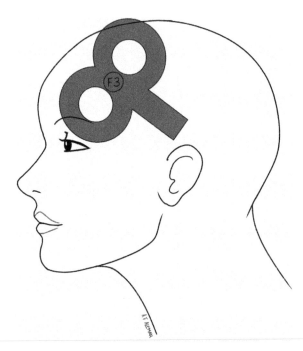

Fig. 15.1 Illustration of transcranial magnetic stimulation coil placement for treatment over the dorsolateral prefrontal cortex, here targeted as electrode position F3 (in the 10–20 system).

That is, frequencies of 1 Hz or lower are generally considered to be inhibitory (i.e. they reduce cortical excitability of the underlying area), whereas frequencies of 5 Hz and higher are considered to be excitatory (5).

Brain stimulation with rTMS occurs at a certain intensity (in terms of output of the machine) of the magnetic pulses delivered. The intensity of stimulation is usually set at a certain percentage of the motor threshold, which differs between individuals. Motor threshold refers to the minimum strength of the stimulus provided, which is the percentage of the total machine output that is required to produce reliable movement of thumb or fingers. A typical standard is to take as the threshold the intensity of machine output needed that yields movement at least 50% of the time. This is of relevance, as intensities that are considerably higher than the motor threshold of a participant are associated with a higher risk of inducing an epileptic seizure. For safety reasons, the precautions listed in internationally agreed guidelines (6, 7) should be taken into account. When those are followed, rTMS appears to be safe and well tolerated. Motor threshold is known to increase with age, perhaps due to increases in the skull to cortex distance, so higher output may be needed while working with older adults. Several contraindications for TMS should be considered: pacemaker, aneurysm clip, heart/vascular clip, prosthetic valve, intracranial metal prosthesis, personal or familial history of epilepsy, medications that reduce the threshold for seizure, and high alcohol or drug consumption, among others. Many clips are made of non-ferromagnetic material these days so rTMS is still an option in these patients if the clips are magnetic resonance imaging compatible. Pregnant women and young children are generally also excluded from research studies, although they might be subject to rTMS for clinical or therapeutic purposes. Fortunately, since the introduction of the international safety guidelines, occurrence of seizures has been very rare. Other side effects are generally mild. They include transient headache (that responds well to analgesics), local discomfort as a consequence of direct stimulation of the facial musculature, and transient changes in the auditory threshold. Use of earplugs is recommended both for the patient and the treater.

Transcranial Direct Current Stimulation

Over the past decade, methods of non-invasive brain stimulation other than rTMS have also been employed to improve negative symptoms such as apathy. The most frequently studied additional method is tDCS. A handful of trials using tDCS have now been published. Brain stimulation with tDCS involves weak electric fields, with currents of 1–2 mA. The exact mechanisms of action in the brain have not been fully uncovered, but it is known that tDCS modulates spontaneous neuronal network activity. This occurs through a tDCS polarity-dependent shift (polarization) of the resting membrane potential (8, 9). Thus, unlike rTMS, tDCS does not induce neuronal firing by suprathreshold neuronal membrane depolarization, but is rather thought to influence excitatory synaptic efficacy. Cortical activity and excitability may be enhanced through anodal tDCS stimulation, whereas cathodal tDCS stimulation may reduce excitability.

As only a few studies have been published on evaluating tDCS effects on negative symptoms/apathy, we will briefly summarize them here and devote the remainder of this chapter to rTMS. In a meta-analysis, published in 2018 (10), of five studies reporting a tDCS trial for negative symptoms in schizophrenia, a mean weighted effect size of actual stimulation versus sham stimulation was found of 0.50 (95% confidence interval (CI) −0.07 to 1.07; total $N = 134$). A study published in 2019 (11) was almost as large as those earlier five combined, with $N = 100$ participants randomized to real or sham stimulation (95 completed the trial). The authors reported a significant improvement, with response rates for negative symptoms (defined as 20% improvement or greater) of 40% in the real treatment group and 4% in the sham group. More studies are needed though, to be able to evaluate the clinical value of tDCS for apathy. Possible electrode placement could be frontotemporal, for example, the anode located over a point midway between F3 and FP1, corresponding to left DLPFC. The cathode can be placed at a point midway between T3 and P3, corresponding to the left temporoparietal junction.

rTMS Studies of Negative Symptoms/Apathy

Most studies investigating the effect of rTMS on apathy have focused on the broader concept of negative symptoms in patients with schizophrenia. Negative symptoms include the flattening of affect, alogia, avolition, apathy, and social withdrawal. Negative symptoms are very invalidating as they hamper functioning in daily life due to lack of motivation and initiation of action. Approximately 25% of the patients with schizophrenia suffer from severe and persistent negative symptoms. Treatment options of these negative symptoms are limited and often not effective (12). Because of this, researchers have explored other treatment modalities, including neuromodulation (especially rTMS). Indeed, in the past two decades a substantial number of randomized controlled trials (RCTs) have investigated the effect of rTMS (see (10) for a recent meta-analysis).

Rationale for Non-Invasive Brain Stimulation

Evidence from neuroimaging has revealed negative symptoms to be associated with reduced activation of the prefrontal cortex (13), particularly the DLPFC. With regard to mechanisms of action of rTMS, these remain to be fully elucidated. There is evidence that dopaminergic neurotransmission may be involved, specifically for rTMS over prefrontal and motor areas. This has been shown in studies with animal models (14) as well as human studies (15, 16). Specifically, increased dopamine transmission in subcortical areas has been observed, but also in medial prefrontal areas, after TMS.

High-frequency rTMS of the prefrontal cortex can increase local cortical excitability and ultimately improve negative symptoms. More than 20 studies have been published over the past decades on the effect of rTMS on negative symptoms (cf. (10)). Whereas some of those studies found a significant improvement of negative symptoms after rTMS, others failed to find a therapeutic effect. Several meta-analyses have been performed to integrate the quantitative evidence for the effect of rTMS on negative symptoms (e.g. (17, 18)). The latest and largest meta-analysis (10), involving 19 studies with a total $N = 825$, found a moderate treatment effect in favour of rTMS with a mean weighted effect size of 0.64 (0.32–0.96). When excluding statistically defined outliers, the mean weighted effect size was 0.31 (0.12–0.50; total $N = 721$). Although these results are promising, it remains uncertain to the extent to which this positive treatment effect is also clinically meaningful and how durable the therapeutic effects of the rTMS are. Of note, one study found a positive treatment effect after up to 3 months of follow-up (14), but most studies did not have a follow-up or only a short follow-up of up to 2 weeks. Lefaucheur et al. (19) recently classified the evidence level as C, in favour of a possible efficacy of high-frequency rTMS of the left DLPFC on the negative symptoms of schizophrenia. This implies that the international panel involved in that consensus review of rTMS efficacy across disorders considered evidence level A (definite evidence for efficacy) or level B (probable efficacy) not to be in order (as yet). This does not only apply to symptoms of schizophrenia, but also much broader across disorders, with exception of a few such as major depressive disorder, that did achieve level A status.

Mechanisms of Action of Prefrontal rTMS Treatment of Negative Symptoms

As indicated previously, increasing cortical excitability of the prefrontal cortex is the primary rationale of rTMS for negative symptoms. This may occur in different ways, and it should be noted that many details of the mechanism of action underlying rTMS remain to be elucidated. Nonetheless, there is emerging evidence that supports the idea of altering prefrontal excitability and connectivity (see (20)). Studies have shown that rTMS can facilitate dopaminergic, GABAergic, and glutaminergic neurotransmission (21). Delivering high-frequency rTMS over the left DLPFC has an additional, propagated, intermediate effect of enhancing dopamine transmission in the prefrontal cortex, the ipsilateral anterior cingulate, and medial orbitofrontal cortex (22, 23). Pogarell et al. (22) found a reduction in striatal iodobenzamide binding after rTMS, suggestive of a release in endogenous dopamine. In another study, acute rTMS showed striatal dopaminergic effects similar to those of D-amphetamine, a substance known to increase dopamine (23). This may support plasticity-related processes in the brain. In order to investigate the underlying working mechanism of prefrontal rTMS in schizophrenia, several neuroimaging studies have been performed. One electroencephalogram study reported a significant increase in brain activity with the improvement of negative symptoms (24). One combined treatment and neuroimaging study that found a positive treatment effect (25) also found changes in brain activation between active and sham groups during a functional magnetic resonance imaging (fMRI) planning task and a social–emotional evaluation fMRI task, accompanied by changes in brain metabolism during a proton magnetic resonance spectroscopy (^{1}H-MRS) measurement (26). During the planning task, activity in the prefrontal cortex increased and activity in the posterior brain decreased in the active group as compared to the sham group. During the social–emotional evaluation task, rTMS treatment resulted in reduced activation of striato-frontoparietal brain areas. Furthermore, the ^{1}H-MRS measurement conducted among a subgroup of patients revealed increased glutamate and glutamine concentrations in the prefrontal cortex after bilateral rTMS in the active group as compared to the sham group.

A few studies did not find prefrontal changes as a result of rTMS. Two studies combined rTMS treatment with single-photon emission computed tomography scans; both studies did not detect any changes in regional cerebral blood flow (27, 28). In addition, two fMRI studies did not find statistically significant differences in neuronal activation during a working memory task between sham and active rTMS (29, 30). Although results are inconsistent, most neuroimaging studies provide evidence for the underlying rationale of prefrontal rTMS treatment for negative symptoms, namely that it can normalize prefrontal brain activity and metabolism. However, study sizes were small and further neuroimaging research is needed.

Potential Moderators of Effect

Non-invasive neurostimulation with rTMS can improve negative symptoms, but in order to optimize treatment parameters it is important to investigate potential moderators of effect. These moderators of effect include rTMS treatment parameters, such as frequency of stimulation or duration of stimulation, as well as patient characteristics such as duration of illness.

Studies on rTMS treatment of negative symptoms show considerable variation in rTMS treatment parameters (see (17) for an overview). These studies varied in frequency of stimulation, location of stimulation (frontal, parietal, cerebellar vermis), percentage of motor threshold, duration of stimulation, and number of TMS pulses administered. In general, a treatment duration of more than 2 weeks and a higher number of TMS pulses administered seems to be more effective (10). Indeed, there is evidence for impaired cortical excitability, connectivity, and plasticity in patients with schizophrenia in all stages of the disease (31). To improve the efficacy of rTMS it may be necessary to target neural plasticity, for example, by applying a greater number of rTMS stimulations or by increasing treatment duration to enhance treatment response.

Regarding the frequency of stimulation, a few studies have investigated low-frequency (1–3 Hz) stimulation of the prefrontal cortex (e.g. (32)) but failed to find an effect. Other studies investigated the effect of 20 Hz prefrontal rTMS, but did not report significant improvements either (e.g. (33)). Most studies (N = 16) have examined the effect of 10 Hz rTMS, which seems most promising as a majority of these studies (N = 10) found a significant improvement of negative symptoms in the rTMS group as compared to the sham group. A meta-analysis also found a greater effect size in studies applying 10 Hz prefrontal rTMS as compared to other frequencies (10). It should be noted though, that a well-conducted trial in 2015 with a good sample size (34) did not observe any superiority of 10 Hz left prefrontal rTMS over sham in ameliorating negative symptoms. Different high-frequency protocols, such as theta burst stimulation, may have a stronger biological plausibility and are gaining interest among researchers (35). Future research should determine whether such protocols are potentially more effective than 10 Hz stimulation.

The location of stimulation varies in published trials, though the majority of trials have investigated rTMS stimulation of the left or bilateral prefrontal cortex. It should be noted that methodological challenges should be kept in mind: achieving/maintaining blinding in sham-controlled studies can be problematic and different sham conditions (e.g. using a sham coil or rotating a coil with real stimulation at 90 degrees) were employed in different studies.

Other treatment characteristics include type and dosage of medication. Patients with schizophrenia may use high dosages of medication, including antipsychotics, benzodiazepines, and anticonvulsant medication. These medications may interfere with the putative working mechanism of rTMS, namely increasing excitability and neurotransmitter (including dopamine) release in the prefrontal cortex. The vast majority of patients use antipsychotics to treat positive symptoms, but most antipsychotics have high affinity for dopamine (D_2) receptors and thus block dopamine. Indeed, one exploratory study found active rTMS to improve antipsychotic-induced extrapyramidal symptoms, possibly by increasing dopamine release (36). Clozapine is an atypical antipsychotic that has shown to be superior in the treatment of refractory schizophrenia. Clozapine, in contrast to most other antipsychotics, shows only weak antagonism to the dopamine D_2 receptor. Patients with schizophrenia using clozapine may therefore more readily respond to rTMS treatment. Until now, only one exploratory study has been conducted, in a cohort of patients on clozapine participating in the RESIS trial (37). That study ($N = 26$) found a significant reduction of the Positive and Negative Syndrome Scale (PANSS) positive subscale and the PANSS general subscale, but not on the PANSS negative subscale, after active rTMS as compared sham rTMS. More research on the effect of type and dosage of medication on rTMS treatment response is warranted. It is important to maintain a stable dose of antipsychotics during rTMS treatment due to their effect on the motor threshold. If the change in antipsychotics is unavoidable, determining the motor threshold may need to be redone.

Besides investigating rTMS parameters as potential moderators of effect, it is also important to explore patient characteristics as potential moderators. Exploratory analyses in an earlier-mentioned meta-analysis found a higher effect in studies that included younger patients with a shorter duration of illness (10). It may be easier to induce neuroplasticity in younger patients with a shorter duration of illness, and more rTMS studies conducted among patients with a first-episode psychosis are required. Cortical atrophy in older patients could make rTMS less effective, unless the stimulation intensity (in terms of percentage of the motor threshold) is carefully titrated upwards.

rTMS Treatment for Apathy Associated with Cognitive Impairment

Apathy treatment with rTMS has a much scantier literature compared to that of schizophrenia, yet there are lot of similarities and some fundamental differences. There are only two RCTs specifically for apathy associated with cognitive impairment however, there is some literature for apathy related to stroke as well. Mitaki et al. (38) treated post-stroke apathy with rTMS over the supplemental motor area with clinical improvement in apathy accompanied by improved inter-hemisphere connectivity on functional neuroimaging. Sasaki et al. (39) conducted an RCT in 13 patients for apathy that persisted for more than a year after their stroke. After five sessions of rTMS over the region spanning from the dorsal anterior cingulate cortex to the medial prefrontal cortex, the rTMS group showed significant improvement in apathy over the sham group. However, neither of these studies reported durability data.

rTMS for apathy associated with cognitive impairment has lot of similarities with the schizophrenia literature as the DLPFC is the preferred site of stimulation, and similar treatment parameters (10 Hz, 3000 pulses per treatment, 4-second stimulation followed by 26- second intertrain interval) are used. The stimulation strength, however, seems to be higher in studies of apathy associated with cognitive impairment, typically targeting 120% motor threshold, perhaps due to the age of the subjects in the studies. A double-blind, randomized, sham-controlled, cross-over study of rTMS was conducted in nine subjects with apathy and mild cognitive impairment (40). The initial 2 weeks of treatment was followed by a 4-week washout period after which the subjects crossed over to receive the other treatment for 2 weeks. Left DLPFC was stimulated with 3000 pulses at 10 Hz, 4-second train duration, and 26-second intertrain interval at 120% of motor threshold per session five times a week. After adjusting for baseline, there was a significantly greater improvement in the apathy (Apathy Evaluation Scale-Clinician version) (41) with rTMS compared to sham (average intergroup difference 5.9 (95% confidence interval (CI) 0.2–11.6); $P = 0.045$). Apathy improved in all participants during rTMS treatment while mixed results were seen during sham treatment. There was a significant between-group difference in Mini Mental State Examination (3.4 (95% CI 1.9–5.0); $t_{(5)} = 5.75; P = 0.002$) and executive function (Trails Making Test-A) between the arms (−4.6 (95% CI −8.8 to −0.3); $t_{(5)} = -2.74; P = 0.041$). Adverse events were mild and transient and did not differ between the arms (40).

Another double-blind, randomized study of rTMS was conducted in older subjects with Alzheimer's dementia and apathy ($N = 20$) by the same team (42). Subjects received either rTMS or sham treatment (5 days/week) for 4 weeks. The left DLPFC was stimulated with 3000 pulses at 10 Hz at 120% of motor threshold per session. After adjusting for baseline, there was significant improvement in the motivation with rTMS compared to sham treatment (−10.1 (95% CI −15.9 to −4.3); $t_{(16)} = -3.69; P = 0.002$). Additionally, there was significantly greater improvement in Modified Mini Mental State Examination (6.9 (95% CI 1.7–12.0); $t_{(15)} = 2.85; P = 0.012$), Instrumental Activities of Daily Living (3.4 (95% CI 1.0–5.9); $X^2_1 = 7.72; P = 0.006$), Clinical Global Impression–Severity (1.4 (95% CI 0.5–2.3), $t_{(16)} = 3.29; P = 0.005$), and Clinical Global Impression–Improvement (−2.56 (95% CI −3.5 to −1.6), $t_{(17)} = -5.72; P < 0.001$) scores for rTMS compared to the sham at 4 weeks.

Minimal side effects are reported in both the post-stroke and cognitive impairment studies with no seizure in any of the subjects and application site discomfort was the most common side effect. One subject dropped out of the treatment due to non-tolerability of the intervention but incidentally he was assigned to the sham arm (42).

Comparing and Contrasting Effects with Pharmacological Treatments

Although there are no head-to-head studies comparing the effects of rTMS with pharmacological treatments of apathy, the effects seem to be comparable. The improvement in apathy with rTMS might be seen in as few as ten treatments compared with 6–12 weeks of methylphenidate treatment (40, 43, 44). The improvement in apathy in the rTMS Alzheimer's disease study (42) was better than 6 weeks of methylphenidate treatment in the ADMET study and better than the 4 weeks of methylphenidate treatment reported by Padala et al. (43, 44). Average Modified Mini-Mental State Examination scores improved by 7.2 points with rTMS which is greater than that reported with 12 weeks of methylphenidate treatment (43).

Durability data are sorely missing in this apathy literature. Of the three RCTs cited earlier, only one study reported duration data for up to 8 weeks after the treatment (42). In that study some, but not all, gains were retained in the rTMS group. The gains in apathy were clinically significant at 8 weeks after the treatment but not statistically significant. Gains in cognition and function were retained at 8 weeks. Based on these preliminary results, a case could be made for longer duration of treatment or adding maintenance treatments for apathy as is the norm for depression treatment with rTMS (45, 46).

A tDCS study of left DLPFC anodal tDCS in patients with moderate Alzheimer's disease ($N = 40$) was recently completed (47). Unfortunately, it failed to show improvement in apathy. However, there are ongoing studies with tDCS combined with cognitive training and rTMS studies focusing on cognitive impairment in mild cognitive impairment with and without apathy exploring prevention of dementia (48–50).

Conclusion

In conclusion, evidence from meta-analysis of high-frequency prefrontal rTMS suggests rTMS may improve negative symptoms in patients with schizophrenia. This effect may last up to 3 months, but most studies did not measure long-term effects. Neuroimaging studies have found rTMS may induce changes in brain activity in prefrontal and connected brain areas, thereby reducing negative symptoms. Although several studies have found a significant improvement of negative symptoms, it remains unclear if the results are clinically significant. Regarding rTMS treatment parameters, a treatment frequency of 10 Hz, a treatment location of the left or bilateral prefrontal cortex, a longer treatment duration, and a larger amount of total TMS pulses administered seems to enhance effectiveness. Regarding patient characteristics, younger patients with a shorter duration of illness may respond better to rTMS treatment. Further research is needed to investigate the potential benefits of treatment with clozapine on rTMS treatment response. Future studies should also investigate the underlying neural working mechanism and further establish the most effective combination of rTMS parameters.

References

1. Barker AT, Jalinous R, Freeston IL. Non-invasive magnetic stimulation of human motor cortex. Lancet. 1985;1(8437):1106–7.
2. Siebner H, Peller M, Bartenstein P, Willoch F, Rossmeier C, Schwaiger M, et al. Activation of frontal premotor areas during suprathreshold transcranial magnetic stimulation of the left primary sensorimotor cortex: a glucose metabolic PET study. Hum Brain Mapp. 2001;12(3):157–67.
3. Rounis E, Stephan KE, Lee L, Siebner HR, Pesenti A, Friston KJ, et al. Acute changes in frontoparietal activity after repetitive transcranial magnetic stimulation over the dorsolateral prefrontal cortex in a cued reaction time task. J Neurosci. 2006;26(38):9629–38.
4. Speer AM, Kimbrell TA, Wassermann EM, Repella JD, Willis MW, Herscovitch P, et al. Opposite effects of high and low frequency rTMS on regional brain activity in depressed patients. Biol Psychiatry. 2000;48(12):1133–41.
5. Hallett M. Transcranial magnetic stimulation and the human brain. Nature. 2000;406(6792):147–50.
6. McClintock SM, Reti IM, Carpenter LL, McDonald WM, Dubin M, Taylor SF, et al. Consensus recommendations for the clinical application of repetitive transcranial magnetic stimulation (rTMS) in the treatment of depression. J Clin Psychiatry. 2018;79(1):16cs10905.
7. Rossi S, Hallett M, Rossini PM, Pascual-Leone A, Safety of TMS Consensus Group. Safety, ethical considerations, and application guidelines for the use of transcranial magnetic stimulation in clinical practice and research. Clin Neurophysiol. 2009;120(12):2008–39.
8. Priori A, Hallett M, Rothwell JC. Repetitive transcranial magnetic stimulation or transcranial direct current stimulation? Brain Stimul. 2009;2(4):241–5.
9. Paulus W. Transcranial electrical stimulation (tES—tDCS; tRNS, tACS) methods. Neuropsychol Rehabil. 2011;21(5):602–17.
10. Aleman A, Enriquez-Geppert S, Knegtering H, Dlabac-de Lange JJ. Moderate effects of noninvasive brain stimulation of the frontal cortex for improving negative symptoms in schizophrenia: meta-analysis of controlled trials. Neurosci Biobehav Rev. 2018;89:111–8.
11. Valiengo LDCL, Goerigk S, Gordon PC, Padberg F, Serpa MH, Koebe S, et al. Efficacy and safety of transcranial direct current stimulation for treating negative symptoms in schizophrenia: a randomized clinical trial. JAMA Psychiatry. 2020;77(2):121–9.
12. Aleman A, Lincoln TM, Bruggeman R, Melle I, Arends J, Arango C, et al. Treatment of negative symptoms: where do we stand, and where do we go? Schizophr Res. 2017;186:55–62.
13. Gruber O, Chadha Santuccione A, Aach H. Magnetic resonance imaging in studying schizophrenia, negative symptoms, and the glutamate system. Front Psychiatry. 2014;5:32.
14. Ohnishi T, Hayashi T, Okabe S, Nonaka I, Matsuda H, Iida H, et al. Endogenous dopamine release induced by repetitive transcranial magnetic stimulation over the primary motor cortex: an [11C] raclopride positron emission tomography study in anesthetized macaque monkeys. Biol Psychiatry. 2004;55(5):484–9.
15. Strafella AP, Paus T, Barrett J, Dagher A. Repetitive transcranial magnetic stimulation of the human prefrontal cortex induces dopamine release in the caudate nucleus. J Neurosci. 2001;21(15):RC157.
16. Moretti J, Poh EZ, Rodger J. rTMS-induced changes in glutamatergic and dopaminergic systems: relevance to cocaine and methamphetamine use disorders. Front Neurosci. 2020;14:137.

17. He H, Lu J, Yang L, Zheng J, Gao F, Zhai Y, et al. Repetitive transcranial magnetic stimulation for treating the symptoms of schizophrenia: a PRISMA compliant meta-analysis. Clin Neurophysiol. 2017;128(5):716–24.

18. Kennedy NI, Lee WH, Frangou S. Efficacy of non-invasive brain stimulation on the symptom dimensions of schizophrenia: a meta-analysis of randomized controlled trials. Eur Psychiatry. 2018;49:69–77.

19. Lefaucheur JP, Aleman A, Baeken C, Benninger DH, Brunelin J, Di Lazzaro V, et al. Evidence-based guidelines on the therapeutic use of repetitive transcranial magnetic stimulation (rTMS): an update (2014–2018). Clin Neurophysiol. 2020;131(2):474–528 [published correction appears in Clin Neurophysiol. 2020;131(5):1168–9].

20. Eshel N, Keller CJ, Wu W, Jiang J, Mills-Finnerty C, Huemer J, et al. Global connectivity and local excitability changes underlie antidepressant effects of repetitive transcranial magnetic stimulation. Neuropsychopharmacology. 2020;45(6):1018–25.

21. Chervyakov AV, Chernyavsky AY, Sinitsyn DO, Piradov MA. Possible mechanisms underlying the therapeutic effects of transcranial magnetic stimulation. Front Hum Neurosci. 2015;9:303.

22. Pogarell O, Koch W, Pöpperl G, Tatsch K, Jakob F, Mulert C, et al. Acute prefrontal rTMS increases striatal dopamine to a similar degree as D-amphetamine. Psychiatry Res. 2007;156(3):251–5.

23. Pogarell O, Koch W, Pöpperl G, Tatsch K, Jakob F, Zwanzger P, et al. Striatal dopamine release after prefrontal repetitive transcranial magnetic stimulation in major depression: preliminary results of a dynamic [123I] IBZM SPECT study. J Psychiatr Res. 2006;40(4):307–14.

24. Jandl M, Bittner R, Sack A, Weber B, Günther T, Pieschl D, et al. Changes in negative symptoms and EEG in schizophrenic patients after repetitive transcranial magnetic stimulation (rTMS): an open-label pilot study. J Neural Transm. 2005;112(7):955–67.

25. Dlabac-de Lange JJ, Liemburg EJ, Bais L, Renken RJ, Knegtering H, Aleman A. Effect of rTMS on brain activation in schizophrenia with negative symptoms: a proof-of-principle study. Schizophr Res. 2015;168(1–2):475–82.

26. Dlabac-de Lange JJ, Liemburg EJ, Bais L, van de Poel-Mustafayeva AT, de Lange-de Klerk ESM, Knegtering H, et al. Effect of bilateral prefrontal rTMS on left prefrontal NAA and Glx levels in schizophrenia patients with predominant negative symptoms: an exploratory study. Brain Stimul. 2017;10(1):59–64.

27. Cohen E, Bernardo M, Masana J, Arrufat FJ, Navarro V, Valls-Solé, et al. Repetitive transcranial magnetic stimulation in the treatment of chronic negative schizophrenia: a pilot study. J Neurol Neurosurg Psychiatry. 1999;67(1):129–30.

28. Hajak G, Marienhagen J, Langguth B, Werner S, Binder H, Eichhammer P. High-frequency repetitive transcranial magnetic stimulation in schizophrenia: a combined treatment and neuroimaging study. Psychol Med. 2004;34(7):1157–63.

29. Guse B, Falkai P, Gruber O, Whalley H, Gibson L, Hasan A, et al. The effect of long-term high frequency repetitive transcranial magnetic stimulation on working memory in schizophrenia and healthy controls—a randomized placebo-controlled, double-blind fMRI study. Behav Brain Res. 2013;237:300–7.

30. Prikryl R, Mikl M, Prikrylova Kucerová H, Ustohal L, Kasparek T, Marecek R, et al. Does repetitive transcranial magnetic stimulation have a positive effect on working memory and neuronal activation in treatment of negative symptoms of schizophrenia? Neuro Endocrinol Lett. 2012;33(1):90–7.

31. Hasan A, Falkai P, Wobrock T. Transcranial brain stimulation in schizophrenia: targeting cortical excitability, connectivity and plasticity. Curr Med Chem. 2013;20(3):405–13.

32. Schneider AL, Schneider TL, Stark H. Repetitive transcranial magnetic stimulation (rTMS) as an augmentation treatment for the negative symptoms of schizophrenia: a 4-week randomized placebo controlled study. Brain Stimul. 2008;1(2):106–11.
33. Novák T, Horácek J, Mohr P, Kopecek M, Skrdlantová L, Klirova M, et al. The double-blind sham-controlled study of high-frequency rTMS (20 Hz) for negative symptoms in schizophrenia: negative results. Neuro Endocrinol Lett. 2006;27(1–2):209–13.
34. Wobrock T, Guse B, Cordes J, Wölwer W, Winterer G, Gaebel W, et al. Left prefrontal high-frequency repetitive transcranial magnetic stimulation for the treatment of schizophrenia with predominant negative symptoms: a sham-controlled, randomized multicenter trial. Biol Psychiatry. 2015;77(11):979–88.
35. Zhao S, Kong J, Li S, Tong Z, Yang C, Zhong H. Randomized controlled trial of four protocols of repetitive transcranial magnetic stimulation for treating the negative symptoms of schizophrenia. Shanghai Arch Psychiatry. 2014;26(1):15–21.
36. Kamp D, Engelke C, Wobrock T, Wölwer W, Winterer G, Schmidt-Kraepelin C, et al. Left prefrontal high-frequency rTMS may improve movement disorder in schizophrenia patients with predominant negative symptoms—a secondary analysis of a sham-controlled, randomized multicenter trial. Schizophr Res. 2019;204:445–7.
37. Wagner E, Wobrock T, Kunze B, Langguth B, Landgrebe M, Eichhammer P, et al. Efficacy of high-frequency repetitive transcranial magnetic stimulation in schizophrenia patients with treatment-resistant negative symptoms treated with clozapine. Schizophr Res. 2019;208:370–6.
38. Mitaki S, Onoda K, Abe S, Oguro H, Yamaguchi S. The effectiveness of repetitive transcranial magnetic stimulation for poststroke apathy is associated with improved interhemispheric functional connectivity. J Stroke Cerebrovasc Dis. 2016;25(12):e219–21.
39. Sasaki N, Hara T, Yamada N, Niimi M, Kakuda W, Abo M. The efficacy of high-frequency repetitive transcranial magnetic stimulation for improving apathy in chronic stroke patients. Eur Neurol. 2017;78(1–2):28–32.
40. Padala PR, Padala KP, Lensing SY, Jackson AN, Hunter CR, Parkes CM, et al. Repetitive transcranial magnetic stimulation for apathy in mild cognitive impairment: a double-blind, randomized, sham-controlled, cross-over pilot study. Psychiatry Res. 2018;261:312–8.
41. Marin RS, Biedrzycki RC, Firinciogullari S. Reliability and validity of the Apathy Evaluation Scale. Psychiatry Res. 1991;38(2):143–62.
42. Padala PR, Boozer EM, Lensing SY, Parkes CM, Hunter CR, Dennis RA, et al. Neuromodulation for apathy in Alzheimer's disease: a double-blind, randomized, sham-controlled pilot study. J Alzheimers Dis. 2020;77(4):1483–93.
43. Padala PR, Padala KP, Lensing SY, Ramirez D, Monga V, Bopp MM, et al. Methylphenidate for apathy in community-dwelling older veterans with mild Alzheimer's disease: a double-blind, randomized, placebo-controlled trial. Am J Psychiatry. 2018;175(2):159–68.
44. Rosenberg PB, Lanctôt KL, Drye LT, Herrmann N, Scherer RW, Bachman DL, et al. Safety and efficacy of methylphenidate for apathy in Alzheimer's disease: a randomized, placebo-controlled trial. J Clin Psychiatry. 2013;74(8):810–6.
45. George MS. Transcranial magnetic stimulation for the treatment of depression. Expert Rev Neurother. 2010;10(11):1761–72.
46. Janicak PG, O'Reardon JP, Sampson SM, Husain MM, Lisanby SH, Rado JT, et al. Transcranial magnetic stimulation in the treatment of major depressive disorder: a comprehensive summary of safety experience from acute exposure, extended exposure, and during reintroduction treatment. J Clin Psychiatry. 2008;69(2):222–32.
47. Suemoto CK, Apolinario D, Nakamura-Palacios EM, Lopes L, Leite RE, Sales MC, et al. Effects of a non-focal plasticity protocol on apathy in moderate Alzheimer's disease: a randomized, double-blind, sham-controlled trial. Brain Stimul. 2014;7(2):308–13.

48. Nguyen JP, Boutoleau-Bretonniere C, Lefaucheur JP, Suarez A, Gaillard H, Chapelet G, et al. Efficacy of transcranial direct current stimulation combined with cognitive training in the treatment of apathy in patients with Alzheimer's disease: study protocol for a randomized trial. Rev Recent Clin Trials. 2018;13(4):319–27.
49. Padala PR. Transcranial magnetic stimulation for apathy in mild cognitive impairment (TAMCI). Clinical Trials.gov; 2019. Available at: https://clinicaltrials.gov/ct2/show/NCT 03590327?term=padala&draw=2&rank=2.
50. Taylor JL, Hambro BC, Strossman ND, Bhatt P, Hernandez B, Ashford JW, et al. The effects of repetitive transcranial magnetic stimulation in older adults with mild cognitive impairment: a protocol for a randomized, controlled three-arm trial. BMC Neurol. 2019;19(1):326.

Index

For the benefit of digital users, indexed terms that span two pages (e.g., 52–53) may, on occasion, appear on only one of those pages.

Tables and figures are indicated by *t* and *f* following the page number